THE WOMEN'S PROJECT

THE WOMEN'S PROJECT

Seven New Plays by Women

Edited by Julia Miles

Performing Arts Journal Publications
&
American Place Theatre

New York

Library of Congress Cataloging in Publication Data
The Women's Project
Seven New Plays by Women
Library of Congress Catalog Card No.: 80-81997
ISBN: 0-933836-06-0
ISBN: 0-933826-07-9 (pbk)

Design: Gautam Dasgupta

Printed in the United States of America

Contents

To my daughters— Stacey, Lisa and Marya

The American Place Theatre wishes to thank and express its deep gratitude to The Ford Foundation for its funding of The Women's Project and this anthology.

Acknowledgements

I'm deeply indebted to and wish to thank all the participants in The Women's Project: the playwrights, directors, actors, stage managers, designers, and technical staff who made the readings and productions possible, as well as the Advisory Board and other audience members who have supported the Project by their presence and response to the work. I am thankful as well for the enthusiasm and support of the many playwrights and directors who submitted their plays or their expressions of interest, but who we were not able to include in the Project.

The entire first season and most of the second were underwritten by The Ford Foundation, and I especially wish to thank Gayle Counts and Richard Sheldon of the Office of the Arts. Other financial support was gratefully received from the following sources: The Helena Rubinstein Foundation, Inc.; The National Endowment for the Arts Literature Program; The Joint Foundation Support, Inc.; Twentieth Century Fox Film Corp.; Con Edison; International Creative Management; Warner Communications; The Hugh M. Hefner Foundation; and many individual supporters of the Project.

I am grateful also to Wynn Handman and the staff of The American Place Theatre for all their help on the Project, and especially to my assistant Elaine De Leon. I owe thanks also to Gautam Dasgupta and Bonnie Marranca for their work on this book, as well as to Martha Holmes for her photographs.

Last, I want to express my appreciation to the staff of The Women's Project, without whose dedication the work could not have succeeded: to Ellen Madison, the first season to Kathleen Chalfant and Caymichael Patten, this year to Susan Lehman and Amy Ober, and most of all to Gayle Austin whose assistance to me throughout and with the preparation of this book has been invaluable.

Julia Miles

Introduction

In literature, women writers have made a name for themselves as poets and novelists, but who can name the women playwrights? Who are they; where are they today? Historically, the theatre has never been hospitable to women, and so women have not used it as a means of expression. Playwrights need a stage, and the collaboration of directors, actors and designers. Because of this, women, unaccustomed to putting themselves forward, have been reluctant to approach the theatre as a forum for their work.

Although theatre has been most often perceived as an exclusive men's club, there have been exceptions. Rachel Crothers had 27 Broadway productions in the 1920s and 1930s. There is Lillian Hellman. And in the 60s, when the Off-Off-Broadway movement was at its peak, Roslyn Drexler, Maria Irene Fornes, Adrienne Kennedy, Rochelle Owens and Megan Terry were, among others, an important part of it, and of course continue to write for the theatre.

However, in my experience at The American Place Theatre, working with new playwrights from fall 1964 through spring 1978, noticeably few of the plays produced on the main stage were by women. The exceptions were May Swenson, Cecil Dawkins, Anne Sexton, Joyce Carol Oates, Rochelle Owens, Maria Irene Fornes and Elaine Jackson. Most of these women were not, and did not go on to be, predominantly playwrights. One of the plays that spoke deeply to women who came to see it in 1978 was *Fefu and Her Friends* by Maria Irene Fornes, and I realized that there were not many plays that had the effect of revealing a particular reality to women; plays created by women in which women can see themselves.

Around this same time a report by a group called Action for Women in Theatre was brought to my attention. It concluded that only 7 per cent of the playwrights and 6 per cent of the directors in funded non-profit theatres during 1969-1975 were women. Of the plays submitted to the American Place at that time, about 10 per cent were by women. I knew there were many talented women around and these statistics made me aware of the fact that though a few women had achieved success, there were not a sufficient number of them and not enough places for them to apply their talents.

Assuming that the scarcity of women playwrights and directors was due to the lack of prominent women role models, I decided to create a special environment that would welcome women in a professional embrace. I wanted to establish a place that would provide women with the tools of every playwright and director: actors, designers, an audience, a stage, and a production. A place that had, in Anne Sexton's words, ". . . a community, a family for my art."

Of course this idea needed funding to make it a reality, and as sometimes happens when the time is right and you get lucky, events fell into place. I heard from a young woman director working at the theatre that the Ford Foundation had recently made women's issues and programs one of the objectives of the Foundation in all areas, including the arts. I contacted Gayle Counts at the Foundation and after several productive meetings with her and talks with Richard Sheldon, we submitted a proposal in April of 1978 and were notified in September that we would receive an $80,000 grant to begin The Women's Project at The American Theatre that season.

The process of producing plays, conceived at The American Place Theatre by the Artistic Director, Wynn Handman, and part of the established approach here, was adapted by me for The Women's Project. It consists of Rehearsed Readings, Second Step Developmental Work, and Studio Productions. The Rehearsed Readings, directed by women, are read before an invited audience of playwrights, directors, and theatre professionals. The Rehearsed Readings are then followed by a discussion with the playwright, director, and audience. These sessions, as well as the readings, are taped so the writer can have access to them. Follow-up conferences, in which suggestions are made for script revisions are held with me, the staff, the playwright, and director.

The first season twenty rehearsed readings were performed, four were worked on more extensively, and four others were given Studio Productions. Of the plays in this volume, Phyllis Purscell's *Separate Ceremonies* received a second, more fully rehearsed reading and subsequently was optioned for production by another theatre. Rose Leiman Goldemberg's *Letters Home*, Joan Schenkar's *Signs of Life*, and another play by Lavonne Mueller (*Warriors from a Long Childhood*) were done as Studio Productions in the spring of 1979.

During our second season (1979-80), ten rehearsed readings and three Studio Productions were performed. A source of great pride to me was the fact that two of the main stage productions at The American Place this season came from The Women's Project: *Letters Home* and *Killings on the Last Line*. Other projects this season have been the publication of this anthology, an outreach program with the purpose of letting other theatres know about the availability of the specific plays we have worked on, and a Directors Unit which has been collecting statistics on the employment of women directors and beginning to take action to improve those statistics.

I never want anyone to say again, "Where are the women playwrights and directors?" They exist, they are talented, and they are ready to enter the mainstream of theatre. I hope this book will be a step in that direction, that these plays will be read and produced and experienced by a larger audience. The plays are not diatribes—they cover a wide range of subject matter and styles and the concerns expressed in them are universal: the playwrights themselves come from diverse backgrounds.

Joyce Aaron, an actress from the Open Theatre and a director, and Luna Tarlo, a Canadian novelist, wrote *Acrobatics* in order to share and thereby relieve their pain. They transformed their personal chaos into a dramatic work that could be shared with an audience. It is a very personal performance piece for two actresses. The play is about the coming together of two women friends who take up their friendship after a long separation and comfort and strengthen each other through shared aspects of their lives.

Kathleen Collins is a college professor and has written screenplays and short stories. She was working with Gilbert Moses, the director, on a play and was asked to help work on the script. Later, after seeing Saroyan's *Time of Your Life*, she realized that a play was the right form to express her experiences of the family in *In the Midnight Hour*. The play takes place in the early 60s, when an upper class Negro family confronts the changes and traumas of the coming Black Movement and its effects on their lives.

Penelope Gilliatt is an established writer who writes fiction, criticism, a screenplay (*Sunday, Bloody Sunday*), plays, and recently a libretto. *Property* is a one-act play from a trilogy called *Quotations from Other Lives*. It takes place in a room that has three beds and may or may not be a hospital. Peg, the central character, is surrounded by Max, her ex-husband, and Abberly, her present love. All tend one another in an atmosphere of joking, feasts in the night, and good will. The central image of the play is woman as property.

Rose Leiman Goldemberg started writing poetry as a child and always knew "I wanted to be a writer." She has written for television, radio and film as well as the theatre, where she had several productions. She read "Letters Home," edited by Aurelia Schober Plath, Sylvia Plath's mother, and was deeply touched by the love and support of Aurelia for Sylvia. The play explores the questions of each one's responsibility toward the other in the intense struggle between a loving mother and her artist daughter.

Lavonne Mueller began writing poetry in boarding school and has been published. She has also taught, published scholarly articles, written two textbooks, and in 1975 was named Illinois Teacher of the Year. She came to playwriting as a student at the University of Iowa. Her first play was written "to impress my child," and she has written ten plays since 1976. Her plays are mostly about men, she wants to write the "Bovary" for men, but after producing her first adult play, *Warriors from a Long Childhood*, from her twin-war trilogy, and reading her other plays, I asked her to write a play about women. *Killings on the Last Line* is that play and it won a Rockefeller Foundation Playwright-in-Residence Grant. The play focuses on the lives of nine working women in a Chicago reactor parts factory, their fight for survival in 1979, The Year of the Child, and their hopes for the 80s.

Phyllis Purscell was born in Iowa, has been a teacher, and lives with her husband and four children in New Jersey. As a child she was always interested in the theatre, first in acting, then in writing. The Women's Project reading of *Separate Ceremonies* was the first time she had heard a play of hers read. The play reunites a brother and two sisters at the time of their father's death and explores their love and response to him as a continuing presence in their adult lives.

Joan Schenkar was a Literature and Aesthetics major in college and started writing plays when she was living alone on a farm in Vermont. She has worked as a playwright-in-residence with the Open Theatre and has had several plays produced. *Signs of Life* parodies the extreme and theatrical relations between men and women in nineteenth-century America. Its cast includes Henry James and his sister Alice, P.T. Barnum and his freak, "Elephant Woman," and Dr. Sloper, from Henry James's *Washington Square*.

Each of these plays stands on its own, but taken together they provide insight into the mystery and surprise of our experience. Women's plays are often about family and about love, but women also write about war, about death, about loss. The sensibility of the artist should not be equated with the sensibility of gender. Women do write from their particular experience, but they are not limited to their own identity.

Joan Vail Thorne, a playwright as well as director, wrote this concerning the Project:

> The Women's Project gives to me and to all its writers and directors a place to raise their voices *without* apology—not to be heard *above* anyone else, but to be heard! And I think that more and more, with the time and encouragement the Project offers, they will learn to use those voices to explore and evangelize the beautiful and the true, and even the bestial visions to which the feminine principle is heir.

I think that with support and the proper setting women will enter the theatre in increasing numbers and enrich it. I'm pleased to be participating in this process, and to have helped provide a community for the playwrights and directors in The Women's Project.

April 1980   Julia Miles
New York City

Acrobatics

Joyce Aaron and Luna Tarlo

For Sacha, Andrew, Joshua

Characters

WOMAN
GIRL

Acrobatics was given a rehearsed reading by The Women's Project on January 28, 1980, directed by Joanne Akalaitis, with the following cast:

WOMAN . . . . Tessa Kaner
GIRL . . . . Ellen McElduff

There were Two Kings' Children
Who Loved One Another so Dear
But they couldn't reach each other
For the water was much too deep.

Dutch 16th Century Faery Tale.

*Scene in Hilton Hotel room. Girl in bed in nightgown covered with blanket, on her lap a tape-recorder playing rock and roll music. ***

She's wearing an embroidered Mexican night-gown. Girl dancing with the top half of her body.

Time: about 6 p.m. Early evening light.

Buzzer system of bell cuts into music. Girl jumps up to open door. Woman enters, dark glasses, wearing chic pants suit and fur coat, passes girl, saying:

WOMAN: He's crazy.

GIRL: (*Shuts off music, gets back into bed*) I knew he was. When I saw him in that deep-sea-diving outfit, I looked right into his eyes. He looked like a criminal.

*Text projected on back wall. Satie music under text . . . Turning into Janis Joplin. ***

(WOMAN *stands up, opens suitcase, starts to take her clothes out and goes to closet.*)

GIRL: Is that new?

WOMAN: It's all new.

GIRL: Did you eat on the plane?

WOMAN: I'm starving.

GIRL: Let's order up. (*While* GIRL *calls room service and says: "Two chicken sandwiches, wine, coffee, cheese and fruit,"* WOMAN *hangs up the rest of her clothes. She gets undressed while* GIRL *watches in silence.*)

GIRL: Your whole body's changed. It's completely different.

WOMAN: I know.

GIRL: You look terrific, really terrific.

(WOMAN *puts on robe and gets into bed.*)

WOMAN: It came from nowhere. Nothing happened. Nothing I could see, nothing I could touch, nothing. Suddenly it was finished.

GIRL: There was no sign? No clue?

WOMAN: Nothing.

GIRL: I don't believe it.

(*Knock.* GIRL *gets food from front of door. She brings tray over to* WOMAN's *bed and sits down on the edge. They begin to eat.*)

GIRL: I never trusted him. He frightened me. (*Pause.*) I don't mean that. I mean, he was dark, something unfamiliar about him. (SHE *hesitates.*) I didn't want to know him.

WOMAN: His touch was so familiar—like my mother's—my father's— I couldn't resist. I never wanted to. It was like a law of nature. I put my life in his hands.

GIRL: Remember that guy I told you about in Holland? That took me out on his motor bike—I was on the back of it—to an island? I remember falling asleep with my head against his back, riding. It was the only day in my life that I ever felt completely happy. (*Pause.*) Listen to this. (*Takes letter from under pillow.*) "After you left, it was like stepping out of a fairy-tale. Into a world that doesn't believe in fairy-tales. I want you to know that contact with you is a primal desire." (*Pause.*) He never touched me. He never even tried.

WOMAN: His hands always fascinated me. Something about them—a sureness—nothing random about the movements—nothing lost.

GIRL: What do you think of what I read to you?

WOMAN: Read it again.

GIRL: "After you left, it was like stepping out of a fairy-tale. Into a world that doesn't believe in fairy-tales. I want you to know that contact with you is a primal desire."

WOMAN: I don't believe it.

GIRL: What?

WOMAN: That he never touched you.

GIRL: I felt a secret—not an ordinary twist—I had no body— I was nobody. (*Laughing.*) Can you believe this conversation?

WOMAN: Nothing surprises me anymore. You know—? People are crazy.

GIRL: What month is he?

WOMAN: I don't know. I think he's some kind of fish or something.

GIRL: Pisces! He's a Pisces too! March 13.

WOMAN: March 13! The same birthday. You must be kidding.

GIRL: Ayayayayaya—Nobody would believe it. (*Pause.*) But can you believe it? The same day? (*Telephone rings.*) Hello? I know you're having a party. I can hear it through the wall. I like to be alone. I don't want company. I don't drink. Have a good life. Yes, she's my friend. She doesn't drink either. I wanna hang up. Listen, I want to hang up, I'm busy, I'm talking. Would you mind hanging up? O.K. If you won't, I will. (*Hangs up.*) A couple of stockbrokers from Texas. They're looking for women. (*Picks up phone, dials.*) Two double martinis, please.

WOMAN: Gibsons.

GIRL: Gibsons. Y'know Gibsons, with the onions. And some peanuts or crackers or something. (*To* WOMAN.) Peanuts or crackers?

WOMAN: Let's have a little of each.

GIRL: Peanuts and crackers. Yeah. A little variety—you know, spice of life.

(*Knock on door.* GIRL *goes to door, picks up drinks. Both women in the bathroom, the older woman in the bathtub with a Gibson in her hand, the younger woman sitting on the toilet with a drink in her hand.*)

GIRL: Did you talk to him much?

WOMAN: Not much. But one day we were sitting over a meal, talking. And all of a sudden he said—this is my mother's dream, that I would sit and talk to her like this. Are you listening? And I asked him—don't you ever talk to your mother? Never, he said. And then he smiled, it was the first time I'd ever seen him smile.

(GIRL *smiles in mirror.*)

GIRL: Can you believe it? You have to admit it, I didn't look like this the last time you saw me. I look suddenly old. Twenty years older. There are these five lines here. This little line here. (*Points to line above upper lip.*) Five lines here and five lines here. (*Eyes.*) That makes ten lines. The biggest thing are these two purple holes under my eyes. And my neck. But I have to admit I had these since I was sixteen. Everyone thinks I look young. I did look young. You look young. (*Takes a sip of drink.*) I hate my mother's body. She always had that same fat stomach that hung and a deep gash from some operation. She had one nipple burnt off—she wore falsies. Can you believe it?

WOMAN: What happened?

GIRL: Do you think they ever told me?

WOMAN: Did you ever ask?

GIRL: No.

WOMAN: Why didn't you ask?

GIRL: You know—when you're young—it's coming, it's coming—it's all coming. Now nothing's coming. It's all here. I feel like I've aged fifty years since I saw you last. Fifty. You know what I mean?

WOMAN: Jesus, you're still young. Look at me. It was the fact that we didn't talk much that appealed to me. The mystery of not knowing everything appealed to my imagination.

GIRL: I don't know anything anymore. I only know that since I gave up everything—my furniture, my apartment, my dog—and moved into this hotel—it's as if I dream my life and live somewhere else—in my work. (*Pause.*) How do people live without love?

WOMAN: They have their dreams. They never give up their dreams.

GIRL: Do you think it's possible? I think Marilyn Monroe would still be living if she'd had a baby.

WOMAN: What a stupid idea.

GIRL: It wouldn't have kept her going for long. But it might have prolonged her a bit. I had a friend. She was an artist. She had two children. One day she took a train to Westhampton, got into a taxi, went to the beach, and walked into the sea. She was found forty minutes later. Her husband was a professor of religion and philosophy. She used to come and pick me up at the theatre and we'd have coffee together. Oh, I forgot to tell you—she was a professional long-distance swimmer.

WOMAN: Why did she do it?

GIRL: When I tell you what I think—her book had gotten bad reviews. It was autobiographical—the reviews were malicious.

WOMAN: Did you read it?

GIRL: No.

WOMAN: I know a story that's really worse.

GIRL: Forget it.

WOMAN: You know my story is really worse.

GIRL: You know who could kill himself? If the circumstances were right?

WOMAN: Who?

GIRL: That guy in Holland.

WOMAN: What would make them right?

GIRL: No hope.

WOMAN: From what you read he sounds great. Terrific! You better grab him.

GIRL: I don't know if I want him. (*Goes and gets letter and reads:* "*After you left, it was like stepping out of a fairy-tale into a world that doesn't believe in fairy-tales. I want you to know that contact with you is a primal desire.*")

WOMAN: That's all there is. There's nothing else.

GIRL: What about art? (SHE *is making herself up and getting into a costume and wig—rehearsing lines: different styles. Repeated several times. Loud voice.*) I *don't* love you. I never loved you. (*Repeats.*) *You make me sick.* (*Repeats as different stereotype woman characters: Japanese, etc.*)

WOMAN: What are you doing? Do you get nervous?

GIRL: Always. Sick.—"Sick to my stomach." I'll be back as soon as it's over.

WOMAN: What time?

GIRL: As soon as it's over. I'll be back. Arrivederci, ciao!!!

WOMAN: I'll be here. (GIRL *leaves. Lights pop out. Door slams. Lights pop up simultaneously.* GIRL *enters.*) I had dinner with Andy. Listen to this. I wrote it all down. He's a terrific kid. (SHE *takes out notebook from pocketbook.*)

(*Through next section,* GIRL *taking off wig and clothing, gets back into her night-gown and into bed.*)

WOMAN: Andy: Do you think he'll ever write to me, Mom?

> Me: You know him. He doesn't write.

> Andy: I hate writing too.

>> Me: Well, nobody likes it, Andy, but sometimes it's necessary.

> Andy: Hey Mom, wasn't that a cool present?

> Me: What?

> Andy: The gun he gave me.

>> Me: I suppose so, if you like guns. Have you used it yet?

> Andy: You know, Mom, I thought it was real. I mean, it looked real.

>> Me: Oh, so did I. Don't you think that was an odd present, Andy? A flare gun?

> Andy: It was real cool, Mom, real cool, he's a cool guy. Sometimes, I think he really liked me. Mom, do you think he really likes me?

>> Me: He's a strange man.

> Andy: Remember last summer when he picked us up at the plane and took us right down to the dock to show us his new boat? And he asked me to help him? But then when I got in it was like I wasn't there. And you weren't there either, Mom.— It was as if he didn't know us. What was he so angry about, Mom? I'm very sensitive about things like that.

WOMAN: I really love him, he's a terrific kid.

(*Morning.* WOMAN *lying in bed staring at ceiling.* GIRL *under covers.*)

WOMAN: You know, for the first time in my life, I could kill.

GIRL: How would you do it?

WOMAN: With a pistol. It's the only thing that would cure me. One day, I went with him and a friend to someone's estate up in the hills of Sardinia. He began to teach me to shoot. I had six bullets. They each had twelve. He set up a target with a bull's eye and we took turns. I hit the bull's eye two times out of six. They each got one out of twelve. It was thrilling.

GIRL: When was that?

WOMAN: About a month ago.

GIRL: I couldn't kill.

WOMAN: You don't know. What makes you so sure?

GIRL: Oh, I love you—I really love you.

WOMAN: No, I mean it. If I just knew he was dead! He said his work came first. I didn't ask him, he just told me. I felt as if I'd been shot.

GIRL: How did you leave him? The last minute, how was it left?

WOMAN: I don't know.

GIRL: You've lived with this man for three years and you don't know if he's gonna write.

WOMAN: He won't write.

GIRL: I don't wanna love that way. I don't, I don't. I do. I do. That's all I ever wanted. There must be another way to live. Ask me something. Something very important. Ask me anything ... anything. Go ahead ... anything.

WOMAN: How would you do it?

GIRL: (*Viva*) With a pistol. One day he took me up to the country.

WOMAN: What are you doing?

GIRL: (*Viva voice; no emotion, empty voice*) Living from the neck up. Try it. It's a new way of living. In Sardinia with a friend. And he taught me to shoot. He set up a bull's eye. I had six bullets. I hit the bull's eye twice. Everyone hit it once. It was thrilling.

WOMAN: (*Viva*) When was that?

GIRL: (*Viva*) About a month ago.

WOMAN: (*Viva*) I couldn't kill.

GIRL: What makes you so sure you could? (*Telephone;* GIRL *picks it up. Viva.*) Hello. Oh, it's snowing? Yeah, Mom, I love snow. What? No, nothing's wrong, Mom. No, what makes you think there's anything wrong here. Yes, she just woke up too. Listen, Mom, I'm in a rush. I have to go now. Yeah, I'm late. Yeah, I'll talk to you later, Ma—O.K. Ma—Bye Ma. (*No viva.*) See? Isn't it terrific? You don't feel anything? No pain. (*Viva.*) You want some coffee? I am dying for my morning coffee.

(*Both women are sitting on beds with coffee.*)

WOMAN: (*Reading from magazine.*) "We're already dying and we don't even know it." "Trouble may well loom for Los Angeles which sits in a smoggy bowl that often contains 300 feet of air." "Almost every other day, the city's public schools forbid children to exercise lest they breathe too deeply."

(*Silence.*)

GIRL: "In South Africa, for example, a campaign was waged against hippopotamuses. Deemed useless beasts that merely cluttered up rivers, they were shot on sight."

WOMAN: You know what really got me—when he sank his teeth into the jugular vein of a lion or a tiger or something. I read every Tarzan book that was ever published. I would feel my own teeth going in. I could even taste the blood. It was like copper.

GIRL: He reminds me of Tarzan. He's got that mucho macho thing. I can imagine him living in the jungle all by himself. That's funny—that guy in Holland thought of himself as a lonely tiger in the jungle. Isn't that funny? I'm just the opposite. When I was a little girl I wanted to shake hands with every person in the whole world. I didn't want to miss anyone.

WOMAN: I used to imagine somewhere somehow there was a tribe of people that were different from all other people, and that they lived on a tropical island, and one day I would be on a ship and it would be wrecked. And I'd walk on to the beach and I'd find them.

GIRL: I remember walking down the street thinking I would find my real mother. I thought: That's her; she looks like me. She has my nose. Does she recognize me? Then she'd pass by and I'd start all over again with the next person. I'd think: No, that wasn't her. That's her.

WOMAN: I used to feel sometimes that my real parents weren't my parents.

GIRL: I was always following people down the street. You know the kind who look in garbage pails, who talk to themselves. There was this one woman who wore a surgical mask as if she would be contaminated by the air.

WOMAN: (*Reading*) "The planet will warm up. The icecaps will melt. The oceans will rise by sixty feet drowning the world's coastal cities." (*Silence.*)

GIRL: Remember you said you'd put your life in his hands? Do you really believe your life is in your hands? (*Silence.*)

WOMAN: Once you really understand the problems, says Barry Commoner, in one of his gloomier moments, you find that it's worse than you ever expected. (*Pause.*)

GIRL: Dear Dr. Margolis. (*Makes a long, extended baby-cry.— Silence.*)

WOMAN: My primitive self finds them fascinating, not my civilized self.

GIRL: What do you mean—civilized?

WOMAN: I don't believe they're stronger than I am. I don't believe they really protect me. I don't believe they know more than I do—it's only when they're being men—

GIRL: What do you mean—men?

WOMAN: Playing the role—

GIRL: What role?

WOMAN: When he's taking me, forcing me, dominating me—that's when I'm hypnotized. There's a kind of collusion—we collaborate in a myth—

GIRL: What myth?

WOMAN: That he has power over me. Once we step outside he becomes just another person. That's all. Just another person.

GIRL: But then you're always acting. I don't believe in playing roles. Anyhow, what are you talking about? Look what's happening now. The whole world is changing and you're back in the stone age.

WOMAN: I couldn't love just another person. I mean—deeply—let myself be swept away. I might have met someone I could love—but not that way.

GIRL: It's not so easy to be swept away. It's not always so exciting to be swept away. Sometimes, it even hurts to be swept away.

WOMAN: I've met a few women who've been swept away.

GIRL: They were probably pretending.

WOMAN: I believed them.

GIRL: Anyway, it's so easy to pretend. You just lie there and ...

(*Breathe deeply, pant, act.*) I was with a guy once (*Legs up in the air*) and he said to me, "Tell me, tell me, tell me that you want me, tell me, tell me to do it to you now," and I said, "I want you, I want you, do it to me now, do it to me now,"and he said, "say it again." "I want you, I want you, do it to me now, do it, do it, I want you, do it to me now." "Tell me you're coming." "I'm coming, I'm coming." "Tell me again." "I'm coming, I'm coming, I'm coming..." (*Knock on door. Through door you hear:*)

RUTH: "Don't you two ever get outta of there? You oughta get some air."

GIRL: You know me, Ruth.

MAID: Yeah, it's true. When I come in there, she's always laying in that bed. I tell ya ...

GIRL: It's so exciting talking. I could spend my entire life talking about all the possibilities. As long as I don't have to live through them. That's all. What would you do if I told you I was just too old for all this. To start all over—?

WOMAN: I'd understand. (*Pause.*) What have you been doing all day in here, these last few months?

GIRL: Few months—it's my second year in here. I'd come back from the workshop about 3:00, buy a newspaper, come upstairs and make some coffee, get into bed and read a little, nap a little, wake.. up, write some letters, write in my journal, go back to reading, use my vibrator,—get up . . . .

WOMAN: What for?

GIRL: Masturbation. It takes one minute that way. With your hand, it takes twenty. There is an outlet in the hall so I just have to lie on the floor.

WOMAN: Naked on the floor of your hotel room?

GIRL: The orgasm is much deeper and much longer that way. I have two kinds of vibrators.

WOMAN: Two nozzles?

GIRL: Five nozzles. I have to pull down the shades and double lock the door so that Ruth can't get in with the fresh towels. That's all.

WOMAN: It's funny you're not embarrassed saying all this, but feelings seem to embarrass you.

GIRL: When I was little, I used to go into my father's closet and lie on the floor and smell his clothes. You know, when I looked at his jacket hanging on a hook I got that same feeling.

WOMAN: Who's?

GIRL: The guy in Holland.

WOMAN: It's strange about certain images—they stay in your head. Nothing takes them away.

GIRL: Yeah, just looking at his jacket. Maybe because it was so big. He's big. He's tall. I liked that. When I leaned my head against him, on the back of the motorbike—I really felt—

WOMAN: Peaceful?

GIRL: Yeah. The first time, the only time in my life. Isn't that crazy? On the back of a motorbike—with a stranger?

WOMAN: You meet a person, and somehow they get inside you for no reason—they make a place for themselves—for no reason—

WOMAN: (*Looks out window*) Someone's watching us.

GIRL: It's those Texas stockbrokers. (*She gets up and pulls down the shade.*) They're looking for women. (*Screaming.*) Well, I ain't goin' in there, mother fucker—

WOMAN: He used to say, if he wanted to get rid of someone, he'd cut—cut... (*Pause.*) You know, those tribes in Africa that cut out the clitoris—the puberty rites—

GIRL: How do they do it?

WOMAN: With a knife, to cut out a woman's autonomy. (*Pause.*) One day my father took me to a movie—*Things to Come*—you know, H. G. Wells—and I got so excited. When I came out I turned to my father and—oh, I can't bear it—I said, "Let's change the world together Daddy!" And you know what he did? He laughed. (*Pause.*) It was one of his favorite stories about me. (*Pause.*) He took away my power to have any effect on him. He killed it. I couldn't affect him anymore. I remember the feeling. He was like a god and I was on my knees. (*Pause.*) He had no face. He was faceless—and he took his knife and he cut—(my eyes, my mouth)—I couldn't see him, I couldn't feel him—until I was nothing—

GIRL: (*Cowgirl*)—well ya' ain't been killed yet!

WOMAN: I feel ugly.

GIRL: You're not ugly. You look so much better than me, you've no idea—you look so much younger—

WOMAN: I could kill myself.

GIRL: You can always go' back to him.

WOMAN: I'd get killed again.

GIRL: Isn't that funny—that guy in Holland once said to me that to fall in love really—both people have to commit suicide.

WOMAN: (*Disgust*) Maybe it's true. (*She shivers.*)

GIRL: Do you believe me when I say that I'm just too old for all this? To start all over again?

WOMAN: I understand.

GIRL: He's so thin. (*Pause.*) He sleeps a lot. Oh, he's probably crazy. Listen to this, I wrote him a letter. (*She goes to desk, takes out letter, gets back in bed, and reads.*) "Dearest love of mine, I am longing to be with you, close to you, to feel you, to touch you, to see you, to look at you, to want you, to talk to you, to laugh with you, to cry with you, to play with you, to fight with you, to desire with you, to wish with you, to dream with you, to listen to you, to watch with you, to hear with you, to rest with you, to eat with you, to awaken with you, to sleep with you, to seek with you, to find with you, to hunt with you, to wonder with you, to build with you, to destroy with you, to grow with you, to travel with you, to stand still with you, to be strong with you, to be weak with you, to remember with you, to forget with you, to mourn with you, to have joy with you, to be rich with you, to be poor with you, to be all with you, to make love with you, to wait with you, to rush with you, to swim with you, to drown with you, to float with you, to fly with you, to sing with you, to die with you, to live with you, to away with you, to reach with you, to burst with you, to more with you, and more with you, to be free with you, to be bound with you, to be me with you, to be you with you, to be us with you, to be silent with you, to be noise with you, to believe with you, to know nothing with you, to know everything with you, to run with you, to walk with you, to learn with you, to teach with you, to keep with you, to give away with you, to be pieces with you, to be whole with you, to be tired with you, to be an animal with you, to be a leaf with you, to be a tree with you, to be the grass with you, to be the sky with you, to be the dark with you, to be the light with you, to be the stars with you, to be the night with you, to be the day with you, to be the sun with you, to survive with you, to be the one with you, to be the many with you, to be god with you, to be nothing with you, to be everything with you, to be with you, to be with you. . ."

WOMAN: Were you stoned when you wrote it?

GIRL: No.

WOMAN: Why don't you call him?

GIRL: What'll I say to him? He's a stranger. (*Pause.*) I want to call him. I want to. I want to. No, I can't. I just can't.

WOMAN: I'll help you.

GIRL: How? You gonna do the talking? (WOMAN *writes a script*, GIRL *picks up phone, dials. Reading script.*) "Hello, how are you? I was just thinking about you, and I had an urge to call. I just wanted to hear your voice ... I miss you." (*Repeats from "Hello, how are you?" Rehearsing with sincerity.*) "Hello, how are you ... (*Then, phone connection made. Now actual speech. Stilted, cool, nervous speech, building to unnaturalistic.*) Hi. Remember me? How are you? It is cold there? It's freezing here. Snowing. Yeah? It's very cold. Yes, we're having a terrible winter. It was below zero yesterday. I don't know how much—Yea. You sound clear as if you were just around the corner. Do I sound clear too? Yes, it is expensive. O.K. Yes. (*Then, very phony.*) Right, sure. Right, yes, great, yea, great! Yes. Sure. Bye now. Yes. Bye. (*Normal speech.*) What did I sound like?

(*Blackout.*)

(*Women under hair dryers, the following spoken loudly. Lights up.*)

WOMAN: I'll bet there are lots of times when you're not uninhibited.

GIRL: You mean I'm inhibited?

WOMAN: Yes.

GIRL: In bed when I'm naked with a man, I'm inhibited — unless it's dark.

WOMAN: You??

(*They come out from under the dryers.*)

GIRL: Don't think it's fun to have hairs growing out of your breasts and a skin fungus.

WOMAN: Well, what do you think I have?

GIRL: (*Interrupting*) — and rolls of fat —!

WOMAN: But what I have is a deformity.

GIRL: Rolls of fat are not deformities —? (*Pause.*) You know what amazes me? Death!

(*Stage goes black — time lapse — both women in bed — it's dark — 4 p.m.*)

WOMAN: I just thought of something.

GIRL: (*Bright voice*)   I'm up — go ahead — I'm up.

WOMAN: One night, we were out driving and he asked me if there was
anything I wanted specially to do and I said go dancing. He said he
knew a place, but when we got there, some private party was going
on, and they said we couldn't come in. He kept insisting. I began to
feel embarrassed. Finally, we left. We drove for a while and then,
without saying anything, he turned the car around and drove back
and parked. He went to the trunk and got something out and said
he'd just be a minute. He walked away, and after some time, he
came back, and got in the car, and said he couldn't fine the main
line — and I said — what line? — and he said — the electric line —
and I said — What did you want that for? — And he said — I
wanted to cut it — To cut it — And I asked him — Why? — And he
said — Because they wouldn't let us in — I thought it was funny —
you know, funny, and I started to laugh.

GIRL: Why did you laugh?

WOMAN: I thought it was funny — No, not really funny. You know,
funny.

GIRL: I wouldn't have thought it was funny. (*Pause.*)

WOMAN: There was something else.

GIRL: Go ahead!!

WOMAN: One night, we'd been to a country bar, and as we were leaving, walking along this dark lane, a car almost hit us. He watched
the car come to a stop — saw a man get out and go into the bar. He
said, You stay here and signal if you see anyone coming. Then he
walked to the man's car, raised the hood, lowered the hood, and
came back. I saw an object in his hand. What did you do?, I asked.
He said: That man won't drive again. I said: Why did you do it?
Why? He said: He came too close to us.

GIRL: Did he do anything else that was funny?

WOMAN: I never knew if he was serious.

GIRL: What made you think he wasn't serious?

(*Film projected — Love making sequence in black and white during
the following text. Meanwhile, women apply white clown make-up to
faces. Text may be repeated to cover duration of film, ending with,
"What about art?"*)

GIRL: It was the fact that we didn't talk much that appealed to me. The
mystery of not knowing everything appealed to my imagination.

WOMAN: I don't know if I want him —

GIRL: That's all there is, there's nothing else.

WOMAN: What about art?

GIRL: When was that?

WOMAN: What do you mean by civilized?

GIRL: What do you mean by woman?

WOMAN: It isn't always so easy to be swept away. Swept away.

(*Women in bed with white facial masks on.*)

GIRL: Did you ever go down to Mexico to get a divorce?

WOMAN: No, did you?

GIRL: The second time. The first time, I got an annulment. I remember my father sitting up there in front of the judge, saying: I've been a lawyer in Manhattan for thirty years, and I remember that on Thanksgiving Day, 1957, my son-in-law Joel Smarlow sat at dinner with the family and said: When I married my wife, I had no intention of having children — but I told her this only after and not before we were married, and now she claims it was a fraudulent marriage and wants it annuled. (*Laughter.*)

WOMAN: Joel Smarlow — what a name!

GIRL: Joel Smarlow. Joel. Joel, I love you. — David, I love you. Jack, I love you. Charlie, I love you. Jim, I love you. Freddy, I love you. Willie, I love you. Sam, I love you. Homer, I love you. Angelino, I love you. — Would you believe it if I told you I'm just too old for all this to start all over again.

WOMAN: I'd understand.

GIRL: I don't want a domestic life.

WOMAN: You don't have to have a domestic life.

GIRL: I wish my mother was dead.

WOMAN: You make your own life.

(*Cocktail party voice.*)

GIRL: You know what they'd say, they'd say to me — "Oh, Hi, what's new? Haven't seen you around."

WOMAN: Oh, I've been away, living in Holland.

GIRL: Why? What're you doing in Holland?

WOMAN: Living.

GIRL: That's nice.

WOMAN: I like it.

GIRL: What d'ya do with all that famous energy of yours?

WOMAN: I'm in love.

GIRL: Again? What's he do?

WOMAN: He's a hotel-keeper.

GIRL: You're kidding. Oh, underneath he's another genius, right?

WOMAN: Could be.

GIRL: So what next? You gonna settle down, get married and have babies?

WOMAN: I'd like that.

GIRL: Come on. How long do you give this one?

WOMAN: I adore him.

GIRL: I do? Yea, but what are ya gonna *do* in Holland?

(*The following conversation takes place while washing off facial masks.*)

WOMAN: People act as if love is a luxury, not a necessity.

GIRL: Well, it ain't food or shelter. (Pause.) The thing is they act as if they don't believe it — it's out of the question — oh, once it was possible, but not any more, not these days — Times have changed. — but they think they can manipulate it, insert it in, a convenience, you know when they're good and ready and everything's under control, all set — you got your education, you got your diploma, you got your taste developed — you know what kind of furniture you want, you know the kinds of books you like, whether you're a cat person or a dog person, a country person or a city person — whether you're a Mercedes type or an Oldsmobile station wagon type — you're a finished product, see?
   They can take it or leave it, but all you have to do is point your finger and say — You, you're the one for me — It's you — (*Pause.*) But you still believe in it. I can tell . . .

WOMAN: You have to be a revolutionary to love. Love is a revolutionary act.

GIRL: I wish my father was dead. I wish my mother was dead. I wish I could let myself die. (*Pause.*)— And start all over—

WOMAN: "And proceed from the dream outward" —

GIRL: That's Jung, isn't it?

WOMAN: Yeah, I think so. You know, I've always wanted to go to South America.

GIRL: I always wanted to go to India.

WOMAN: You'd get sick there.

GIRL: I wouldn't get sick. Oh, I might get another fungus or something, but I wouldn't get sick.

WOMAN: I used to want to go to Japan.

GIRL: Japan's finished.

WOMAN: What about the North Pole?

GIRL: What would you do there?

WOMAN: I read a wonderful book about Eskimos.

GIRL: I know where I want to go, Indonesia.

WOMAN: Indonesia?

GIRL: What do you say we get out of here and go to a restaurant, and think the whole thing over.

(*Lights out. Satie music on, text projected on wall like the beginning. Text and music remain on as audience leaves.*)

End

In The Midnight Hour

Hour

Kathleen Collins

Author's Note

In the midnight hour dreams that have been sitting on either side of you, dreams you knew nothing about, faces that you have been waiting for for a lifetime, memories you wanted to leave behind, all these things begin to take shape before your eyes in the midnight hour, conversations begin that have everything to do with living, life unbends before your eyes and if it's all a dream then let yourself dream, laugh, take your living into the light, let it come floating out of you and all the things you want to remember will come true in the midnight hour.

Characters

RALPH DANIELS, a man around forty-five.
LILLIE DANIELS, his wife, around the same age.
ANNA DANIELS, their twenty-year-old daughter.
BEN DANIELS, their eighteen-year-old son.
CHRISTINE EDWARDS, a friend of Ben and Anna's, a girl around twenty.
FLOYD HAMILTON, a family friend, a man around forty-nine.
CHIPS, the piano player and family friend, a man around twenty-nine.

The Place: The living room of an unexpected apartment in the middle of Harlem.

The Time: The year is 1962.

Act I: Around nine in the evening.

Act II: Scene 1: Around the midnight hour.
          Scene 2: In the middle of the night.

Act III: The next morning.

In the Midnight Hour was given a rehearsed reading by The Women's Project on February 4, 1980, directed by Billie Allen, with the following cast:

RALPH DANIELS . . . . Richard Gant
LILLIE DANIELS . . . . Zaida Coles
FLOYD HAMILTON . . . . Carl Gordon
BEN DANIELS . . . . Zachary Minor
ANNA DANIELS . . . . Lorey Hayes
CHRISTINE EDWARDS . . . . Christine Campbell
CHIPS . . . . Charles Brown

The play was first read at the Frank Silvera Workshop.

ACT I

A large spacious living room in a New York apartment. Big picture window looking out over the Harlem River. Comfortably furnished but distinctive in that all the furniture—couch, armchairs, tables, complicated wall units with bookcase and shelves for a stereo, etc.,—everything is handcrafted in beautiful, unusual looking wood that has been carefully stained and finished. A baby grand piano fills one corner of the room. At the far right is an alcove with a small dining room table and chairs and an overhanging lamp, again all handcrafted pieces. Everything is comfortable. The room is well-lit, interesting pictures and photographs hang on the walls, there are lots of books and magazines around. It's the kind of space that truly welcomes you, come stay, sit down in an easy chair and read a book, browse through all the magazines scattered around, have some coffee or a drink, play the piano, talk awhile, let's get to know each other, say whatever's on your mind, we're all trying to figure out life as best we can, let's get a little pleasure and truth from each other, enjoy each other for awhile. This is the feeling that the room gives.

When the play opens, RALPH DANIELS *is alone in the room. He's squatting in front of a long, unusual-looking coffee table which he's just finished making. He runs his hand admiringly across the surface, brushes a little more stain into the wood and rubs it down gently. He whistles, talks and laughs to himself while he works. Already we can tell he's a funny man with a droll feeling for the humor and irony of life. Physically he is of medium height, light negro skin, glasses, black crinkly hair brushed away from his face, about forty-five years old. It's around nine o'clock in the evening, Duke Ellington's "Take the A Train" is playing in the background. On this gentle mellow note the play begins.*

RALPH: (*Laughing*) That wood is smooth, yes it is, a beautiful piece of wood there's nothing like it, you take a beautiful piece of wood, a saw, a lathe, a little sanding, and you can make something, anything, and then you have it. Life is craftsmanship you just need the right tools. (*Laughing at his own philosophy.*) You get the right tools and you can make it work, you can make it smooth too, there don't have to be no bumps, nowhere, no sir (*That really makes him laugh*), no indeed, not if you start with the right tools. Life is craftsmanship. Wait till Ben sees that table.

(*He chuckles over that while he puts away his tools, whistles a little of "Take the A Train," mixes himself a little Jack Daniels.*)

I'm in no hurry, this is the time in my time when I'm in no hurry, just after a little bit of the truth, and who's to say the 'A' train will get me there (*He chuckles*), the truth may not stop at 125th Street, might be a local only (*He gets a kick out of his own metaphors*), I'm still in no hurry, I got a lot of stops before then, I'm gonna make everyone of them, this is the time in my time when I'm gonna make every one of them. (*He goes over to the window and looks out.*) Where's Lillie?

(LILLIE DANIELS *comes in, a stunning looking woman around forty-two with real presence and charm. Sometimes her voice and manner can be a little affected for those who know her well but she is always trying very hard to be a real person. This makes her sometimes funny, sometimes genuinely witty and eccentric but even when she fails her beauty always works. She is followed by* FLOYD HAMILTON, *a dapper scholarly looking man around forty-nine.* FLOYD *has a polished urbane manner, the true loner intellectual, master conversationalist and humanist, eager to engage in any kind of dialogue about life, people, events, situations. He's been a close family friend for years.*)

LILLIE: (*Excited*) Floyd's with me, Ralph, he was down at the police station talking about cruelty, I had to drag him away, you should have seen him, Ralph, he had these two bright young Negro cops in the palm of his hand, questioning them about the nature of cruelty, the relationship between the citizen and the police, what they felt their moral duties were that stem from the moral imperative as opposed to their imagined duties resulting from the social imperative, you should have seen their faces it was too much . . . a wonderful scene, just fascinating.

RALPH: (*Laughing*) Old Floyd's always up to his tricks, you need a drink, Floyd.

LILLIE: (*Laughing*) I've got some leftover spaghetti, Floyd, a ham, some baked beans, what would you like?

FLOYD: I don't need much, Lillie, I'm in the presence of generosity and charm, a room in which I can breathe and laugh and have my peace. I never need much of anything when I'm here, Lillie.

RALPH: You old bum, this man's full of it, Lillie, a mouth full of marbles, it's a wonder they let him walk the streets. How's your book coming, Floyd, the final treatise on justice and the humane society, listen, take a look at this you old bum, take a look at . . . Lillie, come in here and take a look at this. (*Pointing to his table.*) Craftsmanship, you old bum, it's craftsmanship we've got to talk about one of these days.

LILLIE: Ralph, it's a beauty, it's really a beauty, wait till Ben sees it, and look what you did with the legs, that's something new, isn't it, you never tried that before.

RALPH: (*Enthusiastic*) I got a new tool, Lillie, it can do incredible things, shape the wood in ways I've never tried. I'm just at the beginning of understanding it, it's got a million attachments, I fit one on and this is what I came out with. Next I'm gonna make that bedside table you want, with a place for the phone and a place for messages and a night light, too. I've got a good sketch worked out, Lillie, you're gonna love it. What do you think of my table, Floyd?

FLOYD: It works, it works. It hangs together with feeling. You knew that when you made it. You've got perfect instincts, nobody can teach you a thing when you're down in that shop, what am I supposed to add.

RALPH: (*Chuckling*) You just got to like it, you old bum. Listen Floyd, you ever use your hands . . . tell me what you ever did with your hands . . . you ever play baseball, hold a bat, catch with a mitt, you ever draw, play the violin, thump on the piano, carve figures out of wood . . . give me an answer, you old bum.

FLOYD: (*A sly smile*) The question's about time, my man, you think it moves faster if you use your hands. Not me. Even in the beginning I had a favorite trick, I could stop and listen. For me that's the best trick. I like your table because it's one of your favorite tricks, that's all.

RALPH: (*Chuckling*) Feed him to the wolves, Lillie, feed him to the wolves. Hey, Floyd, I'm turning it upside down, you know that don't you . . . four times a week I step into that psychiatrist's office and take a look at things, it's like having a whole new set of tools. I can take things apart now, look at them in new ways. I never been so excited in my life. I got something brand new, Floyd . . . (*He looks at* LILLIE) . . . don't I, Lillie.

LILLIE: (*Gently*) You can't stop him these days, Floyd, I don't even know if I can keep up with him. He comes home full of new answers, a new way of looking at things, it's something, Floyd, really something.

(*The door opens, three young people come in led by* BEN DANIELS, *a vibrant young man of eighteen, an unforgettable face, a perfect crossing of* LILLIE's *beauty and* RALPH's *sensitivity. He is so full of energy that the room seems to spin around him. He is followed by* ANNA DANIELS, *his sister, a lively vivacious young woman of twenty not as pretty as her mother nor as handsome as her brother but with an incredible vitality all her own.* CHRISTINE EDWARDS *is behind her, a shy girl, watching, with a strong intelligent face.*)

BEN: (*Snapping his fingers, singing at the top of his voice*) I'm gonna wait till the midnight hour, that's when my love comes tumbling down, I'm gonna wait till the midnight hour, when there's no one else around (*He begins dancing like a maniac, snapping his fingers, laughing*), cause you're the only girl I know and I really really love you so in the midnight hour. (*He lifts* CHRISTINE *up in the air, pulls her to the center of the room.*) Look what I found, an orphan, a stray, Christine Edwards meet my folks ... that's Ralph, my Pop, and that's Lillie, my Mom ... (*He spots* FLOYD) and that's Floyd, our Floyd, the wandering nigger ... (*He circles the room with her*) and this is everything else, the place, the hour (*He cracks up laughing*), this is everything else.

ANNA: (*Laughing, carried by her own enthusiastic wave*) He's been like that all night, standing outside, laughing, while Christine and I just listened to the best speech of our lives, we're converts, ready to lay our bodies down, aren't we, Christine, we're ready, ready. ... (*She's caught between an almost righteous enthusiasm and the humor of herself carrying on like this.*) You should have been there, Floyd, it was the place for you, everything was there: theology, philosophy, sociology, ecstasy, ecstasy carried the day, Floyd, I just had my first encounter with ecstasy, and I'm different now (*Becoming a little serious*), I've added something to myself.

RALPH: (*Laughing*) Good old Anna with her additions and subtractions, it's a pleasure to meet you, Christine, welcome, how did a nice girl like you get sidetracked by two loonies, you came along with the first and the last of the crazies, Christine, and I apologize in advance for what they may say or do in your presence. (*He is affected by her shyness, likes her right away.*) Would you like a cigarette. (*He offers her one and lights it for her.*)

LILLIE: (*Walking over to* CHRISTINE) Hello, Christine.

ANNA: (*Joining them*) She's going to spend the night. I invited her first, but Ben claims she's his guest but I saw her first, we were sitting right next to each other and I wanted to hold her hand, she was the only person there who was feeling the same things I was feeling, she was already my friend before we said hello. (*She hugs her.*)

RALPH: (*Teasing* FLOYD) You need a drink? I never saw a man get more mileage out of sitting still and watching, we should call you the sedentary prince, the kingpin philosopher, but all it amounts to is lechery, cold analytical lechery. (*He chuckles, motions to* BEN.) You know what Floyd said about my table (*Pointing it out to his son with pride*), he called it one of my best tricks, I ought to make him stand on his head for that, see what I did with the legs.

BEN: (*Always direct, always simple*) Yeah. It's a beauty. (*Looking at* FLOYD, *teasing him.*) What do you say, man, give Pop a break.

FLOYD: (*Looking at* BEN *who forces him to be more direct, more honest*) It's a fine-looking piece of craftsmanship.

BEN: (*Cracking up*) You're full of shit, Floyd, that's what I like about you, you're full of shit.

LILLIE: (*Wincing*) Ben . . .

(*He pays her no mind, turns the volume up on "Take the A Train" and begins dancing with* ANNA, *free and easy, full of energy and grace, affection and pleasure.*)

LILLIE: (*Watching them, talking to* CHRISTINE *with a mixture of pride and bewilderment*) They grew up without us, that's what I think sometimes, that they grew up without us, I try and remember where we were when they were growing up, what house we were living in, what was going on at the time, it all happened so fast, and there they are.

CHRISTINE: (*Looking at* LILLIE *admiringly*) But they're happy, that must be all that matters.

(RALPH *shakes his head at his children, walks over to* CHRISTINE *and* LILLIE.)

RALPH: Where do you come from Christine, you a New York girl?

CHRISTINE: No, Boston's my home, that's where my folks live, I'm studying at Barnard.

RALPH: A Barnard girl, you hear that, Floyd, our Christine's a Barnard girl, well what do you know, what year are you in, Christine?

CHRISTINE: This is my second year.

RALPH: A second year Barnard girl, you hear that, Lillie, that's exactly where we wanted Anna to go, but she wouldn't hear of it, went and enrolled at City College, took an apartment on the Lower East Side, Anna has a need to be different, but she can handle it . . . I never worry about Anna . . .

(ANNA *and* BEN *stop dancing.* BEN *changes the record to a strong jazz solo, most likely Ornette Coleman, then wraps himself in the music, his music, like a perfect rhythmic accompaniment.* RALPH *pours himself another drink, offers one to* FLOYD *who refuses.* ANNA *comes over to* CHRISTINE.)

ANNA: You want to see my old room? I keep it just like it was. I didn't take a thing when I moved. It's my history that room. My most personal references are there, all the things I'll need to remember as I move away from here and define myself in the world. (*She takes* CHRISTINE's *hand, they go off.*)

RALPH: (*Mostly talking to himself*) I'd like to live long enough to read Anna's memoirs, that's what she'll do one day, she'll put it all down, that room's like a museum, like she was the careful historian of her time and place in the world. It'll all be there, every memory, every event, I wish I could read it now, at this moment in my time when I can learn things I'd like to borrow her memory, have it tell me about all the years when I was asleep, what did I do, how did I talk, what did I say that gave her such a happy childhood when I wasn't really here.

FLOYD: (*Alert to all that* RALPH *is saying*) It doesn't matter where you were. You settled for the right myths. I'd call it a lucky accident or the instincts of a truly honest man. It doesn't matter. You gave them a perfect smell for kindness and sin.

LILLIE: (*Upset*) He thinks that none of it counts because he wasn't really here.

(*Nothing is said for a moment.*)

RALPH: (*Chuckling*) I've been thinking a lot about my brother Carl. He's a smart man Carl is, when he was nineteen he finished up Phi Betta Summa Cum Laude . . . and some big biochemical firm grabbed him up for research. We never got along the two of us, he was always off with his experiments while I was sitting around playing with horseshoes, I could throw a perfect horseshoe just about every time. One day Carl came out back when I was playing and I said: "Carl, do you think you've got any manual dexterity?" (*He laughs.*) Just where did I come up with a phrase like "manual dexterity." I was so impressed with myself that I said—I could hardly keep a straight face—I said, "Carl, if you stand there a minute I'll give you a real exhibition of manual dexterity."

(*He stands there chuckling to himself,* BEN *starts laughing.*)

BEN: (*Laughing*) You said that to him, you always act like you're afraid of him. I don't like to see the two of you together.

RALPH: I am afraid of him. Carl's a scientist, I got nothing but respect for science.

(*He and* BEN *laugh. There is deep affection between them, the son has arrived at a pretty honest assessment of the father, the father feels little need to defend himself.*)

RALPH: We got nothing in common, me and Carl, nothing. But I got a lot of respect for him, he's an organized man, handsome, correct, drives a beautiful Mercedes, lives in an elegant apartment with marble floors, marble walls, a handsome looking foreigner for a wife, it's a classy life Carl organized for himself. (*He shakes his head not really chuckling this time.*)

FLOYD: You admire him.

RALPH: (*Thinking about it*) He's an impeccable kind of guy. Always played by the rules.

BEN: What's he mean to you?

RALPH: (*Smiling*) I like to shake his hand. Carl's one of the few guys who walks in a room and I want to shake his hand, you know (*He grabs for* BEN's *hand*) give him the firmest handshake I can muster, look him dead in the eye, "good to see you, Carl, how's tricks." (*He and* BEN *crack up.*) I don't know if I can take it any further, he's my brother.

BEN: You do stuff with him like you do with me, go sailing or biking, stuff like that?

RALPH: Never. Carl and me were like two only children.

BEN: (*Laughing*) He's not even your brother.

RALPH: He's my brother alright, same flesh same memory, that's all it takes.

BEN: (*Quietly, thinking about it*) Then I'm luckier than you because I really like Anna. (*He walks over to his mother.*) What are you fixing to eat, Lillie?

LILLIE: (*Flushed and happy*) Floyd's hungry, you're hungry, is everybody hungry?

BEN: (*Hugging her*) Yeah, Lillie, everybody's hungry, now what are you fixing to eat? (*He leads her gently into the kitchen.*)

RALPH: (*Shaking his head, putting his "Take the A Train" record back on*) Never know what he'll recognize next. (*He takes out a cigarette, stands smoking, listening, ruminating in space.*)

FLOYD: (*Half to himself, half to* RALPH) 1944 when I first came to

Harlem, you and Lillie were on Edgecombe Avenue, Anna was just
born, Lillie had dark circles under her eyes, she was very happy but
tired, we'd walk over to Convent Avenue, walk under the trees
down to St. Nicholas park with Anna in the baby carriage. Lillie's
hair was black and shiny, she had a gray lambskin coat, people
took me for Anna's father, you were in the Navy then, first time
you saw her she was six months old, it was fall in those days, I had
a job with the YMCA, politics and Christian morals, big revival
meetings on the Old Ironside campus, I wanted to become a monk,
a religious socialist hidden away in a monastery, wanted to go into
some order, the Society of Jesuitical Thought, the Benedictines,
take the vows, live a thoughtful life, used to walk around in a navy
blue trenchcoat with a navy blue french beret, had a room in those
days on the fifth floor corner of 155th Street and St. Nicholas Terrace with a bed and a typewriter, took my meals in the YMCA
Cafeteria, spent my off hours at the 42nd Street Library doing
research in civilization and the roots of evil, life, science, anthropology, the nature of dialogue, the principles of aesthetics and
morality, religion and ecstatic experience, the structure of the
molecule, biology and human behavior, psychoanalysis and myth,
voodoo witchcraft, telepathic experience, primitive thought and
organization, man and his gods, sin and salvation, the dialectic of
catholicism, christian humanism and ethics, the nature of saint-
hood, creativity and bourgeois materialism. There were places I
went for coffee, places for bourbon and scotch, a little lady named
Mabel Diggs had a place on the East Side where you could get free
drinks just as long as you wanted to talk, met a woman named
Helen who lived in the Village and was passing, we used to stay up
all night and talk, it was fall in those days . . . (*He stops.* RALPH
picks it up like this was the way they always spoke to each other,
half out loud, half introspective and drifting.)

RALPH: (*Chuckling*) Came back from the war a circumspect sailor
still wearing his cap, had no idea what I was supposed to do, who
was to know, who could offer me anything but a job, straight from
the Navy I sailed directly into insurance (*He chuckles*), put on a suit
and tie, polished my shoes, put my token in the subway, somebody
said, Over Here, Daniels, made me a manager, straight from the
Navy, Lillie bouncing a baby in her arms, smiling like a winning
photograph, had no idea what was going on, had to perform every
morning so I made it in insurance. (*He laughs out loud.*) What did I
think I was doing, making it in insurance? Didn't know what I was
doing, took the subway at 125th Street, had an apartment, smiled
at folks, built myself a little shop in the kitchen closet, made Anna
a rocking chair, a cradle for her dolls, didn't know what was going
on, something must have been going on, smoked my cigarettes, took

Anna to the park, got the subway at 125th St. to go into insurance
. . . (*He chuckles definitively*) that's right I was in insurance, I was
making it in insurance. (*He can't stop chuckling.*) Tell me again
what you did in San Bernardino.

FLOYD: It's the one time I tried for the priesthood.

RALPH: And how long were you there?

FLOYD: Seven years from 1949 to 1956.

RALPH: After Helen.

FLOYD: After Helen.

RALPH: And what about Delores?

FLOYD: Saint Delores, in the garden, overlooking the San Bernardino
Valley, in a grove of eucalyptus trees, a Mexican woman with
Helen's middle name, she reminded me of Helen.

RALPH: But you didn't take the final vows.

FLOYD: You know all that.

RALPH: I know I know it, I know the whole story, I ask you again and
again, and you tell me again and again, but it always smells fishy,
there's something wrong with that story, something that's not true,
it's the only story you ever told me that's not true.

FLOYD: (*Laughing*) I always tell it the same.

RALPH: (*Laughing*) That's not the point, you old bum. (*He shakes his
head.* LILLIE *comes in.*)

LILLIE: Who's hungry, are you still hungry, Floyd?

BEN: (*Coming in just behind her*) Everybody's hungry, Lillie, just serve
the food.

(CHRISTINE *comes in, stands in the doorway looking,* BEN *watches
her.*)

CHRISTINE: (*Looking at* BEN) It's really a room, it has paintings and
faded flowers, old photographs and books, I never saw a room like
it. I think Anna's wonderful, very alive and wonderful, you all are.
Very different from anyone I've ever known.

BEN: (*Smiling proudly*) That's because you're old, just a little old lady.

(*They stand looking across at each other, neither one moving from his
spot.*)

CHRISTINE: I saw your room.

BEN: (*Proudly*) My room's the junkyard, scraps of metal, busted tires, screwdrivers, wrenches, old refrigerators and stoves, pieces of driftwood that stand for trees.

CHRISTINE: It feels like you.

BEN: It is me. I can strut around that room with my head above the junk (*He begins to do a series of very funny falls, like a drunk, an acrobat, a silent comedian all rolled into one*), turn cartwheels, somersaults, do the zigzag, the shimmy, stretch out on that bed like a zombie. (*He falls out flat as a board.* CHRISTINE *starts laughing, a raucous, throaty kind of laugh that is somehow out of character. It surprises* BEN *and* RALPH *at the same time.*)

RALPH: Well, what do you know, Christine can laugh, you hear that, Ben, the girl can laugh, what a laugh coming from that serious face, the girl can laugh. Your folks know about that laugh, Christine? (*She looks at him unsure whether he's teasing or not, this makes him want to keep it up.*) Next time you're in Boston you tell your father about that laugh, tell your mother, too, that's the kind of thing a parent should know about. (*He chuckles.*) What you thinking, Christine?

CHRISTINE: I'm not sure.

RALPH: (*Taken with this girl*) You're a serious girl, aren't you, Christine. Don't let that laugh fool anybody, you're a serious girl. Came down from Boston, Boston's a serious place, all the way down to Barnard College, what you studying, Christine, theology, linguistics, anthropology, romance languages, whatever it is it's serious. (*He has an urge to hug her which he restrains.*) Christine's a serious girl.

BEN: (*Suddenly angry*) Cut it out ...

(RALPH *turns around, surprised.*)

BEN: You tease hard, all the time you tease hard now like you want to draw blood.

RALPH: What's that supposed to mean?

BEN: I don't know ... but I don't like it. (*He stalks out the room. You can hear his door slam.*)

RALPH: (*Apologizing in a way to* CHRISTINE) Who ever knows where anger starts, who ever knows what they're really angry about. (*He turns away, goes over to the window.* LILLIE *comes in.*)

LILLIE: What's the matter with Ben?

RALPH: (*Facing the window*) He's angry.

LILLIE: About what?

RALPH: About being eighteen. About falling off the kitchen table when he was two. About the way you wear your hair. About Christine's laugh. About the last time he saw me cry. Who ever knows what anybody's angry about.

LILLIE: He was hungry.

RALPH: I'm sure he still is.

LILLIE: We should have a nice meal. I'd like to hear about the girls' meeting. I think Anna's decided to join the Movement. Everything looks big through her eyes ... (*Drifting.*) I don't even know where I am ... what year are we in, Floyd?

FLOYD: (*Circumspect, amused*) It's 1962, Lillie, you know that.

LILLIE: (*Smiling*) Everything looks so big through her eyes. Ask Ben to come out, Ralph. He gets so angry these days.

RALPH: He'll come out, Lillie.

LILLIE: What are you thinking, Ralph.

RALPH: I was looking at the lights on the river, Lillie. They go all the way up to the bridge. I was wondering how many times I've left this apartment, put my feet on the sidewalk and started walking in some direction. Any direction. Trying to get myself somewhere. (*He chuckles.*) What you thinking, Lillie ...

LILLIE: I was thinking about Anna. She's going to do something on her own soon, different and unexpected.

RALPH: She can handle it, I never worry about Anna.

(ANNA *comes in.*)

ANNA: What's going on?

(*There is no answer.* BEN *comes in playing his flute. He stops when he sees that no one is moving or talking.*)

BEN: (*Still angry*) I don't like to be the first to speak.

RALPH: (*Ruefully*) At this or any other gathering ...

BEN: Floyd should speak. Tell us about the good times in this room, Floyd, the easy dialogues on truth and existence.

RALPH: Floyd comes from a long line of sedentary philosophers ...

BEN: You ever hold a job, Floyd?

FLOYD: Not to my knowledge ...

BEN: How do you live with yourself, man, that's a question I've always meant to ask you.

FLOYD: At best ... an uneasy alliance.

(*That cracks* BEN *up.*)

BEN: (*Laughing*) You never overstate things, do you, Floyd.

LILLIE: (*To* BEN) You used to call Floyd your mentor. (*To* CHRISTINE.) He *was* their mentor, Christine, taught them to think, analyze, discuss ideas and possible solutions. The discussions we've had in this room! Fascinating ... just fascinating! What shall we talk about today, Floyd, give us a subject for today.

ANNA: I'd like to talk about nonviolence.

BEN: You would. (*He grabs an apple and a knife from the table.*) Anna's the new custodian of her time. Come unto Anna all ye who are lowly and poor in spirit and Anna will give you rest.

ANNA: That's mean! (*He doesn't answer, begins peeling the apple, standing, watching.*)

ANNA: (*Turning to* FLOYD) I'd like to talk about the Movement, Floyd, I don't want you to tell me if I'm doing the right thing, but I'd like to hear an argument.

FLOYD: Shall we start as always with a common point of view, a definition of terms. Suppose we agree that the Movement is evangelical politics.

ANNA: Why? Because it's nonviolent?

FLOYD: No, because it believes in the persuasion of righteousness.

ANNA: It is righteous.

FLOYD: That's an evangelical attitude, the religious evangelist says the first necessity is to recognize and acknowledge God, then conversion will follow.

ANNA: I don't want to talk about God, Floyd.

FLOYD: (*Nodding*) The political evangelist says the first necessity is to recognize and acknowledge the righteousness of the cause, then justice will follow.

ANNA: Is that what I am, a political evangelist?

BEN: (*Quietly but not without bite*) You could be anything, an anarchist, a poet, even a saint if you decided to dream that far.

FLOYD: You're committed to persuasion.

ANNA: (*Nodding agreement*) I can accept that. I can accept myself as that ... a political evangelist, a nonviolent soldier ... (*She turns to* CHRISTINE.) What about you, Christine?

CHRISTINE: I'm not sure.

ANNA: But you're planning to join the Movement.

CHRISTINE: I'm thinking about it. But not like that. Not in terms of justice and persuasion. It's more personal for me, more selfish. (*She looks at* FLOYD.) Should you join the Movement for selfish reasons?

BEN: (*Who by now has begun to juggle the knife in the air, trying to catch it each time by the handle end*) Go on, Christine, ask him a few straight questions. Make her one of your pupils, Floyd.

FLOYD: I'm not sure what Christine means.

CHRISTINE: I think Anna really wants to help people. I'm not sure I do, I think I just want to understand things. I mean tonight, listening to all those speeches, I realized I hadn't faced anything about being Negro in this country, that I was living in another world and it seemed very selfish, all my preoccupations seemed very selfish and I thought I shouldn't be satisfied with them anymore.

BEN: (*Stopping for a second*) That's the first honest thing I've heard in a long time.

CHRISTINE: What do you think, Floyd?

FLOYD: The politics of persuasion can tolerate a large degree of self-interest.

BEN: She's not talking about politics, Floyd.

FLOYD: You didn't hear me . . .

BEN: I heard you, my ears were wide open and you're full of shit.

LILLIE: (*Wincing*) Ben!

ANNA: We're talking about justice, Ben, not politics.

BEN: (*Getting angrier*) *You're* talking about justice, Christine's not, she's talking about something else that I don't think either of you can hear.

LILLIE: What did they decide about selfishness, Ralph?

RALPH: I'll keep you posted, Lillie . . .

ANNA: (*To* BEN) I hate when you do that, act like you're the only one who sees the truth.

BEN: You're turning into a politician, you know that, just another goddamn politician.

ANNA: Floyd and I were having a conversation about persuasion.

BEN: (*Shaking his head*) It's not about persuasion. It's about need.

Your need. To hang up banners all over your goddamn life.

LILLIE: Why does Ben have to curse, Ralph, this is a fascinating conversation . . . fascinating.

RALPH: He's angry, Lillie, anger cannot be judged by shits goddamns pisses . . . (*He chuckles.*)

ANNA: (*To* BEN) I think Christine has good reasons for joining the Movement. (*She turns to* CHRISTINE.) If you see how lucky your life has been that's all the more reason for going . . .

CHRISTINE: (*Uncertain*) I don't know . . . you come from such a clear place. It's different for me. I feel bad about a lot of things . . .

ANNA: (*Not understanding, suddenly angry at everyone*) We can't argue anymore like we used to, I wanted to talk about ethics and philosophy, the things I'll need to think about as I go out in the world.

BEN: (*Throwing the knife high in the air*) Preach a sermon, Floyd, yea though Anna walks through the valley of the shadow of death . . . (*He loses control, catches the knife by the blade end, cutting his hand.*)

ANNA: (*Screaming*) No . . . .

BEN: (*His hand bleeding quite a bit*) I missed, that's all. Anyone can miss.

(*They stand looking at each other, then* ANNA *turns away.*)

ANNA: (*Spinning inside a slow private dance*) Once we had something that was almost perfect, funny and sad, once we had each other and we took pictures and smiled and remembered something funny from the day before. Once we had each other and it was good and true, and we took photographs to prove it.

(*Lights go out.*)

ACT II
Scene 1

A few hours later. "Take the A Train" plays softly in the background but maybe instead of Ellington it's Anita O'Day or Carmen McCrae singing it. RALPH and FLOYD are in the living room deep in conversation. LILLIE and ANNA are sitting talking at the dining room table. Both conversations have been going on for awhile and are already inside a certain rhythm. The night still feels young though it must be close to midnight by now. The later it gets the more honest and warm the room becomes, each person getting looser and looser saying more and more easily whatever's on their mind.

RALPH: I'm forty-five.

FLOYD: That's got nothing to do with it.

RALPH: You're forty-nine am I right?

FLOYD: You're right.

RALPH: You don't finish things, Floyd.

FLOYD: They change, I arrive at solutions only to see they no longer apply.

RALPH: Still living in one room in one suit among dirty laundry and books. (*He shakes his head.*) We go back a long way, that's what it comes to, we say to each other, we go back a long way, that's our answer. Not anymore. I'm not gonna say that anymore.

(*They are silent for awhile.*)

ANNA: I can't wait to be old, Momma, eccentric, crazy, dealing in potions and herbs, dressed like some wild gypsy lady who knows everything, sees everything. That's my favorite fantasy that I'll grow old with the power to cast spells and heal souls. (*She laughs.*)

LILLIE: (*Laughing too*) My Momma was like that, never young, never wanted or needed to be young, never cared much for the world. Poppa did. He used to take us to political rallies, YMCA conferences and meetings. But Momma wanted no part of it. I'm busy collecting my memories, she'd say. They knew her in all the antique shops on Third Avenue, a quiet pretty lady but old ... even when we were small we thought of her as old.

ANNA: She's not like you, you go out, join committees, attend meetings, you're too responsible to be eccentric. Tell me more, Momma, I'm gonna miss you.

RALPH: Some memories are evil, squeezed into a pocket of you, to pry them loose is one hell of a job, others are unrecognizable, time has distorted them out of shape ... (*Chuckling.*) You think your mother was a beautician when in actual fact she was scrubbing somebody's kitchen.

FLOYD: (*Laughing*) Myths of color and confusion.

RALPH: That's right.

ANNA: Are you sorry about anything, Momma, are there things you wish had turned out differently.

FLOYD: You opt for psychiatry, I want total absolution, I don't want answers nor explanations.

RALPH: That's why you're catholic, it's another of the things I hold against you, who ever heard of a defrocked colored priest. (*He laughs.*)

FLOYD: It's punishment you want.

RALPH: No, indeed, I'm up. There's a difference between being up and down. These days I'm up. Four times a week I step into Fritz's office and go about the business of labelling my memories. I am not willing to be insane, you are, you old bum, you think it's your just due and penitence or some such dirty logic.

LILLIE: I'm going out, Momma, I'd say. She'd have her tea and shawls her shopping bags spread all over the bed. I'm going out, I'd say. There were tennis courts in those days, people I knew in all the brownstones on Convent Avenue, St. Nicholas Terrace. Private people with well-kept lives dances and supper parties. There were evenings then. Evenings at the Johnson's and the Hall's. Afternoon recitals where Momma had a good time. People who came to call. Poppa was gracious and welcomed good talk. Momma was shy but full of laughter. John Anderson came and asked to marry me. I thought of becoming a social worker. Aunt Jennie went to Smith and majored in philosophy. We were always busy, it was the right time for a certain kind of life.

ANNA: (*Turning slightly away*) Is that all, Momma ... dreams full of longing ...

LILLIE: (*Stiffening*) The memory is perfect ...

ANNA: (*Impatient, perhaps angry*) Isn't there *anything* you wished had turned out differently ...

RALPH: Been crossing 125th Street for eighteen years. Past scenes of needy forgetfulness. Say to myself: I been depressed for eighteen years, never grew accustomed to it, been depressed for eighteen years. Raised my children in spite of it, like it didn't exist. Sent them to private schools, didn't tell them what was going on outside. Used to go for walks with Anna, ride the Staten Island ferry, climb the hills to Convent Avenue, St. Nicholas, Jamal Terrace. Used to go down to Canal Street with Ben, spend the day in all the hardware shops, come home with old wrenches, bolts and screws. This is a piece of wood, I'd say, what could we make with it. That's all I ever said. Didn't tell him what was going on outside. Didn't even tell him who he was. (*Suddenly understanding something.*) That's one of the things I forgot. How was I supposed to tell him ... my son, there may be negro reasons ruining your life ... (*He and* FLOYD *look at each other, laugh oddly.*)

ANNA: (*Crying*) I'm leaving, Momma, going away from this house is like walking away from my energy.

FLOYD: If I could I'd buy you a drink right now.

RALPH: (*Getting a kick out of that*) You don't drink, you don't even go to bars.

FLOYD: I come here, this is my bar, new ideas happen every minute, people come and go, this is the best bar I ever found.

RALPH: Tell my why you don't drink.

FLOYD: I don't drink or smoke or take naps in the afternoon.

RALPH: You live out a full day.

FLOYD: Every day.

RALPH: Why's that?

FLOYD: It's the least I can do.

RALPH: You don't cheat.

FLOYD: I cheat in other ways.

RALPH: For instance?

FLOYD: I don't finish things.

RALPH: You feel bad about that?

FLOYD: I remember it.

RALPH: What's the first thing you do in the morning?

FLOYD: I say my prayers.

RALPH: You confess?

FLOYD: I take stock of the ways in which I cheat.

RALPH: And ask forgiveness?

FLOYD: Yes.

RALPH: Then what?

FLOYD: Then I get up.

RALPH: It's a long time a day, tell me how you cheat.

FLOYD: You never asked me that before.

RALPH: These days I want the truth.

FLOYD: I walk a lot and think.

RALPH: You don't earn a living.

FLOYD: No.

RALPH: You feel bad about that?

FLOYD: No.

RALPH: Any dreams?

FLOYD: I'd like to have a little power, nor would I mind being recognized.

RALPH: And after that?

FLOYD: I might finish things.

RALPH: Tell me what happened in San Bernardino.

FLOYD: They rejected me.

RALPH: Why?

FLOYD: I didn't have correct faith.

RALPH: (*Laughing*) What the hell does that mean?

FLOYD: Even after everything they still had suspicions.

RALPH: You failed as a priest.

FLOYD: I never became one.

RALPH: Were they right?

FLOYD: (*Taking his time, quietly*) Here's the story: an orphan boy from Pittsbuirgh with a West Indian father, no trace of childbirth, a crisp scholastic mind, here's the story: a near-sighted brown boy, a face like a priest, a sullen need to know without touching, here's the story: San Bernardino, a walled-in monastery overlooking the Pacific, saints in the garden smelling of ancient forgiveness, here's the real story: a broken down tale with a girl who was passing, the YMCA, an old stone cross that belonged to my father.

RALPH: No place in time.

FLOYD: No place in time.

RALPH: A careful life.

FLOYD: A careful life.

RALPH: A wish to be invisible.

FLOYD: A wish to be invisible.

RALPH: (*Laughing*) That story's about as phony as a two-dollar bill. There are no negro reasons ruining your life.

FLOYD: There are no negro reasons ruining my life.

(*They look at each other and laugh out loud. We hear a man's voice off-stage.*)

MAN'S VOICE: Anybody about?

(RALPH *moves towards the door.*)

RALPH: (*Yelling in a humorous way.*) We're about. All the inmates together under one roof.

(CHIPS *walks in, he's a young man about twenty-nine, good-looking in a spiffy way, intense, a bit nervous, the stance and manner of a polished street guy.*)

RALPH: Chips.

CHIPS: (*Tipping his hat*) Mr. D. . . .

(*He comes into the room greeting everyone in turn.*)

CHIPS: Mrs. D . . . Anna . . . how you doin' Floyd . . .

(*He heads straight for the piano, sits down and begins to play.*)

CHIPS: (*Playing*) I was over visiting two very lightweight ladies.

RALPH: You were.

CHIPS: (*Playing*) Wanted a little taste of reality.

(ANNA *starts to laugh. They all do. They're familiar with the way* CHIPS *walks in, heads straight to the piano, carries on all conversation from there, but it still makes them laugh.*)

CHIPS: (*Playing*) Actually I've been *dallying* with two very lightweight ladies (CHIPS *is fond of taking apart words*) to *dally* meaning, to play amorously in a trifling, wasteful kind of way. (*He gives his full attention to the keyboard.*)

ANNA: (*Laughing*) Chips walks in, the place becomes a nightclub, a bar, I want a cigarette and drink, I feel like I've got on a long dress split all the way up my thigh. (*She laughs to herself.*)

LILLIE: (*Happy*) Tell me about the ladies, Chips.

CHIPS: (*Playing*) The scene is the following Mrs. D. . . . a once chic apartment now gray and windy, long windows cloudy with smoke, two women the sepia tint of a vanderveer photograph lounging in upright chairs, light comes in through the windows, a hazy filter of low saturation and brilliance, the women giggle, they have that tired look that I love, they no longer straighten their hair carefully, there is a dog somewhere barking in a corner, the women are still in their nightclothes, it's five o'clock in the afternoon, I play the fool, keep my hands in my pockets and smile, they ask me to stay, night comes through the window, they put on one red lamp, we giggle together on the couch, my hands are still in my pockets, the tired lines of their faces glow, I'm happy, a hard foolish happy like a dandy, a fop, a coxcomb, caught in the silly passing of women's time. (*He gives his full attention to the keyboard.*)

CHIPS: They couldn't hold a candle to you, Mrs. D. . . .

LILLIE: But it's beautiful, Chips, it's just like a photograph, I can see everything exactly.

CHIPS: It's for your pleasure, Mrs. D. . . . so what's new?

LILLIE: Anna's going to join the Movement, Ben's found himself a girl, her name's Christine. He's in love. First time in his life. (CHIPS *continues to play.*) Are you playing anywhere, Chips?

CHIPS: I might be. I might be playing in a club in Brooklyn called Ralph's. (*They laugh. For a moment* CHIPS *seems lost in the piano.*) It's early morning, I've been up since four. Can't sleep, as always

I'm restless. I feel like I'm in a small town, around the corner is the only coffee shop. The streets are broad like foreign avenues bordered by trees, I can stroll down the streets for the town has adopted me. In reality it's 125th Street, there are three greasy shops, I order coffee to go from one of them and race back to my room. It's around seven o'clock, I drink my coffee with cigarettes. I feel like I'm in an ageing mansion now broken up into apartments, my neighbors don't mind how late I play, they ask for requests at certain hours of the evening. In reality there is only my room, the building is deserted, I play to broken glass in a dead courtyard. (*He plays as if he were still speaking.*)

ANNA: (*To* RALPH) What's the song in the morning?

RALPH: You used to sing, wake me, wake me, stop the blind girl from crying.

ANNA: Was there snow on the ground?

RALPH: Just a few leaves were falling.

ANNA: Who told the stories?

RALPH: The words were my doing.

ANNA: What day did it happen?

RALPH: All the days of our dreaming.

ANNA: Is time in the memory?

RALPH: Like the end of a sentence.

ANNA: Who smiled when I cried?

RALPH: All the pity I could render.

ANNA: Was I ever afraid?

RALPH: Always just before evening.

ANNA: What did you tell me?

RALPH: Only things that came easy.

ANNA: What nights were the worst?

RALPH: When it came to myself.

ANNA: Is it only our secret?

RALPH: Someone will repeat it.

ANNA: Why were we happy?

RALPH: Who can ever remember.

ANNA: What's the song in the morning?

RALPH: You used to sing, wake me, wake me, stop the blind girl from crying.

ANNA: (*Singing softly*)
this little light of mine
I'm gonna let it shine
this little light of mine
I'm gonna let it shine.

CHIPS: (*Still playing, talking to* LILLIE) I wish I'd been born here, Mrs. D., right in this room.

LILLIE: You come and go like family . . .

(*He nods, answers with a flourish of the keys.*)

LILLIE: (*Remembering*) Anna brought you here.

CHIPS: Anna can smell stray souls.

LILLIE: I wasn't home, you were playing the piano when I came in.

CHIPS: I thought to myself, if that's Anna's mother I can't stand it.

LILLIE: For months you lived in Ben's room.

CHIPS: I could be there still, nothing truly budges me from this place . . . listen to this, Mrs. D. . . .

(*The door opens,* BEN *and* CHRISTINE *walk in.*)

BEN: Chips! How you doin', man . . .

CHIPS: (*Taking a bow from the piano*) Okay . . . okay, man. . . .

BEN: Meet Christine.

(CHIPS *leaves the piano to come meet her.*)

CHIPS: Hello, Christine.

RALPH: Christine's a Barnard girl, Chips.

CHIPS: (*Being charming*) How do you do, Christine, my pleasure to meet you.

ANNA: (*Laughing*) Chips can be all charm and savoir-faire, Christine.

CHIPS: (*Bowing ceremoniously to* CHRISTINE) They do PR for my act.

BEN: (*Laughing*) Come on, man. (*He plays a run on his flute.* CHIPS *retreats to the piano to join him.*)

LILLIE: (*Going over to* CHRISTINE) He took you to his places.

CHRISTINE: Yes.

LILLIE: Places where he walks and plays his flute.

CHRISTINE: Yes.

LILLIE: Places where no one else goes. . . .

CHRISTINE: (*Drawn to speak*) You can see things from them . . . the sun going down, lights coming up, barges and boats, old freight cars and metal girders . . .

LILLIE: A taste in the mouth for a different kind of living.

CHRISTINE: (*Looking at her*) Yes.

(LILLIE *shakes her head.*)

CHRISTINE: Does it make you sad?

LILLIE: I think it does. I don't know why but I think it does.

(RALPH *comes over.*)

RALPH: Tell me about your walk, Christine.

CHRISTINE: It was like nothing I've ever done.

RALPH: Ben's the original drifter.

CHRISTINE: (*Agreeing*) I ask myself what it's like to drift, drift and not remember . . . what would I see that I never saw before.

RALPH: Ben can show you, it's the right question to ask in his presence.

CHRISTINE: You're really friends.

RALPH: We have been. In the past we've been the best of buddies.

CHRISTINE: So many things are happening, my mother and father wouldn't believe this night.

RALPH: You seem to fit in just fine.

CHRISTINE: But I'm not like any of you. I don't play the flute, or speak in symbols and dreams. I don't even know if I'd be here now, except tonight something happened that made me ashamed and very aware of myself.

RALPH: (*Gently*) Scenes of Christine in search of herself. . . .

(*Suddenly she is crying.*)

CHRISTINE: Why does it seem so easy to talk about myself . . .

RALPH: (*Almost touching her*) What's the world like for Christine, I keep asking myself. . . .

(*When* BEN *intervenes, physically separating them.*)

BEN: She doesn't have to answer that.

RALPH: (*Caught up short*) He's angry again, Christine, I apologize in advance for his anger and mine.

BEN: You got questions coming out your ass.

RALPH: (*Nodding agreement*) Truth has become one of my significant themes.

BEN: And you're full of it, you're kissin' Fritz's ass you're so full of it . . .

LILLIE: (*Closing her ears*) Ben!

RALPH: (*Looking only at* BEN) He's angry, Lillie, Fritz says anger is the only truth.

BEN: You got nothin' but an ass crammed full of psychological definitions . . .

RALPH: That's right. Exactly right. I walk down 125th Street now and repeat out loud anger is the only truth. It explains to my satisfaction a multitude of sins.

BEN: (*Taking a step toward him*) You even got yourself some negro reasons . . .

(LILLIE *intervenes, physically separating them.*)

LILLIE: There was a time when your father couldn't walk down 125th Street at all . . . .

RALPH: (*Looking at* BEN) That's right, Lillie . . .

LILLIE: He used to say, my own rage is enough, Lillie, and call a cab before he ever walked out that door

RALPH: (*Looking only at* BEN) You're right again, Lillie . . .

LILLIE: (*Beginning to drift*) I like 125th Street. Cab drivers tell me about their days. Old women show me what's in their shopping bags. I'm not afraid of the wine and confusion.

RALPH: (*Looking only at* BEN) People step aside for you, Lillie.

BEN: (*Pushing his mother slightly in order to get by*) It's not true, Lillie, and you know it, you're really afraid and only like this room. (*He leaves, we hear his door slam again.*)

LILLIE: Why does he make us feel like we're all wearing masks . . .

CHIPS: (*Who has been watching* CHRISTINE, *still playing*) They've already forgotten it was about you.

CHRISTINE: (*Embarrassed*) You come here often and play . . .

(CHIPS *nods, runs his hands across the keys.*)

CHRISTINE: You play all the time.

CHIPS: (*Playing*) That puts you at a disadvantage?

CHRISTINE: (*Embarrassed*) I don't know, I've never talked to music before.

CHIPS: (*Stopping*) Would you like me to stop?

CHRISTINE: No, please don't.

CHIPS: (*Stopping anyway, then rummaging in his pockets*) Now I need a cigarette.

CHRISTINE: If you don't play you need to smoke . . .

CHIPS: (*Lighting a cigarette*) Or drink or run around.

CHRISTINE: Then play.

CHIPS: (*Sitting there smoking, not playing*) Take a room where there's no piano. I walk in, look around . . . no keys. I keep my hands in my pockets playing notes in my head. I ask someone for a cigarette. I'm at a loss for words, my fingers are burning holes in my pockets.

CHRISTINE: Start playing again, please.

(*He touches the keys with relief.*)

CHIPS: (*Playing*) The piano is time passing smooth and easy. The hours go by without harsh or cruel edges to knock me over.

CHRISTINE: Have you ever been in love, was it any different then?

CHIPS: (*Playing*) Here's my idea of falling in love: a woman with a large bedroom, plants, a piano, an old four poster canopy and all. We make love. No sooner do we finish than I reach for the keys, write the last notes of sex, a closing arpeggio to love and slumber.

CHRISTINE: That's lovely.

CHIPS: (*Playing*) You like it.

CHRISTINE: I like to think of ceremonies and dreams, a way of being that never forgets how quickly it will be gone. But you've never found the woman.

CHIPS: (*Playing*) Not yet.

CHRISTINE: You've told me everything, why you play and how you would like to love.

CHIPS: (*Playing*) Then tell me something about you.

CHRISTINE: I was going out with someone until tonight. But early, around six o'clock, he did something I can't remember or explain and now it's over. All my attempts at a love life are futile and embarrassing.

CHIPS: Ben loves you, I can see that already, and that's never happened before, he's only ever loved Anna.

CHRISTINE: I'm not prepared for that ... I came here because Anna persuaded me, I'm not prepared for anything more.

CHIPS: (*Playing*) It could happen anyway.

CHRISTINE: My little ideas have held so far, tomorrow I'll be back in my room.

CHIPS: (*Playing*) Then we should make it long tonight, long past the midnight hour.

CHIPS: (*Playing, singing*)
there's a time near the midnight hour
that's like a dream that's about to flower
you close your eyes and the streets are open
it's like a dream that will not be broken ...

in the midnight hour
in the midnight hour

yes there's a time near the midnight hour
that's like the sun at the end of a shower
you close your eyes and the day's still laughing
and in the streets people wait to start dancing

in the midnight hour
in the midnight hour

it's the only time that I'm free
to really really really be me
it's the only hour in the day
when I can really really start to play

in the midnight hour
in the midnight hour

(*He hums, mumbles to himself, lost in his playing.* BEN *comes in, takes* CHRISTINE *to him.*)

BEN: You want to dance?

CHRISTINE: I've never danced in my life, I'm afraid of it.

(*He takes her by the arm, moves her to him slowly.* CHIPS *notices it, slows down the rhythm of his playing to a mellow, easy pace.*)

RALPH: (*To* LILLIE, *yet watching* CHRISTINE *and* BEN) Would you still be with me, Lillie, if it wasn't so easy to call my name.

LILLIE: I don't know, Ralph.

RALPH: Try and answer the question, Lillie.

LILLIE: Once, maybe twice I thought about leaving.

RALPH: Did you have any plans?

LILLIE: I wanted to be happy again . . .

RALPH: What kind of things did you want to do?

LILLIE: I thought I might find someone with my sense of humor, it was when you were in the middle of things, despair and depression, your hands shook, you never looked at me, only Ben and Anna had access to you, you'd come home, go right into the shop to make them something.

RALPH: I was full of surprises. Remember the trees I made for Anna's bedroom. She wanted to feel she was living in a park.

LILLIE: Ben is skilled with his hands because of you.

RALPH: He had the touch to begin with, Lillie.

LILLIE: Holidays and birthdays you gave special attention.

RALPH: I never objected to a thing.

LILLIE: And the stories you could invent . . . endless adventures that kept them happy till bedtime.

RALPH: It was no trouble for me, Lillie . . .

BEN: (*Dancing with* CHRISTINE) We'll sleep on the couch. I've lots of things to tell you.

CHRISTINE: I should sleep in Anna's room, it's only right.

BEN: (*Laughing*) I like you, I don't know why but I like you. (*He holds her, they dance.*)

LILLIE: I guess it was around then I thought of leaving.

RALPH: Where to, Lillie, the West Indies, California, Washington, D.C. . . .

LILLIE: An apartment on Riverside Drive.

(*He laughs.*)

RALPH: Then what?

LILLIE: I'd start to have adventures, become funny and eccentric.

RALPH: A real character people could recognize and remember.

LILLIE: Does that sound familiar?

RALPH: All our dreams are familiar, Lillie.

LILLIE: I want people to say ... that odd Lillie Daniels always does things in a different way ...

RALPH: You want people to notice, you have a flair for moments that could be collected on film and you're in love with the charm of things.

LILLIE: (*Realizing it*) I'm not quite real ...

RALPH: You're like a photograph, Lillie. The photograph is true and pretty and speaks well of you. Look at Lillie, it says, take a look at what Lillie's doing now, well what do you know ... (*He chuckles.*)

LILLIE: (*Dreaming*) Long before it's time I step aside for the memory.

RALPH: Take a look at the pictures in this room, Lillie.

(*He makes a sweeping gesture to everyone, locking them in place like the loveliest of photographs. Lights go out.*)

ACT II
Scene 2

It's the middle of the night. As if it were a movie, at certain moments we will literally fast forward into the future. LILLIE, RALPH, ANNA *will appear, having aged considerably. During each of these fast forward sequences,* BEN *must be lit in such a way that it is clear he is dead, but in the moments between just* BEN *and* CHRISTINE *we slip back into the present.*

BEN: Are you awake?

CHRISTINE: I'm awake, I'm wide awake.

BEN: No you're not, you're half asleep, you don't remember what I've been saying.

CHRISTINE: You were in private school, everything was the same as always: stiff and unhappy. But the same.

BEN: Then what happened?

CHRISTINE: You were about to tell me.

BEN: (*Teasing*) I already told you.

CHRISTINE: (*On the alert*) You couldn't have, I'm wide awake!

BEN: (*Laughing*) You're funny, it's not what you say, what you say is always too serious, but your face is funny, I like to tease you. . . .

(*She just looks at him.*)

BEN: You like to climb?

CHRISTINE: I never have.

BEN: What about boats, you know anything about boats?

CHRISTINE: No, nothing.

BEN: Can you swim?

CHRISTINE: (*Shaking her head no*) Ralph taught you those things.

BEN: (*Proudly*) From when I was very small he started and finished things with me.

CHRISTINE: (*Eagerly*) But I can walk, I'm a good walker.

BEN: (*Laughing*) Then we'll walk, drift from here to California.

(*They don't talk for awhile.*)

BEN: Now what was I saying . . . .

CHRISTINE: About private school . . . .

BEN: I want to tell you about that, it's important to me.

(*Just then* LILLIE *comes in. She has aged considerably. She talks and behaves like a sleepwalker.*

LILLIE: (*Sleepwalking ahead of time*) A door was soon to shut so completely on this room and time, take with it the generous hours the coming and going, the talk and music, that belonged to us. . . .

(*She looks around the room.*)

I sat there . . . the room was never too large or small, meals were easy to prepare. We were eager and clear, a holy feeling that life would leave us be . . . fascinating, eccentric, a lie to all the sad tales collected before our eyes. Ralph was on his way. I thought: nothing can stop him, happiness will slip through now, a tiny opening still left for us. My children were the brightest stars I have ever seen. They took life seriously, their faces were open and free. They had in their fingers a sweet and easy pulse for life. They remembered things, did not betray the tiniest memory we had given them. Now when I think of them I bring them here to this room. They come running through the door, talk and laughter set them apart. Death is nowhere about . . .

(*She looks around the room. Light comes up on* BEN *stretched out on the couch. She laughs lightly with relief.*)

You look the same, same wonderful face and brow. I couldn't believe you would change. In all my dreams you're always the same, you come charging into the room laughing and singing, lift me in your arms, spin me around, how's Lillie you shout, has my Lillie been behaving herself . . . Put me down you bully I say put me down and don't start any of that cursing . . . .

(Her body twists in grief.)

> I don't let myself wake up . . . I lay still . . . keep my eyes shut, hold on as long as I can to the sound of your laughter bouncing through this room . . .

(She leaves quickly. BEN *and* CHRISTINE *continue as if she had never been there.)*

BEN: Duffy was my best friend, he and a little short kid named Bucky Rogers, other than that the school was a proper prison. I didn't like it, but it didn't matter. Are you awake?

CHRISTINE: *(Sleepy)* Of course I'm awake, it's still early.

BEN: This thing about Duffy and Bucky Rogers, Ralph and Lillie have never heard it, Anna knows something only because she saw me right after it happened and she remembers the look in my eyes. *(He shakes her.)* Where are we?

CHRISTINE: *(Waking up)* We're in your house, it's late at night and we're not sleepy. Now tell me, tell me . . .

(RALPH *comes in, sleepwalking in the night, an entirely different voice and manner.)*

RALPH: *(Remembering things ahead of time)* Here's the trick, here's how it all turned out, and it's funny, too, there's no lack of humor in this one and I want you to laugh right along with me. I was on my way down the street, I was going at full speed four times a week religiously like a convert to the habit of confession. I was passing all the stops at breakneck speed on my way to the bottom where all puzzles are solved and truth ties the thing together. It was a Thursday, the third of my four weekly visits, and I was open like a sore. Fritz had taken me down to a fine swollen state where all my memories bled, dissolved, and the hard kernel of dreams came popping to the surface. He was just about to put me back together, a man in a new image, free from rage and insurance. . . .

(He gets a kick out of that.)

> It was late in the afternoon, the best hour for bleeding the soul, the door opens, I nod to a man in black who tips his hat, another soul just released from the bleeding hour or so it seems, go to take my place when he turns and asks if I'm a patient of the good man Fritz. I am indeed, I admit freely. An enthusiastic fool who's holding on to him for life. Ready and willing to be reconstructed in his image, I am presently a man bleeding from stem to stern, only Fritz can plug up the holes, I add proudly, when he informs me of his death, by suicide, by his own hand, somewhere in the middle of a night I walked through with my arms around my soul. He died. That is the

laugh and the humor, the surprise ending to my efforts to get out of insurance.

(*He chuckles, finds himself looking around the room.*)

Now where am I, out of this room, that's for sure, with a fifth of Jack Daniels and my saw.

(*He laughs. Light comes up on* BEN *stretched out on the couch.*)

What do you know. I been looking for you. You look the same. Exactly. No different than I remember you. What's there to say between us. The shop of course. I got things to show you as always, the statement between is not finished. You look the same. Same stern and wonderful face. I keep the memory of you in all the things I make but I've looked forward to this meeting for a long time, the one thing from which I do not hide nor drink too much.

(*He chuckles.*)

How have you been my boy.

(*He is crying.*)

How the hell have you been.

(*He walks off quickly.* BEN *and* CHRISTINE *continue as if he had never been there.*)

BEN: (*Laughing*) Every afternoon it was me, Walter Duffy, and Bucky Rogers, that's what got me hooked up with those guys, I got a kick out of saying their names.

CHRISTINE: They could have been cowboys.

BEN: Yeah. We played paddle ball on the court behind the school. Duffy had a sleigh, a fantastic sleigh, I invited them up here to the hills behind St. Nicholas and Convent, great streets for sleighing, I said.

(ANNA *comes in, sleepwalking in her time. Unlike the others, she sees* BEN *immediately, speaks directly to him alone.*)

ANNA: I keep notes on the old days.

BEN: (*Speaking only to* CHRISTINE) The snow was packed a mile deep, no cars anywhere, I was fifteen . . .

ANNA: My notes begin: in the early period of my life we lived in a room where we danced, learned truth and forgiveness, bathed in the people who came and went. It was a happy time, life was clear, a gentle prism that surrounded us on all sides.

(*She looks around the room.*)

I wish you could tell me what happened. The light that shone on me is gone . . . now when I remember all is sad and quiet, a cushion of ice has fallen and the numbness is refreshing to the me that I became. I cannot apologize nor remember too closely . . . as if in all the dying and the dying I shivered and froze, lost the full memory of my charm, took off the mask of this room.

BEN: (*Speaking only to* CHRISTINE) I'm in the snow with Walter Duffy and Bucky Rogers, I notice they don't look too happy, I don't know why, I think the snow's a gas, I try not to think about it. I'm fifteen, I don't know who I am, they keep looking at me like I had new eyes, a new face, I can tell I'm smiling a lot, I can always tell when I'm smiling big because my lips start to hurt and my jaws get tight. I was smiling big. Snow was falling. Fat patches slapping me across the face. It was a gas, I grab the sleigh away from Duffy, start cruising down the hill, looking around, looking around, dumb ofays . . . what's the matter with you guys, never been to Harlem before, well take a look, here we are on 141st Street and Convent Avenue, best sliding hill in Harlem and you guys acting like rabbits . . . then I knew . . .

(*He snaps his fingers.*)

knew everything. I'm fifteen been walking around private schools, around fancy ofays thinking I was cool, took one more look at their faces, the little rabbits, handed Duffy his sleigh, it's getting late, you guys better get going. I thought of Ralph whistling in his shop, how come he never told me who I was, thought of Lillie reading her books dreaming we could be anybody . . . anybody . . .

(*He gets up torn by a kind of violent anger.*)

I wondered where Anna was, what meeting she was at, what banner she was waving now . . . I was so ashamed, so ashamed of myself, who did I think I was, who the hell did I think I was. . . .

(*He is beside himself.*)

ANNA: (*Crying, becoming hysterical*) I tried *everything* after this room: love, babies, a whole patchwork of feelings and images, other seasons hastily embarked upon . . . a rapid journey out of this time . . .

BEN: (*Shaking* CHRISTINE *violently*) Are you asleep . . .

(*She is, stirs restlessly as if struggling still to keep awake. He turns away, puts on some music begins to dance in an insane kind of way.*)

ANNA: (*Hysterical, screaming at him*) Now when I remember your face it's always at the midnight hour. My children are asleep, cigarette smoke hangs in the air, the dead anger in me wants somewhere to go. I put on our music and dance.

(BEN *dances by himself. The lights go out, first on one, then on the other.*)

ACT III

Early the next morning. BEN *is looking out the window.* CHRISTINE *stirs. He walks over to her and shakes her slightly until she's awake.*

BEN: You didn't hear anything I was saying.

CHRISTINE: (*Defensively*) I did, I remember you were in the snow with Walter Duffy and Bucky Rogers.

BEN: Then what?

CHRISTINE: I have it in my dreams. I just have to remember them.

BEN: (*Laughing*) You're cute and funny and I'm crazy about you.

CHRISTINE: (*Smiling*) I don't know what to say.

BEN: Let's go for a walk, before anyone wakes up. Okay? You like to walk.

CHRISTINE: (*Proudly*) I'm a good walker.

BEN: (*Laughing*) You are, you never deserved a spanking or punishment of any kind. (*He hugs her.*) We'll walk. All over.

(*He is very happy, they leave.* FLOYD *comes in looking a little dishevelled and sleepy, goes to look out the window where he stands for awhile, watching, talking out loud.*)

FLOYD: Those two should get married, she could persuade him to do something again, maybe go back to school, get his high school diploma, go on to some college in the woods where he could read, write his poems, make things. Those are her dreams, she dreams of being happy.

(LILLIE *comes in.*)

LILLIE: What are you mumbling about, Floyd.

FLOYD: Happiness, Lillie, dreams of happiness. Ben's taken Christine for a walk.

LILLIE: She's a nice girl, honest and serious. The first real girl to come along for Ben. I like her. I'll fix you some coffee. (*She goes off.* FLOYD *stands at the window.*)

LILLIE: (*Calling in*) Chips is asleep in the hall in Ben's sleeping bag, curled up like a baby.

FLOYD: No one wants to leave, Lillie.

LILLIE: (*Calling in*) I'm going to call this place LILLIE'S BOARDING HOUSE OF STARS, everyone who comes here is a star in their own right. (*She comes in.*) I love mornings.

FLOYD: I know you do. (*She laughs.*)

LILLIE: I'm a star. Every morning I have perfect thoughts that no one ever had or could have in life except me.

FLOYD: I believe you Lillie.

LILLIE: Ben's a star, he wants an open life with only freedom and truth.

FLOYD: That he does.

LILLIE: What's going to happen to him, Floyd . . .

FLOYD: I can't say, Lillie, he's adamant about a great many things.

LILLIE: And angry . . . no one knows how or when the anger started, he won't talk about it.

FLOYD: Maybe Christine knows.

LILLIE: (*Smiling*) Was that your dream of happiness?

FLOYD: It was. . . .

(*She laughs quietly. No one speaks for awhile.*)

LILLIE: (*Closing her eyes*) What's going on right now, Floyd.

FLOYD: (*Who is still looking out the window*) The scene exactly as I see it . . .

LILLIE: (*Her eyes closed*) Yes.

FLOYD: There's a man coming down 125th Street. It's a windy day, he's heading towards the East River, the barges, and the rain. Buildings are being demolished, another man's getting out of a taxi, he's wearing a checkered coat and hat, he tips his hat to a cop standing on the corner. Three Jehovah's Witnesses are singing Must Jesus Bear the Cross Alone and All the World Go Free. There are people huddled in doorways, three boys are playing in an abandoned lot, a man just wiped his penis and put it away, a woman sits staring out the window at him, bemused and laughing. How's that Lillie.

LILLIE: (*Eyes still closed*) That's what's going on right now?

FLOYD: And every hour both glorious and sad.

(*Again there is silence, this time interrupted by the sound of a woman singing off-stage.*)

LILLIE: (*Opening her eyes*) Who's singing, Floyd?

WOMAN: (*Singing off-stage*)
where there's glory
bounded glory
you will find it
in the sky

where there's hatred
strife and sorrow
you will meet it
passing by

in the memory
of your Jesus
life is sad and
full of sin

but if you will
meet him walking
peace will find you
joy and bliss

WOMAN: (*Speaking off-stage*) Nothing but demonstrations all over the world, east and west, to the north and south, nothing but people marching on their own two feet, banners waving, flags flying, the whole world is demonstrating, colored, white, chinese, and asian flu, nothing but people marching on their own two feet.

LILLIE: (*Yelling off-stage*) My daughter's one of them, waving the banner of her time, she's one of them.

(*The woman repeats her song, slowly it begins to die away as* LILLIE *comes back in the room singing.*)

LILLIE: (*Singing*) Where there's glory bounded glory you will find it in the sky. (*She has a terrible voice and cannot sing for long, but she is still excited and uplifted in spirit.*) Something's always waiting for us, Floyd, that woman just lifted my morning. I'm not a believer, but I want to get down on my knees. (*Which she does.*) What's the prayer you'd say over me, Floyd?

FLOYD: I say it everyday, Lillie.

LILLIE: Say it now.

FLOYD: It's long, Lillie, and complicated. . . .

LILLIE: Why? Because I'm a sinner . . .

FLOYD: (*Laughing*) An enthusiastic woman must always sin, Lillie, and is always in need of forgiveness.

LILLIE: (*In a childish voice*) Bless me, Floyd.

FLOYD: (*Embarrassed*) I'm no priest, Lillie.

(RALPH *comes in in his pajamas.*)

RALPH: (*Oblivious to the scene*) Did you write down your dreams, Lillie?

LILLIE: (*Still on her knees*) I forgot, Ralph.

RALPH: (*Still oblivious*) Dreams are everything, Lillie, I was flying across 125th Street on a pair of roller skates, like my own private chartered plane, men were pissing in the street, a dog tried to crawl up my leg, I landed wide awake and free and here I am. (*He chuckles, sees for the first time that she's down on her knees.*) What are you doing, Lillie . . .

LILLIE: Floyd is teaching me how to pray, Ralph, you want to join me?

RALPH: No thanks, Lillie, I'm in good hands. Science is on my side.

LILLIE: (*Insisting in a childish way*) I want Floyd to give us his blessing.

RALPH: (*Gently*) What will it symbolize, Lillie, what's the picture you have in mind.

LILLIE: That we were once in a state of grace.

RALPH: I'll drink to that, Lillie. (*He gets down on his knee.*) It's a nice picture, and you look fervent and sincere in the telling. Say a prayer, Floyd.

FLOYD: (*Less embarrassed*) I'm not a priest, Ralph.

(CHIPS *comes hopping in inside his sleeping bag, stops dead in his tracks.*)

CHIPS: (*Nervous*) What's the insane moment for today . . .

RALPH: Lillie wants a picture of herself in a state of grace.

(CHIPS *hops over to the piano, begins to play.*)

CHIPS: Alright. Okay. I can play to that.

(*His hands trip into some new and unheard-of melody.* FLOYD *comes center stage facing the audience.*)

FLOYD: (*Speaking to the audience*) I have my own memories of this room, like a storyteller who comes again and again, looking for the tale that defies the rules, the characters who will tell you only of what is possible in a life, not the ending, the sad coming apart, but the hiding into truth and dreams. A different tale, intruding into life like a clear and unexpected melody. I came to listen, again and again. There was space, light, music, exuberant talk. No one came to call who was not eager for a sudden letting go, a wish to leave behind private wounds and bathe in a clear and simple time. Someone was always up, music was always playing. I tell you it was something, defying for a long and generous hour the strict demands of this and any other tale, standing on its own two feet, refusing loneliness and separation. I tell you it was something, a dance to remember in the midnight hour.

(ANNA *comes in still in her nightgown.*)

ANNA: Why are you all up so early.

(LILLIE *and* RALPH *get up.*)

RALPH: Father Floyd is serving confessional, your mother is turning into a mystic, I'm trying to keep a dog from peeing on my leg. (*He chuckles, sniffs the air.*) I smell coffee, Lillie.

LILLIE: (*Running towards the kitchen*) That's right, Ralph, that's exactly what you smell.

ANNA: Where are Ben and Christine?

FLOYD: They went out for a walk.

RALPH: One thing Ben's women have to learn quickly, they must walk and greet the sun. Christine can do that, she can handle that just fine. What's for breakfast, Lillie. (*He goes off to find her.* ANNA *smiles at* CHIPS.)

ANNA: Not a word to me.

CHIPS: (*Playing*) There hasn't been time.

ANNA: Start now.

(*He begins to play a familiar number.*)

ANNA: (*Laughing*) Scenes of Chips in the morning, sleepy still, but playing his music. Where'd you first learn to play, Chips, tell me the story.

CHIPS: (*Playing, maybe making it all up*) I was raised in a house full of women, mothers, sisters, aunts, nieces, the house was a triumph of women. In their moods and loneliness they flattened me to the keys. I could have played football, basketball, run track. But they needed me there at the keys, pecking away at their loneliness, the last of their dreams.

ANNA: Scenes of Chips and his women.

CHIPS: (*Nodding*) That is how I got started in music and other things.

ANNA: (*Laughing*) Is that a true story.

CHIPS: (*Playing*) It explains things well enough.

ANNA: (*Softly, sadly*) Real scenes of Chips outside this room.

(*He doesn't answer, just keeps on playing softly.*)

ANNA: I'm going south, the next time you hear from me I might be in jail.

CHIPS: (*Playing*) Scenes of Anna on the freedom trail.

ANNA: What do you think?

CHIPS: (*Playing*) Sit down, baby, don't sit-in.

(ANNA *laughs, incredulously.*)

CHIPS: (*Pushing his luck*) What's a nice girl from Harlem doing in Ita Bena Miss-a-pee-pee . . .

(*She can't believe it's* CHIPS *making these kind of jokes.*)

CHIPS: What did the non-violent freedom rider say to the cracker who punched him in the jaw?

ANNA: (*Laughing*) I don't know.

CHIPS: (*Playing*) Just wait till Martin Luther King turns his back.

ANNA: (*Cracking up*) I don't believe it, you've never told jokes, never, and they're terrible, awful, like watching Thelonious Monk turn into Groucho Marx.

(*They both laugh.* CHIPS *grunts appropriately, sends his hands flying Monk-style across the keys.*)

CHIPS: I'm gonna get star billing at the Copa with this act.

ANNA: You should get star billing anyway.

CHIPS: Spoken like a true and loyal fan.

ANNA: What'll you do when you're famous?

CHIPS: (*Playing*) I'll take you to New Orleans, up and down the Bayou, listening to trumpets and moans till six in the morning; post bail in every county jail from Maryland to Mis-a-pee-pee just in case. With you there should always be a just-in-case. Just in case you get the blues and want a new train to ride, just in case you get restless and can't take being happy, just in case you remember you're Anna Daniels from Harlem and what should you do about that. . . .

(ANNA *looks at him, sees for the first time that he's in love with her.*)

CHIPS: (*Aware that she's seen, embarrassed, he hits the keys*) Here comes a funky blues without class or charm.

ANNA: (*Sadly*) Play it for me, Chips. Scenes of Anna always looking in the wrong places.

(RALPH *comes in.*)

RALPH: (*Nervous and excited*) Lillie's out there making a fabulous breakfast. She said to tell you, Floyd, that it's for all her star boarders. Are you hungry, Chips, you think you can pull yourself away from the keys long enough to put a little food in your stomach. Where are your cigarettes, Chips, I'm all out of mine. (*He takes one and lights it.*) How'd you sleep, Chips, you have any dreams, the most important thing to do in the morning is remember your dreams, what'd you dream, Chips.

CHIPS: I got one dream I dream again and again, Mr. D., but it's dirty.

RALPH: There's no such thing as a dirty dream, Chips, dreams are science, you can do anything in a dream.

CHIPS: In the dream I'm playing the piano, okay, when all of a sudden I start to piss, I'm pissing and playing at the same time and I don't know how to stop doing either one.

(ANNA *cracks up.*)

RALPH: That sounds like a dirty dream, Chips.

(*They both laugh.* CHIPS *goes on playing, talking with* ANNA, RALPH *is restless, nervous and edgy.*)

RALPH: (*Talking to himself*) What I want is a drink. (*He laughs.*) What I got is a cigarette in one hand and an empty cup of coffee. I could trade the coffee in for a drink, go buy a newspaper and walk around the block. But I won't. I don't like to leave this room. Even for a drink. (*He chuckles.*) What you thinking, Floyd.

FLOYD: I was dreaming of a big old farmhouse in Upstate, New York.

A place where we could go together.

RALPH: (*Agreeing*) Snow and lots of fireplaces. A little dry sherry for Lillie.

FLOYD: A strategic place to hide when we needed it.

RALPH: You're the master at survival tactics.

FLOYD: Ben could live there.

RALPH: (*Sadly*) He needs a place . . . somewhere to hide when the need comes over him.

FLOYD: We need to find new ways to be.

RALPH: I agree. I agree.

(CHIPS *is fooling around with a new song.*)

CHIPS: (*Singing*)
   you came to call
   when there was no one else around
   and I was searching. . . .

   it felt like Fall
   the leaves were falling to the ground
   and I was dying . . . crying . . .

(*He laughs, looks over at* RALPH.)

CHIPS: You want another cigarette, Mr. D.?

RALPH: What I got is an empty cup of coffee. I'll trade you for a cigarette.

CHIPS and RALPH: (*Together*) What I want is a drink. (*They laugh,* CHIPS *hands him the cigarette.*)

RALPH: You ever try and figure out how many moments there are in a day, Chips . . .

CHIPS: You go on ahead of me, Mr. D.

RALPH: A day is a long time, Chips, much longer than a year or a lifetime. I pay strict attention to a day. Yes sir, a day can do you in faster than anything in history. (*He puffs on his cigarette.*)

CHIPS: (*Still trying out his song*)
   you came along
   the night was falling fast like rain
   and I was crying

RALPH: (*Looking at* ANNA *who is looking at him*) What you thinking, Anna?

ANNA: (*Seeing him clearly*) You're going after something brand new, aren't you, Daddy . . . it's lonely where you are and you're all by yourself, none of us can really follow or understand too well.

RALPH: (*Trying to brush it off*) That's pretty good . . .

ANNA: My Daddy wants to fly, spread his own wings and fly . . . .

(RALPH *starts to cry, suddenly, uncontrollably. He moves towards the kitchen.*)

RALPH: Who wants to give Lillie a hand . . . .

(ANNA *stands there looking around, the door opens,* CHRISTINE *comes running in, hysterical.* BEN *is right behind her.*)

BEN: (*Grabbing her by the arm*) I wish you wouldn't say anything.

CHRISTINE: (*Badly shaken*) You jumped . . . if you'd missed by *that* much it would have been all over . . .

BEN: But I didn't miss . . .

CHRISTINE: (*Still remembering it*) But you could have . . . it was this close . . .

BEN: That's what I felt like doing . . .

(*She is crying.*)

BEN: (*Trying to explain*) It's like suddenly knowing there's an answer. If you want one. Just an answer. Simple and to the point.

CHRISTINE: (*Crying*) I don't want to understand that . . .

BEN: (*Getting angry*) I could take a knife and slit my throat, a bullet and blow my head off . . .

CHRISTINE: (*Out of control*) I don't want to understand that!

(RALPH *comes in.*)

RALPH: Lillie's got breakfast . . . (*He sees* BEN *and* CHRISTINE.) . . . you're just in time . . .

(ANNA *rushes to* CHRISTINE.)

ANNA: Tell me something . . . you want to tell me anything . . .

CHRISTINE: (*Remembering like a bad dream*) There were barges and tugboats, and this beautiful bridge reaching to the sky like a rainbow . . . I watched him scale it . . . going up and up . . .

BEN: (*Furious yet also trying to cut her off*) I could choose a million places. Half-way across the Staten Island ferry, the subway at Grand Army Plaza, a room alone on any street in any city in the fucking world!

ANNA: I don't want to remember you jumping off any bridges . . .

(LILLIE *comes in.*)

LILLIE: There's breakfast . . .

RALPH: (*Still upset from earlier, to* BEN) What's the matter with you, I thought you took Christine for a walk.

BEN: You're crying . . .

RALPH: I'm weeping my ass off . . .

BEN: (*Torn up*) You remember me . . .

RALPH: (*Backing off*) I'm trying to get through a day . . .

BEN: I got things I hold against you now . . .

RALPH: The refrain is always the same: I did the best I could remember . . . (*That almost makes him chuckle.*)

BEN: (*Getting angry*) Everything's your business now, just your business . . .

LILLIE: Let's eat, we should eat . . .

BEN: (*Holding up his fist*) I got you like this!

RALPH: I don't even know who I am.

BEN: For years you go filling in the blanks, all the empty spaces . . .

RALPH: (*Seeing himself*) I can't get through the turnstyle.

BEN: (*Strutting in rage*) And I'm fooling around, fooling around, with a picture of myself that don't mean shit!

RALPH: (*Getting lost in himself*) I can't even tie my shoes.

BEN: (*Hitting hard*) Then the jokes.

RALPH: (*Suddenly hitting back*) They were funny.

BEN: (*Still punching*) And the walks.

RALPH: (*Punching back*) I held your damn hand.

BEN: (*Just punching*) And I'm proud. My cheeks are puffin' with pride. I got my sweaty fingers firm in your hand and I don't let go.

RALPH: (*Attacking*) You tell me, what'd I forget, what damn part of the scenario did I forget!

BEN: (*Exploding*) You made it *easy*, motherfucker . . . left out all the lines you didn't want to say . . . (*Screaming.*) You made it *easy* motherfucker. . . .

RALPH: (*Getting vicious*) We were just two ace boon coons taking a free ride for as long as the trip was offered . . .

ANNA and LILLIE: (*Crying*) Stop it now . . . let's sit down at the table . . . stop it . . .

RALPH: (*Out of control*) I got no wisdom stuck up my ass, I can't even make it to the subway.

BEN: (*Punching, just punching*) That's not my business, it's not my business . . .

RALPH: (*In a dead voice*) That's fucking right and true. Fucking right and true.

ANNA: (*Crying, to* BEN) You always want answers, you want everybody to give you answers . . .

LILLIE: (*Crying*) All of a sudden everybody's angry . . .

(*"Take the A Train" comes up, as at the beginning of the play.* CHIPS *begins to play and sing along with it at a slightly different rhythm. Then the room grows dark.*)

End

Property

Penelope Gilliatt

Characters

ABBERLEY

PEG   MAX

Property was given a rehearsed reading by The Women's Project on
October 22, 1979, directed by Gaby Rodgers, with the following cast:

PEG . . . . Diane Kagan
MAX . . . . Sam Schacht
ABBERLEY . . . . Joe Ponazecki

An arc of pale sand-colored hessian reaching around stage and from floor to beyond eyeview. Three single beds, pinned to floor, equidistant. Iron bedsteads, extremely beautiful. Beige and dark brown blankets, white linen. Small antique tables in polished dark woods beside each character, stacked with belongings. ABBERLEY's *with piles of cigarettes, notepads, lawyer's folders, photographs, a torch, pencils, jar of caramels.* MAX's *a pipe, tobacco, scientific journals.* PEG's *notably more bare, has a few books, playing cards, jar of caramels. All have bottles of pills, booze, glasses, thermoses, radios and earphones. At the bottom of each bed there appears to be a miniature TV facing the people lying on the beds. The machines are actually electrocardiographs. The wire recording from the characters' forearms and calves are not particularly visible for the time being. Characters not in nightclothes. Dressed to be ready at any time for expeditions and undertakings that will not actually occur.* PEG *in a gray and white print and some soft turban or scarf that hides her hair.* ABBERLEY *in white shirt, city tie, black trousers.* MAX *in gray flannel trousers and gray brawny pullover. Bare feet. Shoes and socks by beds, neat. No other furniture. All characters are youngish and healthy. No aging in course of play. Spotlights trained on their beds represent reading lamps. When a character goes to sleep or withdraws from contact, his spotlight snaps off. There is also a perpetual faint natural light in this space where they live immovably together.*

4:45 a.m. Curtain up on the three singing the last bars of a song. Ex-uberant mood. Sound rather soft. Pom-pom-pom, like the Swingles. PEG carries the tune. The waltz that grinds out of carousels (calliope) "When you are in love/It's the loveliest night of the year . . ." The men do a unison dum-di-di bass. Slight shambles. Also triumph.

PEG: Now I want to do the (*Sings: dum-di-di*) bass. Abberley do the tune.

MAX: It won't be any good that way. The two people doing the bass have got to be the same pitch.

PEG: Well, let's try. Abberley. (*Gives him a note.*) Max. (*Gives him a note. They do it.* ABBERLEY *sings with his head down. Looking at the sheets. Concentrated.* PEG *has her head up and neck craned, like a dog baying at the moon.* MAX *does it efficiently and stolidly. Born pipe-smoker.* PEG *is married to* ABBERLEY.)

ABBERLEY: (*Unusual excitement*) Now me with her. It worked fine. We were beautiful.

MAX: (*Pleased*) You mean I do the tune?

(*Another go. Subdued rowdiness. Hot drinks out of thermoses.*)

MAX: What time is it?

ABBERLEY: Getting on for five in the morning.

PEG: (*Eager voice*) Is it Friday?

ABBERLEY: (*Solicitous about her*) No, we've barely embarked on Thursday yet.

(PEG *lies on elbow with her back to him, watching* MAX.)

MAX: I think I'll relax for a while. We had a short night. (MAX *puts on radio earphones and leans back with eyes closed. His spotlight snaps off. He remains faintly visible.*)

PEG: (*Slight panic*) Don't go to sleep. We were having fun.

(ABBERLEY *looks at her back.*)

PEG: He's left us. He's quit. God damn him. Are we over?

(*Dread in* ABBERLEY.)

ABBERLEY: (*Fierce*) No. (*Sad.*) Are we?

PEG: Shall we both take a small pill and sleep it out until later? (*Makes sturdy attempt to staunch the dread. Silence. She takes a pill anyway.*)

PEG: (*Without looking at* ABBERLEY) What could I do to cheer you up?

ABBERLEY: You're going to leave me, aren't you?

(*Silence.*)

ABBERLEY: I know you want to, now.

(*Silence.*)

ABBERLEY: Why?

PEG: It's not as good as it was. I remember when it was wonderful.

(*Silence.*)

PEG: No, wrong ... I put that wrong. I don't mean that anything about yourself and me has fallen off. I mean longer ago than that. Much longer.

ABBERLEY: My dear love, you make yourself sound so old. I can't bear hearing you speak of yourself like that. You're very young.

PEG: I meant very long ago.

ABBERLEY: When you were with your *mother*? Good Christ. We must be better off together than that.

PEG: Don't be Freudian.

ABBERLEY: You're beautiful. Brush your hair.

PEG: Why?

ABBERLEY: I like watching it. Hell, why can't you do as you're told. You know that's what you're supposed to do. (*Continues to sit up and watch her for his own pleasure, rapt. But angry voice.*) Let me go to sleep.

(*Pause.*)

ABBERLEY: You're still lying there keeping me awake. Are you going to drop off or not? There are some manners left, not to speak of anxiety. I've got to see you out, haven't I? (*Pause.*) Apart from that, who'd pass up the chance of an idle moment together? Without him? (*Pause.*) All the same, if you're just going to lie there keeping me awake, I've got to go to sleep. (*Grandeur.*) There's a man I should be defending in court all day and it's nearly dawn. (*Lies back.*) It's going to be dawn. You don't know what it's like, trying to go to sleep.

(*Pause.*)

ABBERLEY: (*Hope*) Are you awake?

PEG: (*Wideawake voice*) No.

ABBERLEY: Leave, my darling, if you're going to, I beg of you. (*Pause.*)

What's been the matter? I don't understand.

PEG: We've got too many things.

ABBERLEY: *What?*

PEG: I'm probably wrong. (*Pause. Soft voice.*) Somehow we landed up with too many things.

ABBERLEY: (*Shouts*) I've got to go to sleep. (*Pause.*) How do you expect me to go to sleep after you've told me something like that? What am I to do? Something terrible's going to happen.

PEG: Thursdays are never easy. In fact they're bloody awful. Shall we have some sardines? A headline yesterday said: "Saturday cancelled for lack of support." (*Pause.*) I suppose it was a sporting event. A social event. Badminton. (*Excited.*) Gliding. Jam bottling. (*Pause.*) What a shame. *Saturday* unsupported. That's the best one.

ABBERLEY: (*Shouts*) Shut up, I can't hear what you're thinking. (*Pause. Loud voice.*) I can hear you thinking something awful.

PEG: What could I do to stop you troubling?

ABBERLEY: Promise me not to—(*Pause.*) I could kill you for making me ask you that. One has no right.

PEG: Shall I come into your bed?

ABBERLEY: No room.

PEG: Are you all right?

ABBERLEY: That's my business.

(*He is gazing at his machine. So is she.*)

ABBERLEY: Get the sardines. Sardines would be nice. (*Pause.*) They wouldn't be forlorn, would they?

PEG: (*Firm voice*) Eating in the night is never forlorn.

ABBERLEY: True. Then let's have caramels and you won't have to go away.

(PEG *starts to kick her sheets off.*)

ABBERLEY: (*Panic*) Don't.

PEG: You can't stop me.

(ABBERLEY *sighs, lies back, pulls the sheet up to his chin and pretends to sleep.* PEG *opens a drawer and gets out a nail file from a manicure set. The noise alerts* MAX. *Watches her. Anxiety. She gets out of bed and works on the screws pinning the legs to the floor. Her wires show.*

On all fours, she turns her machine around in MAX's *direction, and ours.* MAX *watches intently. Green track of pulse-beat bouncing like a ping pong ball.* ABBERLEY *talking over her as soon as she leaves bed.*)

ABBERLEY: (*Terror*) You can't do that, you'll come unplugged, we can't do it, in our condition, not fair, we can't be expected. Now I can't see your set. Damn you, what if you've stopped, how'm I supposed.

(ABBERLEY *gets out of bed himself. Stands with back to her with hands in pockets, looking at wall.*)

PEG: (*All fours*) Stop pretending there's a window.

ABBERLEY: I'm thinking.

PEG: No you're not, you're feeling, I can tell. (PEG *tries to go over to* ABBERLEY. *Wires won't reach him. Stands at nearest point to him. Arms slightly forward.*)

PEG: I thought if I could push them together.

ABBERLEY: You're supposed to be someone I look after.

(*Silence.*)

ABBERLEY: (*Rage*) Your energy. O.K., I know it's a miracle, yes. I'd be grateful for it if I were dead. I know it's the best thing that ever happened to me.

PEG: Well?

ABBERLEY: But I can't deal with it. Dear God. (*Pause.*) Rest His soul. (*Pause. Turns round, sees her machine now facing her bed again and in his view. Watches. Relief, then boredom.* MAX's *eyes not removed from it.* ABBERLEY *leans against his bedhead. Tries radio earphones.*)

ABBERLEY: They're talking about *food* on the *music* program. "Noncaloric." (*Disgust. Attention.*) "Flaming kebab tonight on Excalibur's sword." (*Takes off earphones.*) Putting out announcements like that before *breakfast.* (*Lofty.*) What's going on out there? (*Gets back into bed.*) Excalibur. Show-off. I can't stand pushy food. I like your food.

(*Pause. Watches her, back on her hands and knees. Urgent voice.*)

ABBERLEY: I'm hungry. (*Pause.*) Girls shouldn't do things like that.

PEG: Well, you help, then.

ABBERLEY: (*Seigneurish*) I'll get a carpenter tomorrow.

PEG: (*Contemptuous voice*) Tomorrow!

ABBERLEY: What's tomorrow done?

PEG: What guarantee?

ABBERLEY: Darling, tomorrow comes over the hill in hordes, like the Chinese.

PEG: *You* believe that? Old black-heart? (*Sits back on heels.*) What a good day.

ABBERLEY: I was only trying out the idea. (*Pause.*) I seem to believe it as long as you're still going.

(PEG *goes back to work. Men's gazes on her machine.*)

ABBERLEY: (*Rage*) Why won't you ever do what I say? That bed is pinned to the floor for a purpose.

PEG: Don't be religious. (*Pause.* ABBERLEY *looks for something by his bed.*) What are you doing now?

ABBERLEY: My pen's gone. (ABBERLEY *shines his torch at her bedside table.*) You've got my ballpoint pen.

PEG: I didn't know it was yours. No ballpoint can be *your* ballpoint. Ballpoints are *people's*. (PEG *sits on the edge of her bed.* ABBERLEY *knows it without looking.*)

ABBERLEY: Now what is it?

PEG: Darling, go to sleep.

ABBERLEY: How can I when you're wanting to move the bed and I don't want you to? I've given you all this. We've got all this. It isn't enough for you, and I hate you for it, and I want you to go before you decide to leave me, and I love you, and how am I expected to stand being cooped up with him.

PEG: Yes.

ABBERLEY: Yes what?

PEG: That's what it's like.

ABBERLEY: (*Rage*) You're too young to decide that. You're mine. (*Shouts.*) Where am I to live?

PEG: We've no choice.

ABBERLEY: You're where I live.

PEG: I'm here.

ABBERLEY: You're mine.

PEG: Things have changed.

(*Silence.*)

ABBERLEY: You've no business. You're too young.

PEG: I feel as old as the hills.

ABBERLEY: (*Weeps*) I decide.

(*Silence.*)

ABBERLEY: Could we have your lamp off? It's too bright. You will use 150 watt bulbs. (*Hatred of beautiful room.*) Like living in a bleeding watch factory. (*Looks at* MAX.) Of course, there are times when he's company. As technologists go.

PEG: (*Attentive voice*) Do you think your eyes need seeing to?

ABBERLEY: You can't do this.

PEG: I'm in love with him.

(ABBERLEY *whips head away. Pause.*)

ABBERLEY: I'll kill you.

PEG: I could go to a hotel for a bit.

ABBERLEY: Perhaps you won't have to go far.

(*Lights snap off. Lights snap on. Nothing displaced, Much time passed. They look the same.* ABBERLEY *talking cheerfully to* MAX. PEG *asleep. Her spotlight off.*)

ABBERLEY: A lot to be said for it. No more upset nights. A man needs time to hide himself. Where is she?

PEG: (*Voice from semi-dark*) I'm here.

ABBERLEY: (*To* MAX) How is she?

MAX: Fine.

ABBERLEY: I wanted to remind her about her driving license. It's expired and she never remembers.

MAX: (*Impatient*) You can always find us, God knows.

ABBERLEY: (*Chatty*) She came back for her books. She took a painting someone gave us as a wedding present. I'll have to get the wall repainted. The place is a wreck. (*Hand gesture at serene emptiness. No change, ever.*)

MAX: She told me she didn't take a thing?

ABBERLEY: (*Impatient voice*) The paint's a completely different color underneath. Nasty patch. I'll never get anything the same shape. I'm supposed to be a lawyer. I haven't got time to go traipsing around art galleries. Where is she?

MAX: She should be at the dentist's all day tomorrow.

ABBERLEY: Her teeth are perfect.

MAX: She has four impacted wisdom teeth.

ABBERLEY: No decay?

MAX: I'll ask her, if you like. It's not the usual thing we spend time on.

ABBERLEY: (*Addressing himself to his electrocardiograph; loud voice*) Scientists are pompous asses. (*To* MAX, *shouting, immediately.*) As if you hadn't both got all the time in the world. (*Polite voice.*) Could we all meet and talk some day?

MAX: What the hell else do we do?

ABBERLEY: I meant, meet formally. It might make the difference? (*Pause.*) I want to give her a Christmas present. I thought it would go with her hair. As long as you don't mind. A cowhide rug. For you both, really.

MAX: (*Startled*) Then what color is cow?

ABBERLEY: Have you forgotten? *All* cows are *brown.*

MAX: *Some* are black and white. (*Pompously.*) Brown—scarcely—can scarcely be said to match fair hair.

ABBERLEY: *Fair?* Her hair was always brown. Quite a dark brown.

MAX: It's touched up. Tinted. What we used to call dyed. Longer ago, what we used to call helped.

ABBERLEY: She never dyed her hair when she was living with me.

MAX: It's gone gray. You haven't noticed. Peroxiding it seemed a hopeful idea. She did it after she'd been ill.

MAX: (*Rage*) Nothing is ever wrong with her. She's as strong as a horse. Nothing was ever wrong with her in our day. She was going to outlive everyone.

(*Pause.*)

MAX: (*Helping*) Fine woman.

ABBERLEY: (*Gritty*) Girl.

(MAX *humors him and reads a book.*)

ABBERLEY: I suppose I should get somewhere to live. I really do need a place. This (*Hatred*) well-bred—nothing.

MAX: It isn't bad, though.

ABBERLEY: No. (*Pause.*) Nice of you.

MAX: Excuse me for asking, but what did you chat about when you were alone? I don't find chatting very easy. (*Pause.*) You've noticed.

ABBERLEY: You're necessary. It seems. (*Gracious.*) No reflection on you. (*He gets out his flashlight.*) Do you mind?

MAX: Please.

(ABBERLEY *goes over towards* PEG's *bed, trailing his wires. Studies her face in torchlight. Returns to his own bed.*)

MAX: O.K.?

ABBERLEY: Exactly the same.

(*Pause.*)

MAX: Do we really have to go through this nightly ritual?

ABBERLEY: It's not the easiest hour.

MAX: Do you find science fiction helpful?

ABBERLEY: Sodium amital.

MAX: Could I have some?

(ABBERLEY *throws the bottle. They take a pill each.*)

MAX: Cheers. Down the hatch.

ABBERLEY: Life has its rewards.

MAX: What did you talk about? In the old days. Hard to say.

(*Pause.*)

ABBERLEY: We just *talked*. Sometimes we spoke our minds, sometimes not. What are you asking? You could have heard it all if you had the ears. We had quite a lot of laughs. She played the mouth organ. She liked that. I gave her a ridiculously expensive mouth organ one Christmas, much like a cocktail cabinet. Etcetera, etcetera. I know her very well. We never ran out of things to say. Is that what you mean? (*Glee.*) Are you in a blue funk about running out of things to say?

MAX: What *sort* of things did you talk about?

ABBERLEY: Well. (*Pause. Haughty.*) Heavens, man. (*Pause.*) There was food, for instance. (*Pause.*) And her childhood, for another thing. She had a foul father. We had many a cheerful chat about that. He used to swing her by the leg to fortify her character.

MAX: (*Shakes head; earnest*) Those methods never work.

ABBERLEY: And I suppose you could say it was.

MAX: What?

ABBERLEY: Fortified.

MAX: (*Upper hand*) *What*? She's as weak as a kitten. I've never heard her argue back in her life. Can't you hear her teeth chattering in the night?

ABBERLEY: (*Not listening, smoking*) Yes, she's a salty fighter. There's one who knows how to whip up trouble and find out where you stand. That's the thing. Spine. You can rely on her for that.

MAX: Stop using the present tense.

ABBERLEY: (*Patient*) Look, we still live together, don't we? We're still stuck in this place. (*Warm.*) Couldn't you murder it? If you weren't here, Peg and I could have beaten it.

MAX: My dear Abberley.

ABBERLEY: Don't you my dear Abberley me. You're a technological grease-swabber.

MAX: You don't know a thing about her any longer. I don't believe you ever did. She's a mouse. She's also getting long in the tooth and she's subject to migraine.

(ABBERLEY *puts his hand to his head for a second.*)

ABBERLEY: I'm the better judge. We were married for the formative period.

MAX: She always told me you didn't believe in Freud.

ABBERLEY: No, it was *her* that didn't. (*Pause.*) Is that right? It's all screwed up.

MAX: She forgets too.

ABBERLEY: Oh, *no*. Her memory is impeccable. Except for dates.

MAX: Not now. (*Kind.*) She's changed, you see. It only proves my point.

(*Lights snaps off. Lights snap up.* PEG *still in semi-dark. Some other dawn.*)

ABBERLEY: Where is she now? Max? Where now?

MAX: She's supposed to go into the hospital.

ABBERLEY: Save us, what for?

MAX: Just a check-up.

ABBERLEY: When I left her—no, say, say, to put it another way, why not be kind, second husband, after all, when she left me for you, when she quit, she left in perfect repair.

MAX: Well, she's fallen into rack and ruin now.

ABBERLEY: You can't have looked after her. (*Frantic.*) You'll be telling me she's got arthritis next.

MAX: Rheumatism, a bit.

ABBERLEY: Oh no, oh no. (*Pause.*) It's not right.

MAX: I never understand what you liked about her. She always says she irritated you. She says she behaved like hell to you.

ABBERLEY: (*Withdrawn*) It isn't like that at all.

MAX: Wasn't.

ABBERLEY: All right. I probably didn't pay enough heed. At the time. That's crossed my mind.

(ABBERLEY *gets out of bed, trailing wires, and looks at her cardiograph. Sits on the floor for a bit, watching it. Tries to get near her, but the wires won't let him closer than the bedside table. He looks at her pills.*)

ABBERLEY: She's got plenty of phenobarbital. We won't run out. (*Pause. Rage as he tries again to reach her.*) Rheumatism!

MAX: It's to be expected.

ABBERLEY: (*Shouts*) No. (*Soft voice.*) You can't be looking after her. Everything about her has always worked.

MAX: You talk about her like a landlord.

(ABBERLEY *turns his back and goes to his bed.*)

MAX: Temper about the roof falling in. Woodworm. Dry rot. Maintenance. Power failure. Fuses. Normal wear and tear. To be expected, to be expected. (ABBERLEY *can't stand it.*)

ABBERLEY: *You've let it happen.* You've let her wear out.

(*Pause.*)

ABBERLEY: She's beautiful. You should look at her. Young.

MAX: I *live* with her. She's showing the normal signs of middle age. You don't grasp. People deteriorate.

ABBERLEY: (*Snoring*) Peg?

MAX: I call her Margaret.

ABBERLEY: Good God. (*Pause.*) Does she answer to it?

(MAX *gets up and sits on the edge of his bed and smokes a pipe. Pause.*)

MAX: Do you think we should be making more of an effort, or is this as good as one can manage? Considering what's against us?

ABBERLEY: We might listen to the radio for a time. Both of us.

(*Silence for a short while.* ABBERLEY *alone listens to his radio earphones.* MAX *sits thinking.* ABBERLEY *takes off earphones.*)

ABBERLEY: It's nice to be able to talk, isn't it?

(MAX *walks over towards* PEG *and looks at her. It means unplugging his wires from his body. Done casually. That sort of man. He kisses her.* ABBERLEY *watches. Solicitous. Nods. Gets anxious about* MAX.)

ABBERLEY: Would you mind turning your cardiograph around a little so that I can see it?

(MAX *swivels set. Dead screen visible to us.* ABBERLEY *watches.* MAX *plugs himself in again. Normal graph.* ABBERLEY *relieved.*)

ABBERLEY: How's sex, if I may ask?

MAX: Fine.

ABBERLEY: Good. (*Pause.*) I—she must have said this to you.

MAX: She doesn't talk unpleasantly about you. Or give anything away. Is *that* what you thought? (*Pause.*) If so, I'll wake her up. I won't be party to you bitching yourself on the sly. You can do it with her as a witness, so there. (MAX *holds still.*)

ABBERLEY: I'm a difficult man. Naggy. I could never stand the worry of her taking her wires off. (*Pause. Recollection of that terror.*) So you might say sex was a bit thin in this two thirds of the room.

MAX: That's anxiety. (*Patronage.*)

ABBERLEY: I'm furious with you about her teeth. What have you been doing to her? Any operations you haven't told me about? (*Acidity, over great fear.*)

(PEG *wakes up. Her spotlight snaps on. Cheery mood.*)

PEG: Hello, my loves. Oh Christ, it's Sunday. Shall we have an aspirin at once? We'll need a bit of cheering up.

ABBERLEY: (*To* MAX, *serious, after scrutiny of* PEG.) She's exactly the same.

PEG: No.

ABBERLEY: (*Hiding face*) You mean there's sign of toll.

MAX: Of what?

ABBERLEY: Toll.

(*Pause.*)

ABBERLEY: How dare she suffer? You're lying again. I remember her. There wasn't a cloud. She was the sunniest girl I ever knew. Even in the mornings, heaven help me, when burbling isn't exactly welcome. (*Pause.*) Primarily, she belonged to me. Therefore, ultimately. (*Pause.*) She *cannot* have changed.

PEG: (*Robust*) I'm long in the tooth and short in the breath. How about a drink before dawn breaks? (*Moved.*) Nice to be together, isn't it? (*To* ABBERLEY, *making herself.*) Darling, I have changed. You won't like my hair, for a start. I've got thin. I'm not what I was.

ABBERLEY: (*Shouting*) You're exactly the same. You haven't changed. *He's* let you go, if there's any question of it.

PEG: What month is it? October?

ABBERLEY: (*To* MAX, *quick pick-up*) There, see what I mean? I know her backwards. See why I had to remind her about the driving license? Does she keep the insurance premiums up? On her jewelry? I didn't give her enough. Nothing much. But she wouldn't like it to be gone.

(PEG *is playing patience on her lap. Smile at* ABBERLEY. *We can see some bits of jewelry in her night-table drawer. She is wearing some beads now, hidden for the moment under her clothes.*)

MAX: It's November. It'll be her birthday before we can turn around. Feel free to give her anything you like. We don't go in for presents.

(PEG *smiles again at* ABBERLEY.)

PEG: (*Looking from one to another; speaking brightly to close the gaps, as if at a party*) So it's getting near Christmas. Is Christmas worse because of the activity, do you think, or because of God? It *can't* be the activity, can it? (*Pause.*) What are the lucky creeps doing out there? (*Pause.*) The thing that makes me believe in God is that there's a special kind of weather on Sundays. Only on Sundays. Muggy. Gives you a headache. There must be a God.

MAX: That's mood, my love, not weather, and the mood's because the shops are closed. (*Sucks pipe.*)

PEG: That's a housewifeish thing to say. (PEG *makes a noise at her-*

self: brr, shaking head. Packs up the patience and goes toward MAX*'s bed.*) I expect I woke up at the wrong time. It'll be all right.

(MAX *gets up and takes off* PEG*'s hood. Long blonde hair falls out. She plaits it. Her beads show.*)

MAX: Who gave you those beads?

PEG: They're the ones I always wear.

(ABBERLEY *has looked away from her hair. Sad. But pleased about the beads. She sits on the bed and watches him.*)

PEG: Are you all right?

ABBERLEY: Fine.

PEG: How's Ronnie?

ABBERLEY: Fine.

PEG: How's George?

ABBERLEY: Fine.

PEG: How're Joe and Lil?

ABBERLEY: Fine.

PEG: Is Bob fine?

ABBERLEY: Fine.

PEG: Who else is fine?

ABBERLEY: Most of us. (*Pause.*) What have they done to your teeth and your bones? What are these migraines?

PEG: Thy wife, goat or mansion.

ABBERLEY: What?

PEG: Nothing.

ABBERLEY: You sound tired.

MAX: She isn't tired.

ABBERLEY: Stop translating for her. *We lived together.* We had a *life.*

PEG: You don't know me any more. You won't look. You do too much remembering.

ABBERLEY: I don't remember a thing about you. I don't remember the clothes you wore, or your beautiful hair, or the sardines, or the mouth organ. I recall nothing. I haven't owned you for ten years. Sixteen?

PEG: (*To* MAX) Stop him.

ABBERLEY: I gave up the title to you.

PEG: Max, help.

ABBERLEY: Dyeing your hair. Which side of the bed do you sleep on now? (*To* PEG.)

MAX: I sleep on the right hand side of my particular bed. When we share it. The right, seen from the head end.

ABBERLEY: So she's on the left. You've tried to change everything about her. She was on the track, don't you see? I don't believe she's better off. I have an idea of her. You're trying to take it away with all these dentists and bone-men and switching her side in bed. Does she still drink tea all the time?

MAX: Yes.

ABBERLEY: (*To* PEG.) I told you you should take the Georgian teapot.

PEG: (*Tender voice.*) I told you I couldn't be cumbered. (*Pause.*) How is . . .

ABBERLEY: What?

PEG: Our teapot.

(*Immediately after this line, while* PEG *and* MAX *begin to speak to each other,* ABBERLEY *takes off his watch and looks at it. Notes time carefully. Puts watch on table and records the time on a pad.*)

MAX: (*To* PEG) If we weren't having a civilized drink together I'd bash you for that *"our teapot."*

(PEG *hums.*)

PEG: These are the middle years.

ABBERLEY: In a part of Greece, a remote part, a man who kills another man immediately takes over the dead man's wife. The care of her. The property. The sexual rights.

MAX: (*To* PEG.) Make him shut up. What about all humming again?

ABBERLEY: (*Pursuing his own pointed anthropology and wanly fostering academicism*) It's an intelligent union of heroics and economics. From the point of view of the man left alive.

PEG: (*To* MAX) Dear, you can see he is making an effort. Should we have a game?

(MAX *attends to the eternal pipe. Silence.*)

ABBERLEY: (*To* PEG, *accusing, grieved*) You've got other aches by now,

I suppose.

PEG: I'm falling apart. The whole fabric. I need a relief fund. (*To* MAX.) Why don't you draw something?

ABBERLEY: I'd better leave you together. Not that one can move. (*To* PEG.) You're no further off than you were, I suppose.

PEG: (*Pause*) The way I might have cared for you. The people I could have done things for. The place used to be lousy with them. Shall we have a drink? I don't feel very well.

ABBERLEY: You've let her rot away.

PEG: (*To* ABBERLEY) Are you frightened of dying at the moment?

ABBERLEY: Of you being ill. (*Looks at* MAX, *covertly.*) Shh. Not now.

PEG: (*To* MAX) I'm sorry. (MAX *shakes head. Smiles.*)

ABBERLEY: We're not doing badly. We're having a drink. (*Pause.*) My dear, the time we had—it wasn't what we meant. Some. Not enough of it.

PEG: No. (*Pause.*)

(ABBERLEY *looks at his own cardiograph for a time. Then turns it to audience, away from himself,* MAX, PEG. *Gets back into bed and looks at* MAX's *machine instead.* PEG *speaks to air in outrage.*)

PEG: I can't see it. He must know I worry if I can't see it. How dare he not know that?

MAX: Oh dear, now you're going to get upset.

ABBERLEY: Don't get upset. Would you like one of my pills?

PEG: I'm *not* upset. Yes, I would. (*To* ABBERLEY.) Are you all right?

ABBERLEY: Fine. (*Throws pills to her.*) Would you like my solitaire board? I've got too many things. My eyes hurt. I've got earache. I wish it would buck up and be Monday. Lousy dump. (*Pause.*) Perhaps I could yet do better. Scrap the thing so far and begin another. Something I could bring to a decent conclusion. One gripes and holds off and bangs the pillows and thinks the real thing is to come and then one starts to lose the thread. My dear friends, this is it, yes? This. I realized that at a particularly good moment, at 5:48 this morning. I took account of the time. Something pleasant happened . . . Peg, I've grown immensely fat. You may not notice it under the sheets. Clean sheets' a great comfort, eh? (*Laughs.*)

PEG: Getting old has its funny side, I grant you that.

ABBERLEY: Would you do me the goodness of turning your electro-cardiograph around to me? In honor of our—past. Away from him. Until it's light.

(PEG *turns it round to him, crawling to bottom of bed.*)

ABBERLEY: Can we switch the lamps off?

(*Spotlights snap off. Pale light through scrim wall.* MAX *reads by a flashlight under the sheets.* PEG *crawls back to do the same.*)

ABBERLEY: You still have a very nice rump. The rump is often the first to fail.

(*We see the three cardiographs recording.* ABBERLEY's *faces us; the other two face him, diagonally visible to us.* ABBERLEY *watches them.*)

ABBERLEY: Thank you.

End

Letters Home

Rose Leiman Goldemberg

Based on Sylvia Plath's *Letters Home*
Selected and edited by Aurelia Schober Plath

Author's Note

Sylvia Plath was already recognized as a brilliant poet when she took her own life, at thirty, in 1963. Since that tragedy, and in part because of it, the interest in the details of Sylvia's life and death has kept pace with the growing interest in her work. But few biographers have bothered to consult the person who knew Sylvia best and longest. In 1975, in an effort to set the record straight, Aurelia Plath published a huge volume of her daughter's letters home, with spare but meaningful commentary. Every word of the play was drawn from that book. It seemed crucial to me that the real words of this mother and daughter be heard because so much fiction had been written about them. All letters, all dialogue, all words are masks, so the limitations of using the words of the book were only of degree.

Letters Home was not a reading; it was perfomed fully, acting out events as they were told. Actors and director must constantly explore, and finally pinpoint: What exactly is happening at each moment? When that was done with clarity, the whole leaped to life.

Letters Home is really two plays: one takes place in the mind of Aurelia: Sylvia's life and their fight to save it. The other takes place here and now, in this audience, as Aurelia, in telling and remembering her story, struggles for and achieves understanding: she is alive and her brilliant child, who needed—and had—her love, is gone.

In its first production, we looked for the details of the lives of the two women, and found that they were often together when apart, and apart when together, and so we let them range in and out of each other's "space." They were where Aurelia remembered them, or wanted them to be, for the interior play (the Sylvia play) is in Aurelia's mind. The play is always a dialogue: Aurelia always hears Sylvia; Sylvia is always aware of Aurelia. This merging and separating of the two women is deep in the form of *Letters Home*, and must be talked about and worked on in rehearsal. They speak the same words, but with different meanings; they do the same actions, often with different intent. They were one and different, as all parents and children, all lovers, are.

Humor is essential to the play. All the recognitions of "how it is" between parent and child must be offered to the audience so they can laugh. The more they share this laughter, the more powerful the play becomes, and the more Aurelia can share in gratitude and relief her feelings about her daughter.

In the "duets" it is not intended that the audience hear every word of each actor. These are chords sometimes, solos with accompaniment sometimes, rounds sometimes. The levels must be carefully worked on, the legatos must be smooth, the tempos exact. As in any music, the instruments must play responsively together.

Letters Home owes more than most plays to the imagination and devotion of its first director, Dorothy Silver, and to the actors who so brilliantly originated the roles, Doris Belack and Mary McDonnell; as well as to the faith of its producer, Julia Miles, and the staff of The American Place Theatre. But most of all *Letters Home* is indebted for its very life to the courage, dignity, and strength of Aurelia and Sylvia Plath.

Martha Holmes

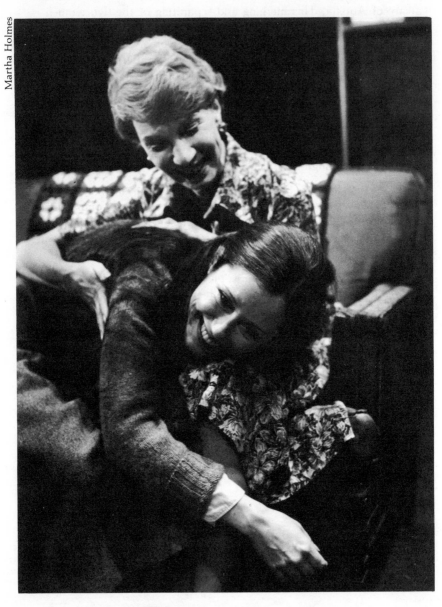

top: Doris Belack; bottom: Mary McDonnell

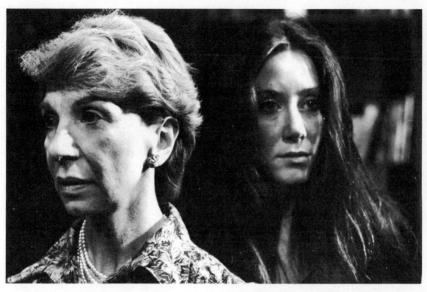

left: Doris Belack; right: Mary McDonnell

Characters

AURELIA
SYLVIA

Letters Home was given a rehearsed reading by The Women's Project on March 19, 1979. It was performed as a studio production May 31 through June 10, 1979, and opened as a full production at The American Place Theatre on October 12, 1979. It was directed by Dorothy Silver, with sets by Henry Millman, lighting by Roger Morgan, costumes by Susan Denison, and the following cast:

AURELIA . . . . Doris Belack
SYLVIA . . . . Mary McDonnell

ACT I

A light picks out AURELIA. *She moves forward uncertainly. She is an amateur, in a strange place. Who are these people? What will they think of her?*

AURELIA: (*To the audience, uncertain*) My first thanks go to my son Warren J. Plath, and his wife Margaret, whose approval, moral support, and assistance encouraged me to undertake this project.

Deep gratitude is owed to each member of my understanding, loyal family.

I am deeply grateful to Ted Hughes for generously giving me the copyright for this selection from Sylvia Plath's letters.

This book is dedicated to my grandchildren: Frieda and Nicholas, Jennifer and Susan.

(*It means: "I am a woman who above all knows never to forget her children." At the mention of* SYLVIA'*s children,* FRIEDA *and* NICHOLAS, SYLVIA *is there.*)

AURELIA: (*With more assurance*) It may seem extraordinary that someone who died when she was only thirty years old left behind six hundred and ninety six letters, written to her family between the beginning of her college years in 1950 and her death, early in February 1963. We could not afford long-distance telephoning though, and Sylvia loved to write.

SYLVIA: (*Softly*)
Dearest Mummy,
Well, only five minutes till midnight, so I thought I'd spend them

writing my first letter to my favorite person. If my printing's crooked, it's only because I drank too much apple cider tonight!

(*She laughs.*)

Dear Mummy,
The most utterly divine thing has happened to me!

Dear Mother,
Just got your Sunday letter this morning, so I thought I'd drop you a line. Your letters are utterly fascinating and they mean so much.

Dear Mum . . .

Love, Sivvy.

AURELIA: Throughout these years I had the dream of one day handing Sylvia the huge packet of letters. I felt she could make use of them in stories, and through them, meet herself.

SYLVIA: God, today is lovely! My cold is still runny, but with plenty of sleep and nosedrops. . . . By the way, do you suck those buffered penicillins, or swallow with water? I don't want to kill myself! (*A dark note.* AURELIA *doesn't miss it.*) Cheerio! Sivvy.

AURELIA: She could taste again the moments of joy and triumph, of sorrow and fear . . .

SYLVIA: Just to think I'm almost 18! . . . life slipping through my fingers like water . . . Little time to stop running . . . have to keep on like the White Queen to stay in the same place.

Can you make any sense out of this? Maybe you can analyze the ramblings of your child better than she can herself.

AURELIA: Throughout her prose and poetry, Sylvia fused parts of my life with hers. So I feel it is important to lead into an account of her early years by first describing my own.

As is often the case in a family having European roots (ours were Austrian), my father made the important decisions during my childhood. However, in the early 1920s, financial catastrophe overtook our family.

SYLVIA: (*Softly*) Dear . . .

AURELIA: My father, broken in spirit and blaming himself most unjustly for his very human error . . .

SYLVIA: (*Softly*) Dear . . .

AURELIA: handed over the reins of management to my mother.

SYLVIA: (*Overlap*) Mummy.

AURELIA: Although my father spoke four languages, he and my mother spoke only German at home. I too spoke only German. How isolated I felt at recess as I stood by myself in a corner listening to the other children shouting, "Shut up!"

SYLVIA: The wave of homesickness hit when I walked into my room, empty and bare. Gosh, I felt lonely!

AURELIA: When I went home at the end of the school day and met my father, I answered his greeting proudly with "Shut up!" His face reddened. He took me across his knee and spanked me. Weeping loudly, I sobbed out, "Papa, was bedeutet das?" *What does that mean?*

SYLVIA: So much work I should have done, and my schedule looked so bleak and unsurmountable . . .

AURELIA: He realized I had not understood what the words meant . . .

SYLVIA: I have now snapped out of my great depression—the first real sad mood I've had since I've been here.

AURELIA: He was sorry, hugged me, and asked me to forgive him.

SYLVIA: Now I come to the most thrilling part! . . .

AURELIA: From that time on we spoke English at home. Father was our teacher, and mother and I studied together.

SYLVIA: Whom should my eight hundred and fifty dollars come from but Olive Higgins Prouty! Good heavens, she is responsible for all this! (SYLVIA *steps toward* AURELIA, *holds out her hands.*) It is an Indian summer day—blue skied, leaves golden, falling. So I sit here, sheltered, the sun warming me inside. And life is good. Out of misery comes joy, clear and sweet. I feel that I am learning.

AURELIA: (*Close now, like girl friends*) In my junior year in high school, the world of American and English prose and poetry burst upon me, filling me with the urgency to read, read! I lived in a dream world . . .

SYLVIA: I'm being stretched, pulled to heights and depths of thought I never dreamed possible.

AURELIA: . . . a book tucked under every mattress, a book in the bathroom hamper. "What's RiRi doing? Oh, she's reading again."

SYLVIA: If only I can weld the *now* into art and writing later on! . . . like animals storing up fat and then, in hibernation or relaxation, using it up.

AURELIA: I completely identified with the characters in a poem or story.

SYLVIA: If only I'm good enough to deserve all this!

AURELIA: My evergrowing wish became to open to other young people this wonder—to teach.

SYLVIA: I just can't stand the idea of being mediocre!

AURELIA: It was the beginning of my dream for the ideal education of the children I hoped to have some day.

SYLVIA: The question is, shall I plan for a career (I hate the word!) or should I major in English and Art?

AURELIA: Fortunately my mother was most sympathetic, and read my literature books too, saying cheerily—

SYLVIA **and** AURELIA: (*Different tones*) "More than one person can get a college education on one tuition."

AURELIA: I remembered that vividly when *my* daughter went to Smith.

SYLVIA: You are listening to the most busy and happy girl in the world! I have just been elected to Alpha Phi Kappa Psi, which is the Phi Beta Kappa of the Arts. Also I think I will get at least one sonnet published in the erudite *Smith Review* this fall.

None other than W. H. Auden, the famous modern poet, is to come to Smith next year. (Imagine saying "Oh, yes, I studied writing under Auden!") Your happy girl, Sivvy.

AURELIA: In 1929, after teaching English for the year following my graduation, I decided I would return to the university to earn a Master of Arts degree. Dr. Otto Emil Plath taught the course in Middle High German.

SYLVIA: (*At the mention of Otto: a darker note*) This is a period of sterility emotionally.

AURELIA: I had met Professor Plath briefly, a very fine-looking gentleman with extraordinarily vivid blue eyes.

SYLVIA: . . . blue skied, leaves golden . . .

AURELIA: I remember the last day of classes at the university very clearly. When I went to say good-bye, Professor Plath played about with a pen on his desk for a bit. Professor Haskell and his wife had invited him to spend the next weekend at their farm. Should I care to join him, he would appreciate it.

SYLVIA: (*Withdrawing*) My date last night . . . looked rather old.

AURELIA: I learned much about Otto Plath that weekend.

SYLVIA: I feel that I'm cut off from all mankind . . .

AURELIA: He astounded me by telling me that he had married over fourteen years before.

SYLVIA: I don't even know how I can last one week!

AURELIA: He and his wife had soon separated.

SYLVIA: I feel like putting my head on your shoulder and weeping from sheer homesickness.

AURELIA: Were he to form a serious relationship with a young woman now, he would obtain a divorce.

(*They speak simultaneously.*)

He thought my thesis proved we had much in common and he said he would like to know me better.	SYLVIA: My face is a mess, all broken out; my tan is faded, my eyes are sunken . . .

SYLVIA: If I could be pretty, I wouldn't mind so much!

Boys are strictly secondary in my present life. I find myself numb as far as feeling goes. All I'm trying to do is keep my head above water, and emotions are more or less absent or dormant for the while. It's a good thing to have one less distraction.

(*It means: I would not do as you have done.*)

AURELIA: Our friendship developed and deepened. We dreamed of projects jointly shared, involving nature study, travel, writing.

SYLVIA: Life looks so bright when you're rested and well.

AURELIA: I enjoyed teaching until January 1932 when Otto and I were married in Carson City, Nevada.

                                        SYLVIA: Your bewildered Sivvy.

AURELIA: Then I yielded to my husband's wish that I become a full-time homemaker.

SYLVIA:
Dear Mother,
I was up in my room talking with a lovely girl [she's one of the people I really can tell things to]—(*This hurts Aurelia; Sylvia rattles on.*)—expounding on the misery and inferior feeling of being dateless this weekend. Bill asked me out, but I refused—he just isn't my sort, no spark—when the phone rang. It was Louise. Three

boys had just dropped over and would I go out tonight. So I threw on my clothes, all the time ranting on how never to commit suicide, because something unexpected always happens!

Turned out that my date was a *doll*. I now feel terrific! What a man can do! Love, Sivvy.

AURELIA: (*Seriously*) As soon as I was certain I was pregnant, I began reading books related to the rearing of children. I was totally imbued with the desire to be a good wife and mother.

(*Bookish* AURELIA! SYLVIA *laughs.*)

SYLVIA: What a man can do!

AURELIA: I quietly followed the "demand feeding" accepted as modern today and labeled old-fashioned in the 1930s. Both my babies were rocked, cuddled, sung to, recited to, and picked up when they cried!

SYLVIA: (*Soft irony*) Dear Mom.

AURELIA: Sylvia was born October 27, 1932, a healthy, eight-and-a-half-pound baby. At a luncheon that day, her father told his colleagues, "I hope for one more thing in life—a son, two and a half years from now." Warren was born April 27, 1935, only two hours off schedule, and *Otto* was greeted by his colleagues as "the man who gets what he wants when he wants it."

SYLVIA: I have been rather worried about a friend of mine.

AURELIA: Social life was almost nil for us as a married couple.

SYLVIA: Dear Mummy,

AURELIA: My dreams of "open house"...

SYLVIA: My physical exam...

AURELIA: for students and the faculty ...

SYLVIA: consisted in getting swathed in a sheet and passing from one room to another...

AURELIA: were not realized.

SYLVIA: in nudity!

AURELIA: All had to be given up for THE BOOK, a treatise on *"Insect Societies."*

SYLVIA: My height is 5' 9" ...

AURELIA: We worked together on this ...

SYLVIA: my weight 137 pounds.

AURELIA: I did the reading and note-taking . . .

SYLVIA: I took such pains . . .

AURELIA: he rewriting and adding his notes.

SYLVIA: to get my ears and heels in a straight line . . .

AURELIA: Then he handed the manuscript to me to put into final form.

SYLVIA: that I forgot to tilt up straight. The result was, "You have good alignment, but you are in constant danger of falling on your face!"

AURELIA: Otto insisted on handling all finances, even to the purchasing of meat, fish and vegetables.

The age difference between us, Otto's superior education, his long years of living in college dormitories or rooming by himself, all led to an attitude of "rightful dominance" on his part. At the end of my first year of marriage, I realized that if I wanted a peaceful home, and I did, I would simply have to become more submissive, although it was not my nature to be so.

SYLVIA: Physically, I want a *colossus!* Mentally, I want a man who isn't jealous of my creativity in other fields than children. Graduate school and travel abroad are not going to be stymied by any squalling, breastfed brats. I've controlled my sex judiciously, and you don't have to worry about me at all. The consequences of love affairs would stop me from my independent freedom of creative activity, and *I don't intend to be stopped*. Love, Sivvy.

(AURELIA *nods. She understands. A moment, then.*)

AURELIA: The year after Warren's birth, Otto began to draw more and more into himself.

> SYLVIA: Dear Mother, I have been rather worried about a friend of mine . . .

(*A duet now,* AURELIA *leading.*)

AURELIA: He was losing weight, was continually weary, and easily upset by trifles.

> Her usual gaiety has been getting brighter and more artificial as the days go by.

He steadily refused a physician, pushing aside all such
suggestions from me, my family, and his colleagues.

So yesterday, after lunch, I
made her come up to my
room. At first, she was very
light and evasive, but at last
her face gave way and melted.

He told me he had diagnosed
his own case and that he
would *never* submit to
surgery.

It seems that since Thanksgiving she hasn't been able to do
her work, and now she can only reiterate, "I can *never* do it,
never."

I understood the significance
of what he said, for he had
recently lost a friend who had
succumbed after several
operations to . . .

. . . lung cancer!

She hasn't been getting enough
sleep . . .

. . . but has been waking up
early in the mornings, obsessed by the feeling she has to
do her work, even if she can
only go through the motions,
that if she could do the work,
nothing would matter.

I even telephoned my family
doctor in Winthrop.

But her parents were either
deceiving her into thinking she
was creative or really didn't
know how incapable she was.
I got scared when she told me
how she had been saving
sleeping pills and razor blades.

I sensed Otto's unspoken
diagnosis: lung cancer.

Oh, mother, you don't know how inadequate I felt!

From this time on . . .

I talked to her all afternoon.

I have been thinking of writing a note to her parents, telling them a bit of how tired she is and how she needs rest.

. . . it was heartbreaking to watch a once-handsome, powerfully built man lose his vigor and deteriorate physically and emotionally.

For her mother kept telling her she was foolish and could do it all.

Appealing to him to get medical diagnosis and help only brought on explosive outbursts of anger.

But her mother couldn't really see how incapable the poor girl is of thinking in this state.

One morning in mid-August, 1940, Otto stubbed his little toe against the base of his bureau. That afternoon I asked to see his foot. The toes were black, and red streaks ran up his ankle. There was no protest this time as I rushed to telephone my doctor. "Diabetes mellitus." The announcement burst upon me like a clap of thunder. So this was his illness, not cancer at all, but an illness which, treated in time, could be lived with and controlled!

From that day on life was an alternation of hope and fear.

Maybe it's none of my business, but I love the girl and feel very inadequate and responsible.

On the nurse's first day off, Otto suggested that I get out into the sun with Sylvia. She and I ran along the beach together for only about a half hour.

(Directly to AURELIA *now.)*

... *Inadequate* ...

On my return, I found Otto collapsed on the staircase. Somehow I half dragged, half carried him to his bed. (It was a Wednesday, the doctor could not be reached!) I gave Otto his insulin injection; he was so exhausted. In the middle of the night he called me, feverish, shaking from head to foot with chills, bed clothes soaked with perspiration. All the rest of that night I kept changing sheets, sponging his face, holding his trembling hands.

... *and responsible* ...

As tears streamed down my face, I could only think, "All this needn't have happened; it needn't have happened!"

SYLVIA: If *you* were her mother, she would be all right.

AURELIA: The next day the doctor came. Amputation from the thigh of the gangrened foot and leg would be necessary to save Otto's life. As I handed Dr. Loder his hat, he murmured, "How could such a brilliant man be so *stupid!*"

SYLVIA: If *you* were her mother. If you were ...

AURELIA: *(With gathering speed)* On October 12, the amputation was performed.

On November 5, when I left Otto his condition was serious. My telephone was ringing when I returned home. It was Dr. Loder. An embolus had struck in a lung and caused my husband's death as he slept.

SYLVIA: If *you* were her mother she would be all right!

*(*AURELIA *nods; she understands the accusation.)*

AURELIA: I waited until the next morning to tell the children. When Warren awoke, I told him as quietly as I could that Daddy's sufferings had ended. Warren sat up, hugged me tightly. "Oh, Mummy, I'm so glad *you* are young and healthy!"

SYLVIA: Inadequate. Responsible.

Then I faced the more difficult task, telling Sylvia, who was already reading in her bed. She looked at me sternly for a moment, then said woodenly, "I'll never speak to God again!"

(*On* AURELIA's *"looked at me,"* SYLVIA *turns away.*)

SYLVIA: (*Wild*) "I'll never speak to God again!"

SYLVIA: (*Wooden*) There is the sort of person who has problems and never tells them to anyone, there is the sort of person who has problems and tells them to one understanding person, and there is the sort of person who fools everyone, *even herself*, into thinking there are no problems, except those shallow material ones which can be overcome.

(*On "even herself"* SYLVIA *turns directly to* AURELIA.)

AURELIA: (*Slowly distinctly*) I told her that she did not need to attend school that day if she'd rather stay at home. From under the blanket which she had pulled over her head came her muffled voice, "I *want* to go to school."

SYLVIA: (*Remembering*) "I want to go to school!"

(*Then, an apology.*)

SYLVIA: For all my brave, bold talk of being selfsufficient, I realize now how much you mean to me—you and Warren and my dear Grampy and Grammy! I am glad the rain's coming down hard. It's the way I feel inside. I love you so.

AURELIA: After school, she came to me, red-eyed, and handed me a piece of paper. In shaky printing stood these words. I PROMISE NEVER TO MARRY AGAIN.

SYLVIA: (*An explanation*) I love you so!

I signed at once.

SYLVIA: (*Irony*) What a superlative mother you have been to me!

AURELIA: I looked at the rumpled "document" I had just signed, and *knew* that unless I should have the opportunity to marry a man I respected, loved, and trusted to be a good father to my children, and whom the children wanted for their father ... I never *would* marry again.

SYLVIA: I wonder if *I* will ever meet a congenial boy.

AURELIA: This was the explanation I gave Sylvia, as a college student. "That document never kept you from marrying again, did it?" ... I assured her that it had not.

SYLVIA: (*Quickly*) All this leads up to my date last night. I told him how I like to write and draw and know people more than just on the surface. He was rather overwhelmed by the fact that I could be so intelligent and yet not be *ugly* or something!

This weekend I went out Saturday with Bill.

I will ask for Mondays off, because there is nothing I'd rather do than see Dick.

Love, love, love, Sivvy.

AURELIA: "Love, love, love ..."

When I viewed Otto at the funeral parlor, he bore no resemblance to the husband I knew, but looked like a fashionable store manikin. The children would never recognize their father, I felt, so I did not take them to the funeral.

What I intended as an exercise in courage, for the sake of my children, was interpreted years later by my daughter as "indifference." "My mother never had time to mourn my father's death."

(*A deep hurt. She shrugs it off, goes on.*)

My husband had no pension. His five thousand dollar life insurance had to be used to pay his medical and funeral expenses.

In the summer of 1942, I was invited by the dean of Boston University to develop a course in Medical Secretarial Procedures.

At the small salary of eighteen hundred dollars a year, it was providential.

SYLVIA: I don't want you to worry about things, Mummy. I am learning a lot.

Now that the hardest twenty years of your life are over you deserve all the returns you can get.

P.S. I *will* grow up in jerks, it seems, so don't feel my growing pains so vicariously, dear!

(*It is an apology, and* AURELIA *accepts it with joy.*)

AURELIA: All the girls at Haven House were invited to Maureen Buckley's coming-out party!

SYLVIA:
Dear Mother,
How can I ever, tell you what a unique, dreamlike and astounding weekend I had!
Saturday afternoon, at two p.m., about fifteen girls from Smith started out for Sharon, Connecticut. Marcia and I drew a cream-colored convertible (with three other girls and a Dartmouth boy). Picture me then in my navy-blue . . .

AURELIA: (*Adding in*) bolero suit . . .

SYLVIA: and versatile brown coat, snuggled in the back seat of an open car . . .

AURELIA: *Snuggled?*

SYLVIA: whizzing for two sun-colored hours through the hilly Connecticut valley! The foliage was out in full tilt, and the hills of crimson sumac, yellow maples and scarlet oak that revolved past . . .

AURELIA: the late afternoon sun on them . . .

SYLVIA: were almost more than I could bear. At about five p.m. we rolled up the long drive to "The Elms." God! Great lawns,

AURELIA: huge trees on a hill

SYLVIA: with a view of the valley, distant green cow pastures,

AURELIA: orange and yellow leaves . . .

SYLVIA: A caterer's truck was unloading champagne at the back.

AURELIA: *Champagne!*

SYLVIA: We walked through the hall, greeted by a thousand living rooms, period pieces, rare objects of art everywhere. Marcia and I and Joan Strong.

AURELIA: (a lovely girl)

SYLVIA: had the best deal—a big double bed and bath to ourselves. We lay down under a big quilt for an hour in the gray-purple twilight, conjecturing about the exciting

AURELIA: unknown!

SYLVIA: evening fast coming.

Joan, Marcia, and I were driven in a great . . .

AURELIA: black . . .

SYLVIA: Cadillac, to the Sharon Inn, where a lovely buffet supper was prepared.

AURELIA: After supper . . .

SYLVIA: another hour of lying down.

AURELIA: Scarlett O'Hara before the ball!

SYLVIA: And then the dressing! Up the stone steps, under the white colonial columns of the Buckley home. Girls in beautiful gowns clustered by the stairs.

Everywhere there were swishes of taffeta, satin . . .

AURELIA: silk!

SYLVIA: I looked at Marcia, and we winked at each other. Walking out in the patio, two stories high, with the elm treetops barely visible through the glassed-in roof . . .

AURELIA: Remember Mrs. Jack's patio?

SYLVIA: The same! Vines trailing from a balcony . . .

AURELIA: fountains playing . . .

SYLVIA: Balloons, Japanese lanterns, tables covered with white linen. A band platform built up for dancing. I stood open-mouthed,

AURELIA: giddy,

SYLVIA: wanting so much to show *you*! If you had seen me! I looked

AURELIA: beautiful!

SYLVIA: Even daughters of millionaires complimented my dress! About nine-thirty we were standing in fluttering feminine groups, waiting for the dancing to begin. I began to wish I had brought a date, wondering if I could compete with all the tall, lovely girls there. Let me tell you, by the end of the evening, I was so glad I hadn't!

The whole Senior Class at Yale was there! Maureen's brother is a senior.

AURELIA: (Ten children in the Catholic family, all brilliant, many writers.)

SYLVIA: A lovely tall hook-nosed freshman named Eric cut in. Turned out we both loved English.

Back to the floor with Carl,

AURELIA: the philosophy major,

SYLVIA: who asked me to Cornell weekend. I refused.

AURELIA: Nicely!

SYLVIA: Next I had a brief trot with the Editor of the *Yale News*. No possibilities there! About then the Yale Whiffenpoofs sang.

AURELIA: Now, suddenly . . .

SYLVIA: A lovely grinning dark-haired boy cut in. "Name?" I asked. "Constantine." He was a wonderful dancer, and twirled so all I could see was a great cartwheel of colored lights. Turned out his father was a general in the Russian Caucasus Mountains! I danced steps I never dreamed of and my feet

AURELIA: just

SYLVIA: flew! A tall boy, who claimed his name was "Plato," did the sweetest thing! In the midst of dancing he said, "I have a picture I want to show you." So we

AURELIA: crossed . . .

SYLVIA: through the cool, leaf-covered

AURELIA: patio . . .

SYLVIA: the sound of the

AURELIA: fountains

SYLVIA: dripping, and entered one of the many drawing rooms. Over the fireplace was a Botticelli

AURELIA: Madonna!

SYLVIA: "You remind me of her," he said.

AURELIA: (*It is happening to* her *now*) I was really touched!

SYLVIA: Imagine meeting such fascinating, intelligent, versatile people! And saving best to last, my Constantine. He cut in, and we danc-ed. . .

AURELIA: (*Taking the lead, awkwardly, tenderly*) and danced. Finally

SYLVIA: we were so hot . . .

AURELIA: and breathless

SYLVIA: that we walked out on the lawn. The night was lovely,

AURELIA: stars, trees big and dark—

SYLVIA: —so guess what we did—

AURELIA: (*Dancing*) Strauss waltzes!

SYLVIA: You should have seen us swooping and whirling . . .

AURELIA: over the grass . . .

SYLVIA: with the music from inside

AURELIA: faint and distant . . . Imagine, on a night like that, to have a

SYLVIA: (*Adding in now*) handsome . . .

AURELIA: perceptive . . .

SYLVIA: male kiss your hand,

AURELIA: tell you . . .

SYLVIA: how

AURELIA: *beautiful* you were! I asked him what

SYLVIA: happened . . .

AURELIA: when a woman got old, and her physical beauty waned, and he said in his lovely

SYLVIA: liquid

AURELIA: voice, "Why she will always be beautiful to the man she married, we hope."

SYLVIA: (*Takes the lead again*) I asked if I could tell him my favorite poem. I did . . .

AURELIA: and he loved it! Oh,

SYLVIA: if you could have heard the wonderful way he talked,

AURELIA: about life and the world.

SYLVIA: Imagine! I told him teasingly not to suffocate in my long hair and he said,

AURELIA: "What a divine way to die!"

(*Mother and daughter laugh together.*)

SYLVIA: Probably all this sounds absurd and very silly. But I

AURELIA: never

SYLVIA: expressed myself so clearly and lucidly,

AURELIA: never felt

SYLVIA: such warm, sympathetic response. There is sudden glorying in womanhood, when someone kisses your shoulder and says "You are charming . . .

AURELIA: beautiful . . .

SYLVIA: and most important,

AURELIA: *intelligent!*"

SYLVIA: It was striking five when I fell into bed beside Marcia. I dreamed . . .

AURELIA: exquisite dreams!

SYLVIA: Brunch at Buckley's at one p.m. on a gray, rainy day, the most amazing repast brought in by colored waiters in great copper tureens. Scrambled eggs, coffee . . .

AURELIA: sausages . . .

SYLVIA: a sort of white farina . . .

AURELIA: Lord, what luxury! Back here . . .

SYLVIA: I can't face the dead reality. I still lilt and twirl

AURELIA: with Eric, Plato, and my wholly lovely

SYLVIA: Constantine!

AURELIA: under Japanese lanterns,

SYLVIA: and a hundred moons twining in,

AURELIA: dark leaves . . .

SYLVIA: music spilling out and

AURELIA: echoing yet

SYLVIA: inside my head. *To have had you there!*

AURELIA: In spirit!

SYLVIA: To have had you

AURELIA and SYLVIA: *see me!*

SYLVIA: (*A change of tone*) I've got to work and work! My courses are frightening. I can't keep up with them! See you the 19th.

AURELIA: Love,

SYLVIA: love,

AURELIA: love,

SYLVIA: Sivvy.

(AURELIA *turns to the audience again.*)

AURELIA: These were the days when we still were together enough to enjoy long talks about books, music, paintings—how they made us feel. For we shared a love of words and considered them as a tool to achieve precise expression in describing our emotions, as well as for mutual understanding.

SYLVIA: Dearest-Mother-whom-I-love-better-than-anybody,

AURELIA: Between Sylvia and me there existed . . .

SYLVIA: You are listening to the most busy and happy girl in the world.

AURELIA: as between my own mother and me

SYLVIA: Honestly, Mum, I could just cry with happiness.

AURELIA: a sort of psychic osmosis, which, at times, was very wonderful,

SYLVIA: The world is splitting open at my feet like a ripe, juicy watermelon!

AURELIA: and comforting. . .

SYLVIA: If only I can work, work, work to justify all my opportunities. Your happy girl, Sivvy.

AURELIA: at other times, an unwelcome invasion of privacy. Understanding this, I learned, as she grew older, not to refer to previous voluntary confidences on her part.

SYLVIA: Today I got a letter confirming my job. I really hope I can earn a lot of money.

(*At the mention of money, another color.*)

AURELIA: The Belmont Hotel, Cape Cod. June 11, 1952.

SYLVIA: Your amazing telegram . . .

AURELIA: announcing five hundred dollars, *Mademoiselle* prize for "Sunday at the Mintons',"

SYLVIA: came just as I was scrubbing tables in the shady interior of the Belmont dining room. I was so excited that I screamed and actually threw my arms around the head waitress who no doubt thinks I am rather insane! Anyhow, psychologically, the moment couldn't have been better. I felt tired. Also, I just learned since I am completely inexperienced, I am not going to be working in the main dining room, but in the "side hall" where the managers and top hotel brass eat. So, tips will no doubt net much less. I was beginning to worry about money when your telegram came. God! To think "Sunday at the Mintons" is *one* of *two* prize stories to be put in a big national slick!!!

AURELIA: The first thing I thought of was: Mother can keep her intersession money and buy some pretty clothes and a special trip or something!

SYLVIA: At least *I* get a winter coat and extra special suit out of the Mintons.

AURELIA: Both Sylvia and I were more at ease in *writing* words of appriciation, admiration, and love than in expressing these emotions verbally—and thank goodness, write them to each other we did!

SYLVIA: So it's really looking up around here, now that I don't have to be scared stiff about money.

AURELIA: I held off

                                      SYLVIA: Even if my feet kill me

because,

                                        after this first week,

as she entered her late teens,

                                        and I drop 20 trays, I will have the beach, boys to bring me beer, sun,

her response to my spoken praise would be,

                                        and young gay companions.

"Oh, *you* think I'm wonderful (or look lovely)

                                        What a life!

because you're my

Love, your crazy old

mother!"

daughter.
Sivvy.

June 15, 1952.

*(The beginning of the terrible
time.* AURELIA *knows it.)*

Dear Mother,
Do write me letters, Mummy,
because I am in a very
dangerous state of feeling
sorry for myself. Just at present, life is awful. I am exhausted, scared, incompetent,
unenergetic and generally low
in spirits. Working in side hall
puts me apart, and I feel completely uprooted and clumsy.
But as tempted as I am to be a
coward and escape by crawling back home, I have re-
solved to give it a good
month's trial. Don't worry
about me, but do send little
pellets of advice now and
then.

June 17, 1952.

SYLVIA: Dear Mum,
It's my week's anniversary
here, and I am celebrating the
beautiful blue day by spending
my morning hour on the
beach. Needless to say, I am in   *(Up and down.)*
a little more optimistic mood
than when I wrote you.

AURELIA: I've got an idea for a
story for *Seventeen* called, of
all appropriate things, "Side   *(And* AURELIA *tries to keep her
Hall Girl." I even have a   up—)*
heroine named Marley who is,

of course,

SYLVIA: *me!*

AURELIA: I should be able to sit
down in a few days,

SYLVIA: and send it to *you* to type
and get notarized.

AURELIA: Would I like to win a
summer at Breadloaf!

SYLVIA: But that is really a dream,
because *boys* usually win
those things, and my style   (*—and down; a terrible seesaw.*)
needs to mature a lot yet.

AURELIA: As for side hall, I figure I deserve a "bad break," what with
all my good fortune winning prizes and going to Smith. I just don't
care what people think about me as long as I'm always open, nice,
and friendly.
Love to you all,
Sivvy, your Side Hall philosopher.

June 25, 1952.

SYLVIA: Just a note to let you know I'm still alive. Never, it seems to
me, has work worn me out so much. In spite of everything, I still
have my good old sense of humor, and manage to laugh a good
deal of the time. I have definitely decided to come home August 10.
I will have stayed two months, slaved for two hundred dollars, and
will need a good month to recuperate physically and mentally.
With all my important and demanding school offices, I can't afford
to crack up. Now I'm always so tired that I just can't *retain*
anything except what kind of eggs people like for breakfast. Well,
tell me what you think of my schemes.
Your

AURELIA: *maturing* . . .

SYLVIA: Sivvy.

(*Now, a roller-coaster "down."*)

SYLVIA: Brace yourself and take a deep breath—not too nice.

AURELIA: (*Bewildered*) God, will I be glad to get home for a few days of rest.

SYLVIA: I am sorry to have to admit it, but I am in a rather tense emotional and mental state.

AURELIA: The crux of the matter is my attitude toward life—hinging on my science course.

SYLVIA: I have practically considered committing suicide to get out of it; it's like having my nose rubbed in my own slime. It just seems that I am running on a purposeless treadmill, behind and paralyzed, dreading every day of the horrible year ahead when I should be revelling! I have become really frantic; small choices and events seem insurmountable obstacles, the core of life has fallen apart . . .

AURELIA: I wonder why? Why?

SYLVIA: It affects all the rest of my life; I am behind in my Chaucer unit, feeling sterile in creative writing . . . Everyone else is abroad or falling in love with their courses. I feel I have got to escape this, or go mad!

AURELIA: I don't even *want* to understand it, which is the worst yet.

SYLVIA: It seems to have no relation to anything in my life. I have wondered, desperately, if I should go to the college psychiatrist,

AURELIA: try to tell her how I feel about it,

SYLVIA: how it is obsessing all my life, paralyzing my action in every other field. Life seems a mockery . . .

AURELIA: I can't go on like this!

SYLVIA: Luckily I haven't gotten sinus yet; that would be another form of escapism. When one feels like leaving college and *kill*ing oneself over one course . . . ! Every day more and more piles up. I hate formulas, I don't give a *damn* about valences,

AURELIA: artificial atoms and molecules,

SYLVIA: I am letting it ruin my whole life! I am really *afraid* to talk it over with a psychiatrist, because they might make me drop my activities and spend half my time pounding formulas and petty mathematical relationships into my head, when I basically don't want to learn them! To be wasting all this year of my life,

AURELIA: *obsessed* by this course, *paralyzed* by it,

SYLVIA: Oh, Mother—! Life is so black, anyway. Everything is empty, meaningless. How could I ever persuade the college authorities, how could I convince the psychiatrist? My reason is leaving me!

Everybody is happy, but this has obsessed me from the day I got here.

AURELIA: (*Frantic*) I am driven inward, feeling hollow. No rest cure in the infirmary will cure the sickness in me!

SYLVIA: Love, your hollow girl, Sivvy.

(*Then, relief, exasperation, laughter.*)

AURELIA:
Dear Mother,
Well, the world has a miraculous and wonderful way of working. You plunge to the bottom, and you think that every straw must be the last. Then you break your leg, and the world falls like a delicious apple in your lap!

If a hideous snowy winter with midyears and a broken leg is heaven, what will the green young spring be like? How can I bear the joy of it all!

Much overflowing love,

Your own Sivvy.

SYLVIA: Today I had my too-long hair trimmed just right for a smooth pageboy, and got, for twelve ninety-five, the most classic pair of silver pumps. With my rhinestone earrings and necklace, I should look like a silver princess. God, how I wish I could win the *Mademoiselle* contest.

AURELIA: I got two villanelles back from *The New Yorker* today.

SYLVIA: Got back the *Mademoiselle* manuscript today. I don't see how I have any sort of a chance if I just write one or two stories and never revise them or streamline them for particular market. I want to hit *The New Yorker* in poetry and *Ladies, Home Journal* in stories and—

AURELIA: Birthday Greetings! My present is following news. *Harper's Magazine* just graciously accepted three poems for one hundred dollars in all. *Mademoiselle* sent ten dollars for runner-up in third assignment.
Best love to you, Sivvy.

SYLVIA: I dedicate this *Harper's* triumph to you, my favorite person in the world! Can't you just hear the critics saying, "Oh, yes, she's been published in *Harper's*"? When I am rich and famous I will hire you for my private secretary and babytender, and pay you scandalously high wages, and take you on monthly jaunts in my own shocking pink yacht!

AURELIA: (*More softly*) Letter to Warren; written about May 12, 1953.

SYLVIA: You know, as I do, and it is a frightening thing, that mother would actually kill herself for us if we calmly accepted all she wanted to do for us. She is an abnormally altruistic person, and I have realized lately that we have to fight against her selflessness as we would fight against a deadly disease.

AURELIA: (*Painfully*) My ambition is to earn enough so that she won't have to work summers in the future.

SYLVIA: After extracting her life blood and care for twenty years, we should start bringing in big dividends of joy for her. Really, you and I have it good. Food, clothes, best schools in the country—our first choices, all sorts of prizes, etc.

Just hope the world doesn't blow up and queer it all before we've lived our good hard lives down to the nub.

AURELIA: (*Desperately cheerful; a last chance*) Telegram to Sylvia from *Mademoiselle*:

Happy to announce you have won a *Mademoiselle* 1953 Guest Editorship! You must be available from June 1 through June 26. Please wire collect.

SYLVIA: (*Overlap, excited*) Dearest Progenitor,

I've already sent in the names of four writers: J.D. Salinger; Shirley "*The Lottery*" Jackson; E.B. White of *New Yorker* fame; and Irwin Shaw. Hope one of those luminaries consents to be—

AURELIA: The two days at home between her last examination at Smith and her departure for New York were crammed with frantic activity, including—

SYLVIA: (*Overlap*)
New York, NY.
June 4, 1953.

Dear Mother,

So incredibly much has happened so fast! Gardens, alleys, the rumbling Third Ave. El, the UN with a snatch of the East River, at night at my desk a network of lights, the sound of car horns like the sweetest music . . . I love it!

AURELIA: Whooshed up to the sixth floor. Spent morning with other Eds filling out endless forms. Talked with Fiction Editor, Jobs and Futures Editor, fabulous Editor-in-Chief. Afternoon—rewrote poetry squibs. Assignments announced. I'm Managing Ed. At first I was disappointed at not being Fiction Ed, but now I see how all-inclusive my work is—

SYLVIA: I love it!

AURELIA: Affairs scheduled include fashion tours (e.g., John Frederics hats), UN and *Herald Trib* tours, movie preview, City Center ballet, TV show, dance at St. Regis Roof. Love, Syrilly.

SYLVIA: I sometimes wonder who is me.

AURELIA: I have been very ecstatic, horribly depressed, shocked, elated, enlightened, and enervated. I want to come home and vegetate in peace this coming weekend, with the people I love around me for a change.

SYLVIA: I can't talk about all that has happened this week . . . I am too weary, too dazed. I have, in the space of six days, toured the second largest ad agency in the world, seen television, heard speeches, gotten ptomaine poisoning from crabmeat the agency served us in their "own special test kitchen" and wanted to *die* very badly for a day! Spent an evening in Greenwich Village with the most brilliant, wonderful man in the world . . . who is *tragically* a couple of inches shorter than I! Spent an evening fighting with a wealthy, *unscrupulous*

AURELIA: (*Wonderingly*) Peruvian delegate to the UN at a Forest Hills tennis club dance—spent Saturday

SYLVIA: in the Yankee Stadium with all the stinking people in the world, watching the Yankees trounce the Tigers, having our pictures taken; getting lost in the subway and seeing

AURELIA: (*Softly in horror*) deformed men with short arms that curled

AURELIA and SYLVIA: (*Together*) like pink, boneless snakes

SYLVIA: around a begging cup stagger through the car, thinking to myself all the time that Central Park Zoo was only different in that there were bars on the windows. Oh, God, it is unbelievable to think of all this at once! My mind will split open!

AURELIA: *I love you* a million times more than any of these slick admen, these hucksters, these wealthy beasts who get "dronk" in foreign accents all the time.

SYLVIA: Seriously, I am more than overjoyed to have been here a month; it is just that I realize how young and inexperienced I am in the ways of the world.
Your exhausted, ecstatic, elegiac New Yorker, Sivvy.

AURELIA: My mother and I met a tired, unsmiling Sylvia on her return from her month in New York City. I dreaded telling Sylvia the news that had come that morning: she had not been accepted as a student in Frank O'Connor's short-story writing class.

I knew Sylvia would see it as a rejection of her as a competent or even promising writer, despite all the writing honors and publications she had to her credit. At this point, success in short-story writing was her ultimate goal, and Sylvia was too demanding of herself.

AURELIA: Sylvia's face in the rear-view mirror went white when I told her, and the look of shock and utter despair that passed over it alarmed me.

SYLVIA: (*Bitterly remembering*) "By the way, Frank O'Connor's class is filled; you'll have to wait for next summer before registering again."

SYLVIA: (*A new color; cool, ironic*)   Belknap House
                    McLean Hospital
                    Belmont, Mass.
                    December 28, 1953

Dear E.
I don't know just how widely the news of my little scandal this summer traveled in the newspaper but I received letters from all over the United States, from friends, relations, perfect strangers and religious crackpots—and I'm not aware of whether you read about my escapade, or whether *you* are aware of my present situation. At

(*A duet between mother and daughter now, each telling her side.*)

AURELIA: (*Strongly*) From that point on, *I* was aware of a great change in her; all her usual joie de vivre was absent. My mother tried to reassure me that this was no doubt temporary, a natural reaction to the strains of the last year.

There had been no respite at all, so we encouraged her to "just let go and relax." We packed picnics and drove to beaches in New Hampshire and Massachusetts. At home, she would sunbathe, always with a book in hand, but never reading it.

After days of this, she finally began to talk to me, pouring out an endless stream of self-deprecation, self-accusation. She had no goal, she said. As she couldn't read with comprehension anymore, much less write creatively, what was she going to do with her life? She had injured her friends, "let down" her sponsors—she went on and on.

Sylvia's self-recrimination even extended to reproaching herself for one of the two prize-winning stories in *Mademoiselle*. She felt it had been unkind to a young friend, one of the two characters in the story.

any rate, I'm prepared to give you a brief resume of details.

SYLVIA: I worked all during the hectic month of June.

(*Then more softly, a jumble of words*) in the plushy air-conditioned offices of *Mademoiselle* magazine helping set up the August issue. I came home exhausted, fully prepared to begin my two courses at Harvard Summer School, for which I'd been offered a partial scholarship. *Then things started to happen.*

I'd gradually come to realize

(*On and on*)

that I'd completely wasted my Junior year at Smith by taking a minimum of courses (and the wrong courses at that), by blufffing my way glibly through infrequent papers, skipping by with only three or four exams during the year, reading nothing more meaty than the jokes in *The New Yorker* and writing nothing but glib jingles in an attempt to commune with W. H. Auden.

I had gaily asserted that I was going to write a thesis on James Joyce (when I hadn't even read *Ulysses* through thoroughly once!) And take comprehensives in my senior year, when I wasn't even familiar with the most common works of Shakespeare, for God's sake!

(*Wilder*).

To top it off, all my friends were either writing novels in Europe, planning to get married next June, or going to med. school. The one or two males I knew were either proving themselves genii in the midst of adversity, or were not in the market for the legal kind of love for a good ten years yet, and were going to see the world and all the femmes fatales in it before becoming victims of wedded bliss.

In an effort to pull herself together, Sylvia, who had by this time decided not to attempt any courses at Harvard Summer School, felt that some form of scheduled activity would keep her from feeling that the whole summer was being wasted.

Anyhow, to sum up my reactions to the immediate problem at hand, I decided at the beginning of July to save a few hundred dollars, stay home, write, learn shorthand, and finesse the summer school deal.

(*Heavy irony.*)

You know, sort of "live cheap and be creative."

Her plan was that I should teach her shorthand for an

hour each morning so that she could "get a job to support my writing—if I can ever write again."

One unforgettable morning, I noticed some partially healed gashes on her legs.

Truth was, I'd counted on getting into Frank O'Connor's writing course at Harvard,

Upon my horrified questioning, she replied, "I just wanted to see if I had the guts!" Then she grasped my hand—hers was burning hot to the touch—

(*Low, on and on*)

but it seemed that several thousand other rather brilliant writers did, too, and so I didn't; so I was miffed, and figured if I couldn't write on my own, I wasn't any good anyhow.

and cried passionately, "Oh, Mother, the world is so rotten! I want to die!"

It turned out that not only was I totally unable to learn one squiggle of shorthand, but I also had not a damn thing to say in the literary world; because I was sterile, empty, unlived, unwise, and UNREAD. And the more I tried to remedy the situation, the more I became unable to comprehend ONE WORD of our fair old language.

"Let's die together!"

I took her in my arms, telling her that she was ill, exhausted, that she had everything to live for and that I would see to it that she wanted to. We saw our own doctor within an hour; she recommended psychiatric counseling.

And the long summer of seeking help began.

The first psychiatrist:

I began to frequent the offices and couches of the local psychiatrists, who were all running back and forth on summer vacations. I became unable to sleep; I became immune to increased doses of sleeping pills, I underwent a rather brief and traumatic experience of badly given shock treatments on an outpatient basis.

He insisted that a series of shock treatments would be *beneficial.* I felt so inadequate, so alone. A kind neighbor took Sylvia and me to the hospital for the treatments; it was she who sat with me, holding my hand as we waited for Sylvia to reappear, for though I had pleaded to accompany her, I was *not allowed to do so!*

Pretty soon, the only doubt in my mind was the precise time and method of committing suicide.

The consultants with the referred psychiatrist, an older man, gentle and fatherly, gave me a ray of hope. He prescribed sleeping tablets, which he told me to administer each night— and which I kept locked in a metal safety case.

(Her voice rising.)

(Low.)

Sylvia still talked to me constantly in the same self-deprecating vein, becoming very agitated at times as she noted the approaching date of the fall term of college.

The only alternative I could see was an eternity of hell for the rest of my life in a mental hospital, and I was going to make use of my last ounce of free choice and choose a quick clean ending. I figured that in the long run it would be more merciful and inexpensive to my family;

(Then with great clarity, and passion)

instead of an indefinite incarceration of a favorite daughter in the cell of a State San, instead of the misery and disillusion of sixty odd years of mental vacuum, of physical squalor, I would spare them all by ending everything at the height of my so-called career, while there were still illusions left among my profs, still poems to published in *Harper's*, still a memory at least that would be worthwhile.

(Same tone as "live cheap and be creative.")

(Deeply troubled, reliving it.)

Well, I tried drowning, but that didn't work.

On August 24, a blisteringly hot day, a friend invited us to a film showing of the coronation of Queen Elizabeth II. Sylvia said she wanted to stay home with her grandparents, but urged me to go.

So I hit upon what I figured would be the easiest way out.

*(*AURELIA *looks at* SYLVIA, *who smiles dazzlingly. When* AURELIA *turns away, the smile fades.)*

She looked particularly well this day.

Her eyes sparkled, her cheeks were flushed. Nevertheless, I left her with a sense of uneasiness, feeling that her buoyancy was contrived.

I waited until my mother had gone to town,

I found it difficult to concentrate

(Now SYLVIA *takes the lead)*

(More softly)

my brother was at work, and my grandparents were out in the backyard. Then I broke the lock of my mother's safe, took out the bottle of fifty

on the slow-moving, archaic ceremony on the screen, and in the middle of it I all at once

found myself filled with terror
1such as I had never experienced in my life. Cold perspiration poured down me; my heart
pounded. I wanted to get out of
my seat and rush from the theater. I forced myself to remain
quiet until the close, then begged my friend to drive me home
at once. Propped against a bowl
of flowers on the dining-room
table was a note in Sylvia's
handwriting: "Have gone for a
long walk. Will be home tomorrow."

The nightmare of nightmares
had begun.

The report of Sylvia's disap-
pearance which I phoned to the
police, was issued over the
radio. Then I discovered that
the lock to my steel case had
been broken open and the bottle of sleeping pills was missing.

At noon on the third day

he dashed from the table. "Call
the ambulance!"

He had found his sister, returning to consciousness in the
crawl space beneath the downstairs bedroom.

(*Open pain, passion.*)

In minutes she was car-
ried into the ambulance,

sleeping pills, and descended
to the dark sheltered ledge in
our basement, after having left
a note to mother that I had
gone on a long walk and
would not be back for a day or
so. I swallowed quantities and
blissfully succumbed to the
whirling blackness that I
honestly believed was eternal
oblivion.

My mother believed my note,

sent out searching parties,
notified the police, and, finally, on the second day or so,
began to give up hope when
she found that the pills were
missing.

My brother finally heard my
weak yells

a nightmare of flashing lights,
strange voices, large needles,

and a *hatred* toward the people who would not let me
die—but insisted rather in
dragging me back into the hell
of sordid and meaningless existence!

and we followed to the hospital. When I was allowed to see her, there was an angry-looking abrasion under her right eye and considerable swelling. Her first words were a moaned "Oh, no!" When I took her hand and told her how we rejoiced she was alive and how we loved her, she said weakly, "It was my last act of love."

(An attempt at cool irony again.)

I won't go into the details that involved two sweltering weeks in the Newton-Wellesley Hospital, exposed to the curious eyes of all the student nurses, attendants and passers-by, or the two weeks in the psychiatric ward of the Mass. General, where the enormous open sore on my cheek gradually healed, leaving a miraculously intact eye, plus a large, ugly brown scar under it.

(They are playing together, cello and violin.)

As soon as the news of our finding Sylvia was made public, I received a sympathetic telegram from Mrs. Prouty.

Suffice it to say that by fairy-godmother-type maneuverings, my scholarship benefactress at Smith got me into the best mental hospital in the U.S., where I had my own attractive private room and my own attractive private psychiatrist. I didn't think improvement was possible. It seems that it is.

One of Sylvia's deep concerns throughout her illness had been that she had not proven herself

worthy of the scholarship help
given her.

I have emerged from insulin
shock and electric (ugh!) shock
therapy with the discovery,
among other things, that I can
laugh, if the occasion moves
me (and, surprisingly enough,
it sometimes does), and get
pleasures from sunsets, walks
over the golf course, drives
through the country. I still
miss the old love and ability to
enjoy solitude and reading. I
need more than anything right
now what is, of course, most
impossible, someone to love
me, to be with me at night
when I wake up in shuddering
horror and fear of the cement
tunnels leading down to the
shock room, to comfort me
with an assurance that no
psychiatrist can quite manage
to convey.

(AURELIA *turns to her on "love."*
SYLVIA *motions her away.*)

(*More and more pain.*)

(*Then an attempt at the old gay
bravery.*)

The worst, I hope, is over.

(*Another color.*)
My dear Mrs. Plath:
    It is good news to know that
your general practitioner finds
no trace of psychoses; a neur
osis can be long drawn-out and
requires even more wise handling. Of course Sylvia doesn't
want to see anyone now . . .

I can now have visitors, go for
drives, supervised walks, and
hope to have "ground privi-
leges" by the end of this week,

(AURELIA *understands;* SYLVIA
doesn't want to see her.)

It will take some time, you say,
for her face injury to heal.
(Poor child! I am so sorry!)

You have been through a terrific ordeal, and I know well you are still terribly anxious and beset by all the decisions to be made, and also by Sylvia's suffering.

I wish I could help relieve your anxiety about Sylvia's future, but

I am very hopeful there will be no disfiguring scars left on either her body or soul.
Sincerely, Olive H. Prouty.

freedom to walk about the grounds alone, to frequent the Coffee Shop and the library,

as well as the Occupational Therapy rooms.

I long to be out in the wide open spaces of the very messy, dangerous, real world which I *still love*, in spite of everything.

(*A blazing false smile.*)

As ever, Syl.

(*The two women turn to each other. Blackout.*)

ACT II

SYLVIA: Hello again! Where to begin! I feel that I am walking in a dream.

(Carefully. They are feeling each other out, reassuring each other—making boundaries.)

AURELIA: Sylvia returned to Smith in the second semester, taking only three courses.

SYLVIA: Needless to say, it is simply wonderful to be back.

AURELIA: She was not on scholarship at this time. I wanted her to be free of any sense of obligation and cashed in an insurance policy to meet her expenses. During the first few months we telephoned frequently—more for my peace of mind than hers.

SYLVIA: I am so happy about my thesis on Dostoevsky, and also rooming with Nancy, who is now my dearest friend.

Am still chatting with Dr. Booth, the college psychiatrist, once a week—mostly friendly conversations. I really feel I am an extremely well-adjusted buoyant person, continually happy in a steady fashion, not ricocheting from depths to heights, although I do hit heights now and then.
Love, Sivvy.

AURELIA: Sylvia was welcomed back by her classmates and faculty. Understanding and every possible kindness were given her. She picked up an active "date life," which helped build up confidence, and she said she enjoyed herself "in a casual, hedonistic way."

SYLVIA: I am so happy, so elated! Smith just voted me a scholarship of twelve hundred and fifty dollars!

AURELIA: She made me think of deep-sea plants, the roots firmly grasping a rock, but the plant itself swaying in one direction then another with the varying currents that pass over and around. It was as though she absorbed each new personality she encountered and tried it on, later to discard it. I kept saying to myself, "This is only a stage; it will pass."

Her memory grasped and held to discords, and seemed to have lost recollections of shared childhood joys. Kindnesses and loving acts were now viewed cynically, analyzed for underlying motives.

Then periodically, to our relief, her sunny optimism would reassert itself, and we would be once more showered with affection.

SYLVIA: (*Softly, trying out new new moods like grace notes*) You'll be happy to hear of ... Wonderful letter from ... See you Saturday ...

Tomorrow I have ... I really feel that ...

I love ... I feel ...

SYLVIA: Today I cut because I wrote my first poem—a sonnet—since last May! While I have not got a paying job, I *am* the correspondent to the *New York Tribune*—good experience, even if it doesn't pay money.

Both Sassoon and his roommate claim to be intensely in love with me!

I won one poetry prize this year. Also, just got elected president of Alpha Phi Kappa Psi, a very honorary post with a minimum of work and a solid gold, ruby-studded pin from Tiffany's—minor events compared to the splash last year, but events nevertheless. See you in a week.

AURELIA: This, too, was a very turbulent summer. Sylvia returned from Smith with her hair *bleached*! Although initially shocked, I had to admit, it was becoming.

SYLVIA: It was more than a surface alteration. She was trying out a more daring, adventuresome personality, and one had to stand by and hope that neither she

AURELIA: nor anyone else

SYLVIA: would be deeply hurt.

AURELLA: She strove for

SYLVIA: and achieved

AURELIA: competency in her various undertakings, domestic and scholarly. She would be disarmingly confiding, then withdraw, and I quickly learned that it was unwise to make any reference to the

SYLVIA and AURELIA: *sharing*

AURELIA: that had taken place.

SYLVIA: My main concern in the next year is to grow as much as possible. I need space and solitude. I feel that you will understand.

(AURELIA *nods; she is trying to.*)

AURELIA: The ulcer I had developed during my husband's illness had been quiescent until the time of Sylvia's breakdown. In 1954, in an attempt to recover again, I took the summer off and joined my parents in a rented cottage on Cape Cod. Sylvia visited with friends in New York, attended several weddings, then returned to Wellesley to "keep house."

SYLVIA: I do want you to know how I appreciate time for a retreat of sorts here. Of course the house is lonely without you, but I have to fight for solitude.

AURELIA: "Space and solitude."

I am happy I dyed my hair back, even if it fades and I have to have it touched up once or twice. I feel that this year I would much rather look demure and discreet.

SYLVIA:
Dearest Mother,
Now I think it is time for me to concentrate on the hard year ahead, the last push of my senior year. I know that underneath the blazing jaunts in yellow convertibles I am really regrettably conventional, and puritanical, but I needed to practice a certain healthy bohemianism for a while, to swing away from the gray-clad, basically dressed, brown-haired, clock-regulated, responsible, salad-eating, water-drinking, bed-going, economical, practical girl I had

become—and that's why I needed to associate with people who were very different from myself.

AURELIA: At this time, I was in the Newton-Wellesley Hospital. Sylvia telephoned, telling the nurse that her news would help me more than anything else could. She had been awarded a Fulbright grant to study at Cambridge University!

SYLVIA: I am so happy, so encouraged! Now, just so you can remember it, I'll give you a list of prizes and writing awards for this year:

AURELIA and SYLVIA: (*Passing it back and forth, overlapping*)
$ 30. Dylan Thomas honorable mention for "Parallax," *Mlle.*
$ 30. For cover of novel symposium, *Mlle.*
$ 5. *Alumnae Quarterly* article on Alfred Kazin
$100. Academy of American Poets Prize (10 poems).
$ 50. Glascock Prize (tie).
$ 40. Ethel Olin Corbin Prize (sonnet).
$ 50. Marjorie Hope Nicholson Prize (tie) for thesis.
$ 25. Vogue Prix de Paris (one of 12 winners).
$ 5. *Atlantic* for "Circus in Three Rings."
$100. *Christophers* (one of 34 winners).
$ 15. *Mlle.* for "Two Lovers and a Beachcomber by Real Sea."

(AURELIA *winds it up, truly thrilled.*)

$470.   TOTAL, plus much joy!

SYLVIA: Get well *fast*—can't wait to see you Wednesday. All my love, Sivvy.

AURELIA: I had permission to leave the hospital to attend Sylvia's commencement, and made the trip flat on a mattress in a friend's station wagon. Adlai Stevenson gave the commencement address, Marianne Moore was one of the honorary-degree recipients. And Alfred Kazin waved to Sylvia as she returned from receiving her degree. I was in full accord with her as she later whispered in my ear, "My cup runneth over!"

(*They are one. For a moment. Then—*)

SYLVIA:
Dear Warren,
I know the Fulbright is the best and only thing for me; staying in New England or even New York would suffocate me completely. It does take guts to change and grow. My wings need to be tried.

AURELIA: September 25, 1955.

SYLVIA::
> Dearest Mother,
> London is simply fantastic!

AURELIA: Oh, mother, every alleyway is crowded with tradition, and I can feel a peace, reserve, lack of hurry here which has centuries behind it.

SYLVIA: The days are generally gray, with misty light

AURELIA: and landscapes are green-leaved in

SYLVIA: silver mist

AURELIA: like Constable's paintings.

SYLVIA: I would welcome any cookies!

AURELIA: I have to begin life on *all* fronts again, as I did two years ago, but I have all that experience behind me.

SYLVIA: I can't wait to start meeting the British men!

AURELIA: Don't worry that I will marry some idiot, or even anyone I don't love. I simply couldn't.

SYLVIA: Don't worry that I am a "career woman," either. I am definitely *meant* to be married and have children and a home, and write.

If you only knew how hard it is to have so much strength and love to give, and still not have met anyone I can honestly marry.

I don't know how I can bear to go back to the States unless I am married!

AURELIA: When you think of it, it is so little of our lives we really spend with those we love.

SYLVIA: Met, by the way, a brillant poet at the wild party last week; will probably never see him again, but wrote my best poem about him afterwards—the only man I've met here who'd be strong enough to be equal with—such is life.

AURELIA: The man was Ted Hughes.

SYLVIA: Oh, mother, if only you knew how I am forging a soul!

AURELIA: The most shattering thing is that I have fallen terribly in love, which can only lead to great hurt.

SYLVIA: The strongest man in the world, ex-Cambridge, brilliant poet, whose work I loved before I met him, a large, hulking, healthy Adam, half-French, half Irish,

AURELIA: with a voice like the thunder of God!—a singer, story-teller, lion and world-wanderer, a vagabond who will never stop. You should see him, hear him!

SYLVIA: He has a health and hugeness. The more he writes poems, the more he writes poems! I am writing poems, and they are better and stronger than anything I have ever done.

AURELIA: I am full of poems; my joy whirls in tongues of words. I have never been so exultant.

SYLVIA: I cook trout on my gas ring and we eat well. We drink sherry in the garden and romp through words. He tells me fairy stories and dreams, marvellous colored dreams, about certain red foxes.

AURELIA: My God,

SYLVIA: this is Eden here, and the people are all shining, and I must show it to you! All my love.
Your singing girl, Sivvy.

AURELIA: If you have a chance, could you send over my *Joy of Cooking*?

SYLVIA: *You must come to England!*

You, alone, have had crosses that would cause many a stronger woman to break. You have borne daddy's long hard death, your own ulcer attacks.

You have seen me through that black night when the only world I knew was NO and I thought I could never write or think again.

You deserve, too, to be with the loved ones who can give you strength. I am waiting for you, and your trip shall be for your own soul's health and growing.

AURELIA: To my complete surprise, three days after landing at Southampton, I have found myself the sole family attendant at Sylvia's and Ted's secret wedding. From Paris I saw them off for "a writing honeymoon on a shoestring" in Spain.

SYLVIA: For the first time in my life, mother, I am at peace. For the first time I am free.

I feel that all my life, all my pain and work has been for this. I see the power and voice in him that will shake the world alive. Even as he sees into my poems and will work with me to make me a woman poet the world will gape at; even as he sees into my character and will tolerate no fallings away from my best self.

AURELIA: In spring, news that Ted's first book of poetry had been accepted was followed by the welcome announcement that Sylvia had been appointed to teach Freshman English—at Smith!

SYLVIA: My most cherished dream is to bring him home with me next
June for a sort of enormous barbeque in Wellesley, to which I will
invite all the neighbors, young couples, and dear people like Mrs.
Prouty, Dr. B., just to meet him before we set out on our world-
wandering; not really wandering, but living and teaching English in
country after country, writing, mastering languages and having
many, many babies.

AURELIA: I know you're fantastically busy, but have two small desperate requests: could you please possibly send my *Joy of Cooking* and
lots more 3-cent stamps. I'm starting to send batches of Ted's
poems out to American magazines. I want the editors to be crying
for him when we come next June.

SYLVIA: He has commissioned me his official agent and writes pro-
lifically as shooting stars in August. I have great faith in his promise; we are coming into our era of richness, both of us, late maturing, reaching beginning ripeness after twenty-five and going to be
fabulous old people!

AURELIA: (*Remembering, cautioning*) "We dreamed of projects, jointly
shared involving nature study, travel, writing."

SYLVIA: We are utterly in love with each other!

Mrs. Sylvia Hughes, Mrs. Ted Hughes, Mrs. Edward James
Hughes, Mrs. E. J. Hughes (wife of the internationally known poet
and genius); and—

AURELIA: (*Same*) "Dr. Otto Emil Plath"...

SYLVIA:
Dearest, dearest Mother,
If only you could see, wherever Ted and I go people seem to love
us.
My whole thought is how to please him.
The joy of being a loved and loving woman; that is my song.

AURELIA: Life is work *and* joy.

SYLVIA: The girls at Smith are *unscrupulous!* I would be absurd to
throw Ted into such hysterical, girlish adulation. I shouldn't have a
minute's peace.

I shall apply for Ted at Amherst.

AURELIA: Oh, he has everything!...

SYLVIA: And I am so happy with him! (*More softly.*) I was most
moved by your account of S.

AURELIA: (The son of a dear friend.)

SYLVIA: He must feel, as I felt, only three years ago, that there is no way out for him. I wish you could somehow use me as an example. Tell him I went through six months where I literally couldn't read, felt I couldn't take courses at Smith, even the regular program. I am sure he is not that badly off.

AURELIA: Get him to go easy on himself.

SYLVIA: I remember I was terrified that if I wasn't successful writing, no one would find me interesting or valuable.

Psychiatrists blither about father and mother relationships when some common sense, stern advice about practical things and simple human intuition can accomplish much. I hope you will adopt him for my sake.

AURELIA: (*Softly*) When he dies, his marks will not be written on his gravestone. If he has loved a book, been kind to someone, enjoyed a certain color in the sea—that is the thing that will show whether he has lived.

Show you love him and demand nothing of him but the least that he can give.

SYLVIA: (*Another color*) Hello, Hello! It must not yet be 6 a.m. in the hamlet of Wellesley, but I thought you wouldn't mind being wakened by such good news.

"*Hawk in the Rain* judged winning volume Poetry Center First Publication." We both jumped about yelling and roaring like mad seals. I am so happy Ted's book is accepted first! Genius will out!

AURELIA: (*Very careful; she will* not *criticize*) From the time Sylvia was a very little girl, she catered to the male of any age, to bolster his sense of superiority.

SYLVIA: I can rejoice much more, knowing Ted is ahead of me!

AURELIA: In her diary she described coming in second in the spelling contest. "I am so glad Don won," she wrote. "It is always nice to have a boy be *first*. And I am second-best speller in the whole Junior High!"

SYLVIA: I have worked so closely on these poems of Ted's and typed them so many times that I feel ecstatic about it all.

What a blessing to wear heels with Ted and still be "little!"

I've been bogged down on two stories I'm I'm working on for the *Ladies' Home Journal*. Well, he took me on a long walk, listened to me talk the whole plot out, showed me what I'd vaguely felt I should change about the end. Last night he read all 30 pages of it, word for word, unerringly pointing out awkwardness here or an unnecessary paragraph there.

Doesn't it all sound heavenly and exciting? Work, work, that is the secret, with someone you love more than anything.

See you in a week!

AURELIA: Sylvia and Ted arrived in Wellesley the last week in June 1957, and were given a catered reception in a large tent in the rear of our small house, attended by more than seventy people. Sylvia was radiant as she proudly introduced her poet husband.

A few days later her brother drove them to a small cottage in Eastham. Here Sylvia prepared her work for the fall semester at Smith College.

SYLVIA:
Dearest Warren,
My ideal of being a good teacher, writing a book on the side, and being an entertaining homemaker, cook and wife is rapidly evaporating!

This is not the life for a writer.

I am sacrificing my energy grubbing over sixty-six Hawthorne papers a week in front of a rough class of spoiled bitches! If I knew *how* to teach a short story, or a novel, or a poem. I'd at least have that joy. But I'm making it up as I go along, through trial and error, mostly error.

AURELIA: It's easier for the men, I think. . . .

SYLVIA: It's Ted who really saves me! He is sorry I'm so enmeshed in this and wants me to write starting this June. How I long to write on my own again! When I'm describing Henry James's use of metaphor, I'm dying to be making up my own metaphors. When I hear a professor saying: "Yes, the wood is shady, but it's a green shade"—I feel like throwing up my books and writing my own bad poems and bad stories! I don't like talking *about* D. H. Lawrence. I like reading him selfishly for an influence on my own life and my own writing.

Ted and I are fermenting plans, hoping to rent a little apartment on the slummy side of Beacon Hill, which we love—work at unrenponsible jobs (for money, bread and experience) and *write* for a solid year.

AURELIA: Very few people can understand this!

SYLVIA: There is something suspect, especially in America, about people who don't have ten-year plans, or at least a regular job. We found this out trying to establish credit at a local store. We fitted into none of the form categories of "The Young American Couple." I had a job, Ted didn't; we owned no car, were buying no furniture on the installment plan, had no charge accounts, no TV . . .

AURELIA: When we are both wealthy and famous, our work will justify our lives.

SYLVIA: God feeds the ravens. I hope *you* understand this better than mother!

AURELIA: The following is from a page of my diary, Sunday, August 3, 1958.

We visited Ruth on Thursday. She had come home with her five-day-old son, a wee, red-faced infant.

I believe I felt Ted withdraw from him—a very young baby can be so raw and weird looking. Sylvia, however,

SYLVIA: opened the curled hand and stretched out the exquisitely finished little fingers; examined the wrinkled petal of a foot—each toe a dot, yet complete with a speck of pearly nail—the whole foot shorter than her little finger.

AURELIA: There was such warmth, such yearning in Sivvy's face, my heart ached for her.

SYLVIA: Every time you make a choice you have to sacrifice something.

AURELIA: Unlike mother, I am a writer, not a teacher.

SYLVIA: After I have written twenty stories and a book or two of poems, I might be able to keep up writing with work or a family . . .

AURELIA: By spring 1959, both writers had published a number of poems and Ted was awarded a Guggenheim grant. They now planned to have a child, whom Ted wished to be English-born. Sylvia concurred in this decision.

SYLVIA: (*Softly*)
Dear Warren,
Ted has . . . Ted and I . . .

AURELIA: On the day they left, Sylvia was wearing her hair in a long braid down her back with a little red wool cap on her head, and looked like a high school student.

As the train pulled out, Ted called, "We'll be back in two years!"

SYLVIA:
Dear Mother,
I have gone through a very homesick and weary period, but once we get a foothold in London, life will become much better.

AURELIA: Wonderful news via telegram, for Ted. The Somerset Maugham Award, just over one thousand dollars, to be spent "enlarging his world-view." We envision the Greek Islands next winter, and all sorts of elegant sun-saturated schemes.

SYLVIA: The first British publisher I sent my new collection of poems to, wrote back within the week accepting them! Amaze of amaze!

The Colossus and Other Poems, by Sylvia Plath.

AURELIA: For Ted.

Went to my doctor again today, and he let me listen to the baby's heartbeat! I was so excited.

I'm going to see if London has diaper service.

SYLVIA: Lots of love from us both.

AURELIA: On the morning of April 1, 1960, at about 3 a.m., the phone at my bedside rang.

"Mother," said a tremulous voice. "Sylvia!" I cried.

"Is it Nicholas or Frieda Rebecca?"

"Oh, Frieda Rebecca, of course! Ein Wunderkind, Mummy. Ein Wunderkind!"

SYLVIA: From where I sit, propped up in bed, I can see her, pink and healthy, sound asleep. "A wonder child." Of course, of course! Alas, she has my nose! On her, though, it seems quite beautiful.

AURELIA: I have never been so happy in my life!

SYLVIA: Ted was there the whole time.

You should see him rocking her and singing to her! She looks so tiny against his shoulder, her four fingers just closing around one of his knuckles. Already she shows a funny independence and temper.

AURELIA: Things seem much calmer and more peaceful with the baby around. Ted will have a study and utter peace by the time I have all my strength back and am coping with baby and household.

SYLVIA:
Dear Mother,
I've been going through a rather tired spell, at the depressing, painful stage of trying to start writing after long silence.

AURELIA: Something odd happened to me today.

SYLVIA: I was walking the baby, the air too cold and windy to go far, and half-dreamily let my feet carry me down a road I'd never been before. Saw a house: FOR SALE, 41 Fitzroy Road, *the street where Yeats lived.* I was so excited that I ran home and called Ted. Well, of course I had visions of a study for Ted in the attic, a study for me, a room for guests (you)—

AURELIA: Ted is much more hesitant than I to commit himself.

SYLVIA: And I am loath to jeopardize

AURELIA: Ted's

SYLVIA: writing. I am thinking of getting a job myself, if

AURELIA: Ted

SYLVIA: would just feed the baby. By the way,

AURELIA: Ted

SYLVIA: has a real desire to take a degree in zoology—a job he could give his heart to, not the fancy literary white-collar work or English teaching which would make him unhappy . . . Any ideas or suggestions?

(AURELIA *shrugs; how can she answer that?*)

I am now working very hard on women's magazine stories. I also have a fine, lively agent, so after I get acceptances here, they'll send any stuff good enough to the *Saturday Evening Post,* etc.

AURELIA: I am very excited that children seem to be an impetus to my writing. As soon as I start selling, I could afford a half-day babysitter to do the drudge-work.

SYLVIA: Oh how I look forward to your coming! My heart lifts now that the year swings toward it! . . . Could you possibly alter your flight to cover August 20? The reason I'm asking is, I discovered today your second grandchild is due about then.

AURELIA:
Dearest Mother,
I feel awful to write you now after changing your plans and probably telling your friends about another baby, because I lost the little baby this morning, and really feel terrible about it.

Ted is taking wonderful care of me. He is the most blessed, kind person in the world.

All weekend, while I was in the shadow of this, he gave me poems to type and generally distracted me.

AURELIA: Actually, the most wonderful thing you could do for us would be to live here with Frieda for two weeks, while we had our first real vacation in France

SYLVIA: with the Merwins.

AURELIA: By now Ted had the use of a friend's study where he could work in quiet, and Sylvia worked there, too, drafting *The Bell Jar*—unknown to me.

SYLVIA:
Dear Mother,
I am working fiendishly at the Merwins' study seven mornings a week, as they are coming home at the end of May, and I've a lot I want to finish before then. I have found that the whole clue to happiness is to have four to five hours perfectly free and uninterrupted to write in, the first thing in the morning—no phone, doorbells, or baby.

AURELIA: I'm trying to get the bulk of my writing done before you come, but even if I work in the mornings, we'll have the whole rest of the day together!

SYLVIA: I think you'll be a lot more comfortable at the Merwins'.

AURELIA: (*Nods; she understands*) In July 1961 I visited them, staying with Frieda while Sylvia and Ted went on a holiday to France. Sylvia was again pregnant, and they were longing to establish a home of their own.

Dear Warren,
On Thursday the two of them took off for Devon, a trip of five hours by car. They have been sending for real estate listings since early spring, and had selected eight places to visit . . .

SYLVIA: all sounding lush!

AURELIA: While they were gone, Frieda decided to cut her twelfth tooth. Neither of us slept much as a result.

Well, Sivvy and Ted returned at midnight Friday,

SYLVIA: exhausted.

AURELIA: Seven of the eight houses were impossible.

SYLVIA: Some actually ruins.

AURELIA: But the third place they saw they fell in love with, and if all is correct legally, I guess they are going to purchase it. It is the ancient

SYLVIA: Yes!

AURELIA: house of Sir and Lady Arundel, who were there to show them about.

The Arundels impressed Sivvy and Ted, and seemed anxious to get people who would have a sense of the historic value of the place.

SYLVIA: There is a Roman mound there!

AURELIA: From Sivvy's description, I gathered the following statistics: The main house has

SYLVIA: nine rooms,

AURELIA: A great lawn in front, a thatched roof—

SYLVIA: —honest! And a "cottage" . . .

AURELIA: that is in great need of repair! I wish I could see it, but Ted and Sylvia are glad (I sense) that the distance makes this impossible. They don't mind *your* seeing it, but said that I would find flaws that they intend to eradicate.

SYLVIA: (*Overlap*) I shall be so happy to start fixing it up!

AURELIA: (*Real concern*) Both Ted's mother and I are loaning them five hundred pounds so they won't be snowed under by the terrible interest rate—

AURELIA: (*It's so much!*) six and a half per cent!   SYLVIA: (*It's so little!*) six and a half per cent!

AURELIA: I was willing to take the whole mortgage at *three* per cent, but—

SYLVIA: (*Quickly*) And now you will have a lovely country house to visit next summer!

Thanks so much. Lots of love, Sivvy.

AURELIA: (*Amused, admiring; they did it anyway!*) Devon, England. September 4, 1961.

SYLVIA:
Dear Mother,
We moved without mishap on Thursday and had a fine, hot, sunny, blue day for it. Ever since, a fog has shrouded us in; just as well, for we have been unpacking, scrubbing, painting and working hard.

The place is like a person; it responds to the slightest touch and looks wonderful immediately.

My whole spirit has expanded.

This is a wonderful place to have babies!

AURELIA: (*Cautioning, the beginning of trouble*) Ted has been driving thirty-five miles to the BBC . . .

Ted had a day in London this Tuesday . . .

SYLVIA: Ted woke up this morning and said, "I dreamed you won a twenty-five dollar prize for your story about Johnny Panic." Well, I went downstairs and found out I had won a Saxton grant for two thousand dollars!

AURELIA: Today came a big Christmas parcel from you with the two *Ladies, Home Journal* magazines.

SYLVIA: I love it!

Recipes in English magazines are for things like "Lard and Stale Bread Pie, Garnished with Cold Pigs Feet," or "Left-Over Pot Roast in Aspic."

AURELIA: I feel so thwarted not to be giving out anything but cards, but we really need to pinch this year to weather the piles of bills for plumbers, electricians, extra heaters, coal, land tax, house tax, solicitors, surveyors, movers . . .

SYLVIA: Small things loom very large.

AURELIA: Oh, saw my doctor. I look forward to my home delivery. Given up all pretence of working in my study. I am simply too ponderous.

SYLVIA:
Dear Mother,
By now I hope you have received the telegram Ted sent.

AURELIA: Our first son, Nicholas Farrar Hughes . . .

SYLVIA: All during the delivery, I felt it would be a boy. Then at five minutes to twelve, as the doctor was on his way over — this great bluish, glistening boy shot out onto the bed in a tidal wave of water that drenched all of us to the skin, howling lustily! It was an amazing sight. I immediately sat up and felt wonderful — no tears, nothing.

AURELIA: Now everything is quiet and peaceful. Ted is heating the apple pie I made to tide us over.

SYLVIA: Oh, how I look forward to your visit!

I long to have a day or two on jaunts with just Ted. We can hardly see each other over the mountains of diapers and demands of babies.

Tell Warren to get a big house with a soundproof bedroom before *he* has a baby.

I am so longing for spring!

(*She begins to sing softly.*)

AURELIA: The ecstasy that followed the birth of Nicholas . . .

SYLVIA: (*Singing*) His eyes are a deep slate-blue . . .

AURELIA: and the blooming of their gardens after the long harsh winter . . .

SYLVIA: Our daffodils and jonquils are wonderful, I have such spring fever, don't want to see another dish or cook another meal! I am dying for you to come, to see it all through your eyes.

I have got awfully homesick for you since the last baby.

All through this, I've not said anything about Warren's engagement. How wonderful! What fun for you to have all the traditional trappings for *one* of your children — diamond ring, Bachrach, a formal wedding —

AURELIA: I am now awaiting Ted's return from a daytrip to London.

SYLVIA: Having babies is really the happiest experience of my life! I would just like to go on and on!

I have the queerest feeling of having been reborn with Frieda, as if my real, rich, happy life only started about then. I feel I'm just beginning at writing, too!

Well, I must get supper for my family. Lots of love from us all. Sivvy.

AURELIA: By June . . .

SYLVIA: Honestly, the reason I have been so slow in writing is that I have said to myself, "I will write tomorrow; then it is sure to be a sunny day and how cheerful I will be." Believe it or not, we haven't seen the sun for *three weeks*.

I have been feeling tired . . . hope the Strontium 90 level doesn't go up too high in milk . . . been very gloomy about the bomb news . . . got awfully depressed reading about the terrifying marriage of big business and the military in America, the John Birch Society, etc.

I seem to need sleep all the time . . . the day a whirlwind of baths, laundry, meals, feedings, and . . .

AURELIA: (*Overlap*) The marriage

SYLVIA: (*Overlap*) I am the busiest and happiest —! My book is due
out! Our daffodils and jonquils —!
Lots of love to you all.

AURELIA: The welcome I received when I arrived in June was heart-
warming.

SYLVIA: This is the *fourth* day in a row of absolutely halcyon, blue,
clean, hot weather.

I have such lovely children and such a lovely home now.

AURELIA: After the first few days, I sensed a tension between Sylvia
and Ted.

SYLVIA: Honestly, the *reason* —

AURELIA: On July 9th Sylvia said proudly, "I have everything in life I
ever wanted: a wonderful husband, two adorable children, a lovely
home"

SYLVIA: "and my writing."

AURELIA: Yet the marriage was —

SYLVIA: No!

AURELIA: the marriage was seriously troubled.	SYLVIA: No!
Ted had been seeing	Never ... seeing.
someone else	
and Sylvia's	Never
jealously	speak to
was very	God
intense.	again!
I thought it best to leave.	
	Leave!

AURELIA: (*Low.*)
On August 4, 1962, the four of them were together, waiting for my
train to pull out of the station. The two parents were watching me
stonily. Nick was the only one with a smile. (*She turns away.*) It
was the last time I saw Sylvia.

SYLVIA: (*Flat, calm now*)
August 27, 1962.
I do not believe in divorce.

Dear Mother,
I hope you will not be too surprised or shocked when I say I am going to try to get a legal separation from Ted.

I have too much at stake and am too rich a person to live as a martyr. I want a clean break, so I can breathe and laugh and enjoy myself again.

Tell no one but perhaps Margaret and Warren of this, perhaps not even them. It is a private matter and I do not want people who would never see me anyway to know of it.

I am in need of nothing and desirous of nothing!

I meant you to have such a lovely stay!

September 23, 1962.
I will try to rent the house and live in the cottage. I want to be where no possessions remind me of the past, and by the sea, which is for me the great healer.

I must at all costs get a live-in nanny, so I can start to write and get my independence again.

AURELIA: (*Eagerly*)
September 24, 1962.
I began to see that life is not over for me! It is the uncertainty, week after week, that has been such a torture. And, of course, the desire to hang on to the last to see if something, anything, could be salvaged.

SYLVIA: It is a beautiful day here, clear and blue.

AURELIA: I got this nanny back for today and tomorrow, a whiz, and I see what heaven my life could be if I had a good live-in nanny.

SYLVIA: I will rent the house for the winter and go to Ireland. I dream of Warren and Maggie! I would love to go on a skiing holiday in the Tyrol with them someday. I just read about it in the paper. And then if I do a novel or two, I might apply for a Guggenheim to go to Rome with the children. Right now I have no money, but if I get the cottage done this winter —

AURELIA: I might even take a London flat, send the children to the fine free schools there and enjoy the London people.

SYLVIA: I went up to London to the solicitor yesterday.

The laws are awful. A wife is allowed one third of her husband's income, and if he doesn't pay up, the suing is long and costly.

Together we earned a fine salary, I earning one third. Now it is all gone. I shall be penalized for earning, or, if I don't earn, have to beg. Well I choose to invest everything with courage in the cottage and the nanny, and *write like mad.*

I must get control of my life!

AURELIA: (*Worried*) It is the evenings here that are the worst. . . .

SYLVIA: I do have to take sleeping pills, but they are, just now, a necessary evil.

AURELIA: I have to get a nanny in the spring. I don't break down with someone else around!

SYLVIA:
Dear Mother,
I don't know where to begin. I just can't take the $50!

AURELIA: I finally persuaded her to do so, monthly, and opened a joint account in a London bank, so she could use it in any emergency — hoping she would consider returning to the United States. We, as a family, were prepared to set her up in her own apartment here.

SYLVIA: America is out for me! If I start running now, I will never stop. I shall hear of Ted all my life, of his success, his genius. I must make a life all my own as fast as I can! The flesh has dropped from my bones. But I am a fighter.
I want a flat in London. The cultural life is what I am starved for . . . I haven't the strength to see you for some time. The horror of what you saw —

AURELIA: (*Anguished*)what I *saw* you see —

SYLVIA: is between us, and I cannot face you again until I have a new life; it would be too great a strain.

I was very stupid, very happy . . . no time to make any plans of my own.

I have *no one.* Stuck down here as into a sack, I fight for air and freedom.

I will need protection. I look to Warren now that I have no man, no adviser.

Everything is breaking!—my dinner set cracking in half; the health inspector says the cottage should be demolished — there is no hope for it. Even my beloved bees set upon me today when I knocked aside their sugar feeder, and I am all over stings!

If I can spend the winter in the sun in Spain . . . Spain is out of the question! I could take the children to Ireland. I must get to London next fall!

Please tell Warren to say he and Maggie will come in spring! In Ireland I may find my soul, and in London my brain, and maybe in heaven what was my heart. Love, S.

AURELIA: These letters were, of course, written under great strain. They are desperate letters, and their very desperation make it difficult to read them with any objectivity. I could not, at the time.

Dear Mother,
I have had an incredible change in spirit; I am joyous, happier than I have been for ages.

My life can begin.

Every morning, when my sleeping pill wears off, I am up about five, in my study with coffee, writing like mad — a poem a day before breakfast. Terrific stuff, as if domesticity had choked me.

I need a bloody holiday.

I miss *brains*, hate this cow life, am dying to surround myself with intelligent, good people. I am a famous poetess here — mentioned this week in *The Listener* as one of the half-dozen women who will last.

SYLVIA
Dearest Warren and Maggie,
I have been through the most incredible hell for six months, and amazingly enough,

AURELIA: the one thing I retain is love and admiration of Ted's writing. He is a genius, and for a genius there are no bonds and no bounds. It is hurtful to be ditched, but thank God I have my own work.

SYLVIA: I think I'll be a pretty good novelist. My stuff makes me laugh and laugh, and if I can laugh now it must be hellishly funny!

Just now I am a bit of a wreck, bones literally sticking out all over and great black shadows under my eyes from sleeping pills, a smoker's hack (I actually took up smoking the past month out of desperation and I practically burned off all my eyebrows!).

Tell me you'll consider taking me (I mean escorting; I'll have money!) to Austria with you, even if you don't, so I'll have that to look forward to. I've had nothing to look forward to for so long!

AURELIA:
Dear Mother,
I am writing with my old fever of 101 degrees alternating with chills.

I need help very much just now. Home is impossible! I can go nowhere with the children, and I am ill, and it would be psychologically the worst thing to see you now. I am a writer. I am a genius of a writer. I am writing the best poems of my life. They will make my name.

SYLVIA: Very bad luck with nanny agency; a bitch of a woman is coming tomorrow from them; doesn't want to cook, do any breakfast or tea, wondered if there was a butler—? Ten pounds a week! If I had time to get a good nanny, I could get on with my life!

I am all right. Could either Dot or Margaret spare me six weeks? I must have someone I love to protect me. The babes are beautiful — though Frieda has regressed. *I cannot come home.* I am full of plans, but do need help for the next two months. I am fighting now against hard odds, and alone.

AURELIA: (*Low*) Fighting now . . .

Mention has been made of my coming home for Christmas. Do you suppose instead there is any possibility of your chipping in and sending me Maggie? Could she come *now* instead of then? I already love her; she would be such *fun* and love the babies. Do I sound mad? Taking or wanting to take Warren's new wife? Just for a few weeks!

AURELIA: Fighting . . .

I need someone from *home.* A defender. I have a fever now, so I am a bit delirious. I work from four to eight a.m. On the next few months depend my future and my health.

I am fine in mind and spirit, but wasted and ill in flesh. I

AURELIA: against hard odds . . . fighting, fighting . . .

love you all. Sivvy.

AURELIA: On receiving the above letter, I cabled Mrs. Winifred Davies, Sylvia's midwife and friend: "Please see Sylvia now and get woman for her! *Salary paid here!*"

SYLVIA: Winifred, bless her, came round last night with some hopeful news! A young nurse nearby would love to live in till mid-December!

The weather has been heavenly — fog mornings, but clear, sunny, blue days after. I have a bad cough and shall get my lungs x-rayed and my teeth seen to. I am writing very good poems. I need time to breathe, sun, recover my flesh.

I love and live for letters.

Dear Warren,
I know what I need, want, must work for.

Please convince mother of this. She identifies much too much with me, and you must help her see how starting my own life in the most difficult place, here — not running, is the only sane thing to do.

AURELIA: (*In anguish*) "fighting ... alone"

I wrote two worrying letters when I was desperate. Do try to convince mother I am cured.

I am a writer and that is all I want to do; have had my first novel accepted (... a pot-boiler and no one must read it!)

Don't tell mother!

Dear Mother,
Will you please, for goodness
sake, stop bothering poor
Winifred Davies! She is busier
than either you or I, and
knows and sees my situation
much better than you can.

She came over this afternoon
and said you sent her some
wire? Please do understand
that while I am very very
grateful indeed for financial
help from people who *have*
money, I want no monthly
dole, especially not from you.
You can help me best by saving your money for your own
retirement.

I am doing a poem a morning,
great things. Don't talk to me
about the world needing
cheerful stuff! What the person out of Belsen wants is
nobody saying the birdies still
go tweet-tweet, but the full
knowledge that somebody else
has been there and knows the
worst.

It is much more help for me to
know that people are divorced
and go through hell, than to
hear about happy marriages.
Let the *Ladies' Home Journal*
blither about *those*.

I know just what I want and
want to do.

I am well liked here, in spite of
my weirdness, I think.

I adore the babies and am glad
to have them, even though
they make life fantastically

difficult now. The worst is that Ted is at the peak of his fame and all his friends—But I can manage that, too.

Dear Mother,
Please forgive my grumpy, sick letters ... I see now just what I need—

(In the form of a "round.")

not professional nannies, who are snotty and ex - pensive, but an adventurous, young, cheerful girl to whom my life would be *fun*. O, it is *ideal*!

AURELIA: ... I see now just what I need— not professional nannies, who are snotty and expensive, but an adventurous, young cheerful girl to whom my life would be *fun*. O, it is *ideal*!

I must be one of the most creative people in the world! I must get back to the live, lively, always learning and developing person I was! I want to study, learn history, politics, languages, travel. I want to be the most loving and fascinating mother in the world—and I shall, in spite of all obstacles, have that, and Frieda and Nick and the Salon I deserve. I shall be a *rich, active woman*!

I must be one of the most creative people in the world! I must get back to the live, lively, always learning and developing person I was! I want to study, learn history, politics, languages, travel. I want to be the most loving and fascinating mother in the world—and I shall, in spite of all obstacles, have that, and Frieda and Nick and the Salon I deserve. I shall be a *rich active woman.*

(SYLVIA *hears how all this sounds to* AURELIA.)

SYLVIA: *(Softer.)* I should love to use your birthday check on a dress. I shall take all my hems up. All my clothes are ten years old! Just wait till I hit London!

Dearest Warren and Maggie,
 The critic of the *Observer* ... says I'm the first woman poet he's taken seriously since Emily Dickinson!

Now can you possibly get mother to stop worrying so much?

Dear Mother,
Now *stop* trying to get me to write about "decent courageous people"! Read the *Ladies, Home Journal* for those! I believe in going through and facing the worst, not hiding from it. That is why I am

going to London this week—to face all the people we know and tell them happily and squarely I am divorcing Ted, so they won't picture me as a poor country wife. I am not going to steer clear of those professional acquaintances just because they know or because I may meet Ted with someone else.

Dear Mother,
I am writing from London, so happy I can hardly speak. I have a place! By an absolute *fluke* the street and the house where I've always wanted to live. Flew to the agents. It seems I have a chance! And guess what—it is *Yeats's house*, with a blue plaque over the door, saying *he lived there!*

AURELIA: (*Softly*) "Love . . .
Sylvia . . . Sivvy . . .
Cyrilly . . .
Your maturing . . .
crazy old . . .

happy . . .

dearest . . .

whom I love better than anybody . . ."

I am now staying with a wonderful Portuguese couple, the girl is a friend of Ted's girl, and they see how I am, full of interest in my own life, and are amazed, as everyone is, at my complete lack of jealousy or sorrow.

I have found a *fabulous* hairdresser . . . and the cut, shampoo and set was only $1.50. I did it on your check. Men stare at me in the street now, truck drivers whistle; it's amazing.
Living apart from Ted is wonderful — I am no longer in his shadow. It is heaven to be liked for myself alone.

AURELIA: The most,

the absolute,

love,

I may even borrow a table for my flat from Ted's girl. I could be gracious to her now . . .

I am so happy,

She has only her high-paid job, her vanity . . . and *everybody* wants to be a writer.

singing,

I may be poor in bank funds, but I am so much richer in every other way. I envy them nothing.

O, he has everything!

My babies and my writing are my life! Wish me luck.
Sivvy.

Sivvy.

(*It is very hard for* AURELIA *to go on.*)

AURELIA: In December she closed the large house in Devon and moved with the children to a flat in Yeats's former home in London, where, for a brief time, she responded excitedly to the cultural stimulation of the city. Then the worst cold, snow-storms, and blackouts in over a hundred years engulfed London for months. Sylvia fought off flu; the children had coughs and colds.

SYLVIA: Someone to love me . . .

In spite of all this, she continued the writing she had started in Devon. She began at 7 a.m. each morning to pour forth magnificently structured poems, renouncing the subservient female role, yet holding to the triumphant note of maternal creativity in her scorn of "barrenness."

to be with me at night . . .

Feeling she needed a backlog of funds to prepare for the sterile periods every writer dreads, she had earlier sent out *The Bell Jar*, under a pseudonym, in the firm belief that this would fully protect her from disclosure.

By the time the novel appeared in London bookstores, she was ill, exhausted, and over-whelmed by the respon-sibilities she had to shoulder *alone*.

SYLVIA:
Dear Mother,
Well, here I am! Safely in Yeats's house! And I can truly say I have never been so hap-py in my life. I just sit think-ing, shall I write a poem, shall I paint a floor, shall I hug a baby? Everything is such fun, such an adventure, and if I feel this way *now*, with everything bare and to be painted—

AURELIA: "What will the green young spring be like? ..."

SYLVIA: (*Disjointed*) ... Clear, crisp blue day ... I arrived here to find no gas stove in and no electricity connected!

... first letter through my door was from my publishers ... Oslo, Norway ... to translate and do ... "Three Woman" and

A. Alvarez ... best poetry critic here, thinks my second book ... should win Pulitzer Prize ...

Everybody ... says you worry if I don't write. For goodness sake, remember no news is good news!

Lots and lots of love to all,
Your happy Sivvy.

... the cement tunnels leading down to the shock room ...

AURELIA: The green

young ...

spring ...

AURELIA: (*Slowly, painfully*) I am in the best of hands. I am slowly pulling out of the flu, but the weakness and tiredness makes me cross.

SYLVIA: (*A new voice*) The weather has been filthy . . . all the heaped snow freezing . . . the roads are narrow ruts, and I have been very gloomy with the long wait for a phone . . . which makes me feel cut off, along with the lack of an "au pair." I did interview a very nice German girl of eighteen . . . but her employer is making difficulties . . . I still need to sew the bedroom curtains, have some made for the big front room, get a stair carpet. It is so hard to get out to shop with the babies.

I have never been so happy in my life.

AURELIA: Still have the babies' floors to paint, the "au pair's," the hall floors and three wood bureaus. *Blue* is my new color, royal, midnight (not aqua). Ted never liked blue.

SYLVIA: Oh, Mother . . .

AURELIA: My German "au pair" is food-fussy and boy-gaga, but she does give me some peace mornings. My solicitor is gathering evidence for a Divorce Petition.

SYLVIA: Your package came today.

AURELIA: There have been electric strikes and every so often the lights and heaters go out for hours; children freeze; dinners are stopped; there are mad rushes for candles . . .

SYLVIA: I am going to start seeing a woman doctor free on the National Health which should help me weather this difficult time. Don't worry about my paying bills. I pay them immediately. Always have. My love to all. Sylvia.

AURELIA: On February 12,

SYLVIA: (*A cry*) Oh, Mother!

AURELIA: (*Struggling to go on*) 1963 . . .

SYLVIA: It is a blue, blue day, blue skied, leaves golden . . .

AURELIA: My sister received a cablegram from Ted, telling us   SYLVIA: falling . . .
Sylvia died yesterday.

SYLVIA: And life is good.

AURELIA: (*Her whole soul naked*)
"I'll ... never ... speak ... to
... God—"

SYLVIA: *No!*

(*A moment, then.*)

AURELIA: No ...

SYLVIA: (*More softly*) No.

AURELIA: (*A decision. To herself,
to* SYLVIA, *to the audience;
gathering resolution, strength*)
November 13, 1949.
As of today I have decided to
keep a diary again—just a
place where I can write my
thoughts and opinions when I
have a moment. Somehow I
have to keep and hold the rap-
ture of being *seventeen*. Every
day is so precious. I feel in-
finitely sad at the thought of
all this time melting farther
and farther away from me as I
grow older. *Now, now* is the
perfect time of my life.

I still do not know myself.
Perhaps I never will. But I feel
free—unbound by respon-
sibility, I still can come up to
my own private room, with
my drawings hanging on the
walls, and pictures pinned up
over my bureau—a room
suited to me, uncluttered and
peaceful. I love the quiet lines
of the furniture, the two
bookcases filled with poetry
books and fairy tales saved
from childhood.

Always I want to be an
observer. I want to be affected
by life deeply, but never so
blinded that I cannot see my

(*A summation of* SYLVIA's *life
and death in which* AURELIA
*comes to understand. She has
done her best. Though much
of this is true of her also, she
is not* SYLVIA. *She has survived. She is strong—*

and learning.)

share of existence in a wry, humorous light.

I am afraid of getting older. I am afraid of getting married. Spare me from cooking three meals a day—spare me from the relentless cage of routine and rote. I want to be *free*—free to know people and their backgrounds—free to move to different parts of the world. I want, I think, to be omniscient. I think I would like to call myself "the girl who wanted to be God" ... perhaps I am *destined* to be classified and qualified. But, oh, I cry out against it. I am I.

I love my flesh, my face, my limbs. I have erected in my mind an image of myself, idealistic and beautiful. Is not that image, free from blemish, the true self—the true perfection? (Oh, even now I glance back on what I have just written—how foolish it sounds, how overdramatic!)

SYLVIA: (*Very softly*) A certain color in ... the sea

Never, never, never will I reach the perfection

Blue

I long for with all my soul.

There will come a time when I must face myself at last. Even now I dread the big choices

love

which loom up in my life. I am afraid. I feel uncertain. I am not as wise as I have thought.

the busiest

happiest

I can now see, as from a valley, the roads lying open for me

sharing girl in the

but I cannot see the end—the

consequences.

Oh, I love *now*, with all my
fears and forebodings,   It is an Indian summer day

for now I still am not com-
pletely molded. *I am strong.*   I feel that I am . . .

My life is still just beginning!

                                          . . . *learning.*

(*Blackout.*)

End

Killings On The Last Line

Lavonne Mueller

To Julia Miles

Author's Note

"If it were desired to reduce a man to nothing—to punish him atrocious-ly, to crush him in such a manner that the most hardened murderer would tremble before such punishment—it would be necessary only to give his work a character of complete uselessness... Let him be con-strained to pour water from one vessel into another, or to carry earth from one place to another and back again, then I am persuaded that at the end of a few days the prisoner would strangle himself or commit a thousand crimes punishable with death, rather than live in such an ab-ject condition and endure such torments."

Dostoievsky
The House of the Dead

Characters

ELLIS, age thirty, from Kentucky.
HIDELMAN, age thirty-two, strong and muscular.
STARKEY, age nineteen, daughter of Mrs. Starkey.
MRS. STARKEY, age fifty-one, mother of Starkey.
BETTY, age sixty, a widow.
QUASHIE, age forty-four, leg in cast, a Bahamian.
JUBA, age forty-five, a Bahamian.
DAY-TRIPPER, age seventy-five, part-time help, a woman.
MAVIS, age thirty-five, union representative.
ELMHURST, age forty-five, floor supervisor.

Killings on the Last Line was given a rehearsed reading by The Women's Project on November 12, 1979, directed by Dorothy Silver, with the following cast:

STARKEY . . . . Ellen Barkin
MRS. STARKEY . . . . Scotty Bloch
MAVIS . . . . Kathleen Chalfant
DAY-TRIPPER . . . . Sylvia Davis
JUBA . . . . Venida Evans
HIDELMAN . . . . Kathleen Gittel
ELLIS . . . . Joan MacIntosh
QUASHIE . . . . Theresa Merritt
ELMHURST and MAN'S VOICE . . . . Jess Osuna
BETTY . . . . Sylvia Short

A revised version of this script will open as a full production at The American Place Theatre in May 1980, directed by Dorothy Silver, with sets by Henry Millman, costumes by Mimi Maxmen, and lighting by Annie Wrightson, and the following cast:

STARKEY . . . . Ellen Barkin
JUBA . . . . Verona Barnes
QUASHIE . . . . Rosanna Carter
MAVIS . . . . Kathleen Chalfant
BETTY . . . . Alice Drummond
HIDELMAN . . . . Marilyn Hamlin
ELLIS . . . . Joan MacIntosh
MRS. STARKEY . . . . Sandy Martin
ELMHURST . . . . Pat McNamara
DAY-TRIPPER . . . . Marian Primont

ACT I

Time: *1979, Year of the Child*
Early morning
Early summer

Scene: *Reactor parts factory*

Place: *Chicago*

Setting: *The stage is divided in two parts. To one side is a large wall of windows, the panels painted black. To another side is a locker area for workers. The upper front of the stage is the machine area where the women work.*

At Rise: *A whistle blows. Then seven women come on stage to their lockers at right. It is early morning and the start of their shift. They are wearing their ordinary clothes. They strip to their underwear and begin to put on white overly large lab coats, white caps, and paper scuff slippers. The lab coats are unaesthetic and give the appearance of janitorial coats.*

The women talk as they are dressing and hanging up their own hats and jackets and scarfs. They also comb their hair and primp.

ELLIS *comes in a few seconds after everybody else but before the whistle stops.* ELLIS *has a sleeping baby strapped to her front. She carries a small portable play-pen which she unfolds. She puts the baby in the play-pen at her side as she dresses.* QUASHIE *and* JUBA *each carry a mesh bag of coconuts and bottles.* QUASHIE *is in a walking cast on her right leg.*

STARKEY: Half-day ta-day.

BETTY: First thang I thought when 'larm went off. Half day.

MRS. STARKEY: We'll make it up.

HIDELMAN: Christ. I'm dead.

ELLIS: Me, too.

STARKEY: Least ever-body's on time.

HIDELMAN: (*To* ELLIS) Yer here. When's the mug woke up. *Kan*-tucky!

ELLIS: I'm woke up.

BETTY: (*Looks to* QUASHIE) Poor Quashie.

QUASHIE: I told you, darlin, I'm all right.

JUBA: (*To* QUASHIE) I hear this foot clump to the ground . . . turn round to see who does make the noise, and look, the body is you.

QUASHIE: I was working in the yard and dropped outside—cracked me leg on the street. I just reached back from the doctor.

JUBA: (*To* QUASHIE) I know your face all right, but don't recognize the foot.

QUASHIE: What is to is must is, and that's the way it is. (QUASHIE *puts her sack down and it lands on* JUBA's *foot.*)

JUBA: (*Good natured*) Woman put she things on me toe with the sack. What you think I name? Sack holder?

QUASHIE: (*Chuckles*) You don't look out, woman, and oh, you easy to put on. (QUASHIE *puts her sack in the locker.*)

ELLIS: (To QUASHIE) That's a real shame, Quashie.

QUASHIE: What is shame to you, is death to me.

HIDELMAN: (*Says to* QUASHIE *as she glares at* ELLIS) Least yer on time.

ELLIS: I was here 'fore the whistle stopped.

(HIDELMAN *wears a silver whistle around her neck. She acts as if she is going to give a large blast on the whistle.* ELLIS *shrinks back and holds her baby's ears protectively.*)

HIDELMAN: (*Dropping the whistle back down hanging from her neck without blowing it. To* ELLIS) So you kin hear.

BETTY: (*To* HIDELMAN *about the whistle*) What's that, Hidelman?

HIDELMAN: My rape whistle.

MRS. STARKEY: Christ. That's like King Kong wearing a rape whistle.

ELLIS: (*Defensive*) I hear.

HIDELMAN: (*Mocking*) Oh . . . it's yer old man that don't.

ELLIS: He's got the double mastoid.

HIDELMAN: . . . right . . . 4-F . . . 'n didn't go ta Nam.

ELLIS: (*Faultering*) He don't like killin people . . . not whole bunches of 'em. . . .

HIDELMAN: My old man, he done two years in Nam . . . him with double hemorrhoids.

STARKEY: Don't start in on that, Hidelman.

BETTY: Not on half day.

HIDELMAN: (*Aside*) Hillbilly! (*She goes back to dressing.*)

ELLIS: (*Proudly*) My cousin . . . his two jaws was wired after Nam.

(HIDELMAN *ignores this.*)

MRS. STARKEY: It'd be nice once 'n a while wear real clothes.

BETTY: It's the job, Mrs. Starkey.

MRS. STARKEY: Jist once, I'd like ta dress like people.

QUASHIE: (*Caustic*) Wid-out dis, they doan know who works. (*Plucks her uniform.*) Folks punchin de clock! Folks movin! That's who, all yuh do.

HIDELMAN: (*She leans over to take off her shoes*) I hate this . . . take off good shoes. (*Displays them before her.*)

BETTY: They're big enough, Hidelman.

HIDELMAN: (*Looking at* ELLIS) And when we ivver get safety fer shit around here, then I'm gonna kick ass with my metatarsal steel-toed billy-kickers.

(JUBA *goes to* HIDELMAN *and slips into* HIDELMAN's *shoes.*)

HIDELMAN: Hey, leave them 'lone.

JUBA: (*Dancing around in them*) Ah goan sport around.

HIDELMAN: (*Following her*) What the hell. . . .

JUBA: If crab no walk, he no see nothin.

HIDELMAN: God-damn!

JUBA: (*Dancing awkwardly in the shoes*) Ah dance sum carnival break-away.

QUASHIE: (JUBA *is dancing around* QUASHIE) What thing yuh do. Give dis womahn fatigue.

(*After a pause.*)

HIDELMAN: (*Holding out her hand*) All right . . . come on . . . nough!

JUBA: (*Dancing around* HIDELMAN) Just stand still darlin. I'll make you look good. Now . . . I bassa-bassa.

MRS. STARKEY: Oh . . . jam with yer bod, Juba.

(*After a few seconds,* JUBA *stops dancing around* HIDELMAN *and takes off the shoes and tosses them toward* HIDELMAN.)

JUBA: Nothin live in them shoes like nothin live in a bad woman.

(HIDELMAN *scowls and puts the shoes protectively in her locker. After a pause.*)

BETTY: (*As she puts on her paper scuffs*) I kinda like those slippers.

JUBA: We suck salt from a wooden spoon. We got to bare it.

QUASHIE: Oh, mahn, a slave is rottin in this land.

HIDELMAN: What I'd give for outdoor work. Git me 18 wheel truck . . . long haul ta Utah or California. . . .

QUASHIE: Hills . . . they take on white in coffee blossom time. Back at "Barbeque Bottom."

HIDELMAN: . . . listen ta the road bein ate up under my wheels. . . .

ELLIS: Plenty people outta work.

STARKEY: I know lotta girls waitress cause there's nothin.

HIDELMAN: Waitress is gotta be the lowest down job . . . I did me that fer five years.

BETTY: I heard to the TV last night, companies is not put in to the Pension what they should.

ELLIS: Sometimes I think we'd better off Social Security.

STARKEY: They're goin broke, too.

BETTY: I seen that 'n Sunday's paper.

ELLIS: Whole country'll go broke then.

BETTY: You live long nough, it'll happen.

MRS. STARKEY: Pension! My God, all innybody talks about.

BETTY: You'll worry soon nough.

MRS. STARKEY: Job bores me.

BETTY: Women down in the "repair pit" . . . they . . .

ELLIS: Be glad ya got a job.

MRS. STARKEY: (*Mocking*) Be glad ya got a job.

HIDELMAN: I wouldn't smart ass, I was you.

MRS. STARKEY: . . . 'n what's that suppose ta mean?

HIDELMAN: Meanin . . . this here da-partment's in fer cutbacks.

ELLIS: (*Scared*) Whole floor? (*She hugs her baby protectively.*)

JUBA: I know sumt'ing in the air cause of that old Elm tree on Independence Avenue. Ah does see white warts all over it.

QUASHIE: Hush your mouth, girl, you always think the worse.

STARKEY: (*Pointing to the machines*) We got us them—fer protection.

HIDELMAN: Machines—they kill off their own . . . 'n bring in different other ones. Maybe some big generator for the whole floor.

STARKEY: (*She goes to a machine and tightens up a gauge*) See that. They need them looked to.

(*They continue dressing.*)

JUBA: Just put my socks on wrong-side-out cause bad luck don't like unfamiliar sides. (JUBA *dramatically turns her socks inside out and then she puts her scuffs over them.*)

QUASHIE: (*To* JUBA) You talk crazy like you don't have no common sense.

ELLIS: (*Weakly*) Where'd ya hear cutbacks?

HIDELMAN: Down to the Twin Taps. Heard myself from Gallagher.

ELLIS: He mighta got mixed up. Floor A has two people ta retire that don't get replaced.

HIDELMAN: Nope.

STARKEY: We kin ask Elmhurst.

BETTY: (*Frightened*) I don't think we oughtta ask nobody.

ELLIS: Betty's right.

HIDELMAN: If one or all of us is goin, I say sooner we know, sooner ta start lookin.

MRS. STARKEY: My God, nobody got notice yit.

BETTY: She's right. All worked up—on half day, too.

STARKEY: (*Happily*) Whole afternoon in the Arcade Room. On company time.

MRS. STARKEY: (*Unimpressed*) Big deal!

HIDELMAN: (*To* MRS. STARKEY. *Caustic*) You got it better somewheres else?

STARKEY: Leave Mom alone. She kin have her own opinion.

HIDELMAN: You know what you kin do with her opinion.

BETTY: No way ta start out a good half day.

MRS. STARKEY: Person ain't suppose ta talk round here.

STARKEY: Come on, Mom. Forget it. What about this afternoon? You promised me electro-ping-pong.

MRS. STARKEY: Sure . . . sure . . .

(HIDELMAN *takes out a small disk which she rubs on the balding top of her head.*)

MRS. STARKEY: Yer gonna rub what's there off.

HIDELMAN: (*Defiant*) Circulating the scalp.

BETTY: That bald spot's from rollers at night.

MRS. STARKEY: (*Lewdly*) It's from thigh burns. (*She snikers.*)

HIDELMAN: I don't go down on no guy. I don't care if he's the Pope.

QUASHIE: (*Lewdly wiggling her tongue*) You need a flamin fire to make a fine sword.

BETTY: Well no little do-hickie's gonna bring back hair.

MRS. STARKEY: Who's do-hickie?

BETTY: You oughta git yerself hair-transplant like on TV.

MRS. STARKEY: She needs "head transplant."

STARKEY: Hair ta-day . . . gone ta . . .

HIDELMAN: (*To* STARKEY) Let's see what you look like at 32.

STARKEY: (*Shocked*) 32. No kiddin. (STARKEY *has heard these ages before, but she is constantly amazed.*)

HIDELMAN: Yah!

ELLIS: (*Innocently*) I got nough hair right now fer five. (*Brushes her thick hair.*)

HIDELMAN: (*She glares at* ELLIS. *After a pause, she goes to* ELLIS) Know how a "billy" parts her hair? (*After a pause,* HIDELMAN *does a semi-squat.*)

MRS. STARKEY: (*Laughs lewdly*) Hidelman, I ain't heard that one.

STARKEY: (*Embarrassed. Looking at her mother*) Mom . . . that's sick.

MRS. STARKEY: (*Laughing appreciatively*) God!

(ELLIS *ignores* HIDELMAN *and tends to her baby. There is a pause. Then* HIDELMAN *drags out a big folded tarpaulin from under her locker. She goes to the working area carrying it. The women follow. They all begin to spread out the tarpaulin on the floor, adjusting it firmly on the floor in front of the machines. They continue talking and spreading and adjusting the tarpaulin until the factory whistle blows.*)

MRS. STARKEY: This ain't gonna do no good.

HIDELMAN: Keeps chemicals on the floor off us.

QUASHIE: You can't trust *inside work.*

BETTY: We don't know fer sure, Hidelman.

HIDELMAN: (*Proudly*) My brother in Army Surplus over ta Lincoln Avenue give me this. Free!

MRS. STARKEY: It's jist ex-tree work.

BETTY: We used ta see when it leaked.

HIDELMAN: (*Disgusted*) Try ta help . . .

BETTY: Machines . . . they used ta clank 'n scream at us. . . .

STARKEY: Chemical spill on the floor don't amount ta anything.

HIDELMAN: Don't give me company shit.

BETTY: (*Looking pensively at machine*) In the beginning, when I started, I cud see ever-thing. Drive shafts . . . pulleys. Now it's all covered up. (*Pause.*) . . . 'n you don't hear you a hum even. Nothin.

(*There is a pause as they work silently on the floor covering. Then, still working.*)

STARKEY: Game's on.

HIDELMAN: In color?

STARKEY: (*Impressed*) Yah.

HIDELMAN: . . . my good color set took back cause I couldn't make payments.

MRS. STARKEY: I don't see me many games 'n color.

STARKEY: I had ta watch hockey down to ma sister's.

QUASHIE: I see them teams hit one nother . . . mess up the head and the face like gungoo soup.

(*After a pause.*)

ELLIS: (*Softly*) Cut backs?

JUBA: Trouble brewing on this floor ifing the Loogaroos don't brew here first.

BETTY: Nobody's gonna hire my age. Who's gonna take 60 years old?

STARKEY: 60? No kidding.

MRS. STARKEY: Sixty . . . fifty-one . . . not this place, 'n some place else.

STARKEY: Fifty-one. God, mom!

MRS. STARKEY: (*Annoyed*) Yah. I'm fifty-one!

JUBA: I don't fear anything ifing that Elm tree stand . . . cause it stood the tornado last year. But this morning it do have white warts on it when I come to work.

QUASHIE: (*Scared*) I have eight pickney—one child back in Mango Bay I call my name for . . . and a man he does yell like a howler monkey.

BETTY: Don't know how old you really are till ya start lookin for 'nother job.

STARKEY: Nobody got notice!

(*The factory whistle blows. It is now time for the machine work. As soon as the whistle blows, ELLIS runs quickly with her make-shift small play-pen and puts it in the washroom. The baby is in a deep sleep on the floor of the play-pen. Then ELLIS returns to the work area. The upper area of the stage has large flat machines painted a medicinal white. There are blue, yellow, green, brown lights blinking when the machines are working properly. The machines must dwarf the people, surround them, overpower them. A large clock hangs down from the ceiling facing the workers. The clock's back is toward the audience. The workers continually look at the clock intermittently throughout the play. When the work day begins, the women go to their respective work areas. Their work consists of pushing a series of eight levers back and forth in a careful monotonous way as they look and check gauges. Before QUASHIE begins, she blows a conch shell before her machine. The shell is on a string around her waist.*)

MRS. STARKEY: (*Wincing. To* QUASHIE) Have ta do that every morning?

QUASHIE: That Jamaician, darlin.

JUBA: This here no place for low-island foolishness.

QUASHIE: That help me mock the "flamin hours."

(*After a pause.*)

BETTY: Gits so, I start this, I git me cluster-headaches.

ELLIS: You need a man, Betty.

MRS. STARKEY: Volunteerin yers, Ellis?

HIDELMAN: We talk bout men . . . long as it ain't bout our husbands.

MRS. STARKEY: Be nice if we was ta have dudes around here.

HIDELMAN: No man's gonna take this pay.

MRS. STARKEY: I'd like ta see me a good looking stud ta the next machine.

ELLIS: Not for what we get.

HIDELMAN: They're makin a killin on us.

MRS. STARKEY: I like a tall dude.

HIDELMAN: If I wanted height, I'd screw a telephone pole.

JUBA: Used to love this man from Potters Cay Dock. A secret Obeah man. He could call up duppies. Him make a picture jump right off the wall and walk on down the street.

QUASHIE: (*To* JUBA) You think you young or what? Mind show-off don't kill you.

JUBA: (*Dreamily*) It make the soul sleep soft.

QUASHIE: Her dry as cane fire.

ELLIS: I like 'em good lookin.

MRS. STARKEY: Good looking guys is lousy in the sack.

QUASHIE: They is good and they is bad in the both.

MRS. STARKEY: Every "looker" I ever knew got it up once a night. And thought he was King Kong.

JUBA: A woman get decent a little and goes up in this world 'n long come a man do bad for her.

ELLIS: You like good lookin hunks, Betty?

BETTY: Last thang I need's a man.

JUBA: Woman . . . she's gonna age fast when a man gits her.

HIDELMAN: Livin all alone. . . .

BETTY: I got me Al's mother.

HIDELMAN: How long kin she last?

BETTY: (*Not cruelly. Matter of fact*) Old thang's ninety. She'll go forever.

STARKEY: Ninety. No kidding.

HIDELMAN: Don't she get social security?

BETTY: She gets me.

HIDELMAN: Jesus! ·

MRS. STARKEY: You oughta let somebody else take her.

BETTY: Who? Al was the only child.

MRS. STARKEY: She's not even yer own.

BETTY: She's tied ta me. "Strings" is my habit now.

JUBA: I need good sorrel wine from Kingston, what I'm askin for.

QUASHIE: You just keep cool. I tell you this even you older woman.

JUBA: (*Indignant*) I elder by two months.

MRS. STARKEY: I need that money back from my brother. So I kin go to
beautician school.

STARKEY: I'm doin engines out ta Dellavon's. I want me the engineer
rating.

MRS. STARKEY: Who cares?

STARKEY: Elmhurst cares. He knows I'm somebody ta call fer maintenance.

MRS. STARKEY: (*Mocking*) Sure.

STARKEY: First openin' fer foreman. You'll see.

MRS. STARKEY: Foreman. At yer age.

HIDELMAN: All we need is nother "pencil-prick."

STARKEY: I a-sisted front-end mechanic for Ford dealership over two
summers.

HIDELMAN: Heeeee . . . llll.

STARKEY: I'm getting me engineer rating. Man's pay.

HIDELMAN: Pig's ass.

(*Suddenly* HIDELMAN's *machine shakes and makes a sputtering sound. It hisses off a light steam that can be seen. The machine "blinks" red and black distress lights which brighten and dim and flicker alternately.*)

HIDELMAN: (*She gives out a yell and jumps back from the steam*) Starkey!

(STARKEY, *without emotion, takes out a special wrench from her pocket and adjusts some bolts on the machine and turns some dials until the machine quits sputtering. There is a mask hanging on each machine.* HIDELMAN *frantically reaches for her mask. She puts it on and starts choking.*)

STARKEY: (*Without emotion. About the mask*) That ain't gonna do no good.

(*Struggling in her mask,* HIDELMAN *finally takes it off and flings it across the floor. The others go on working without alarm as they are used to various kinds of incidents like this.*)

HIDELMAN: (*Coughing*) Shit! Fumes is jist get inside faster with that fuckin thang on. (*Pause. Still coughing. To* STARKEY.) Don't nothin git ta you!

STARKEY: (*Strongly*) I'll git me spooked when generator-control-circuits is showed ground alarms. Not till. An' that ain't gonna happen, Hidelman. We got us back-ups.

HIDELMAN: (*To machine*) Damn monster.

STARKEY: (*Without emotion*) Ordinary machine fatigue.

HIDELMAN: I wanted kilt, I could kill myself.

JUBA: Devil make a "zeppy" on we.

STARKEY: Machines is like us, Juba . . . they have them good 'n bad mixed in.

MRS. STARKEY: I ain't seen the good.

HIDELMAN: First they'll torture us all ta hell . . . 'n then move on in ta take our place.

STARKEY: (*Defensive for machines*) You jist got ta find the right way with 'em. (STARKEY *pats the machine. The machine is fixed now and the lights blink safely. They all continue working. After a pause.*)

HIDELMAN: Long as break-down is kept out of writing—that's all Elmhurst cares bout.

ELLIS: When Mavis talk ta him?

HIDELMAN: Mavis ain't negotiated ta nobody 'n days.

ELLIS: What the hell am I payin dues fer?

HIDELMAN: Mavis don't represent innybody but herself.

STARKEY: Mavis got us the coffee area.

BETTY: She don't get paid bein on Negotiations.

HIDELMAN: Innybody hear her yell ta get off?

ELLIS: What I hear—she's chummy with Elmhurst.

BETTY: She goes to the same church, that's all.

HIDELMAN: Woman sits ever Sunday next ta first line supervisor.

QUASHIE: That Mavis . . . her crazy for truth, like fish drink salt water.

JUBA: This place in for bad times.

BETTY: Mavis got us air vents.

STARKEY: The floor was a sweat box six months ago.

HIDELMAN: It ain't no Ramada Inn now.

STARKEY: We got us regulation air-movement.

JUBA: Take you hands up and flap 'em . . . that's the best fan.

STARKEY: We got air movement twenty-five feet per minute.

HIDELMAN: Don't give me fuckin handbook values. By noon, I'm drippin sweat like a busted radiator.

STARKEY: Company is put them in air-conditioning ta *Shippin.*

HIDELMAN: Not for the women. So the "plastic tapes" on the cartons don't melt.

(Pause. HIDELMAN *slaps the upper part of her machine.)*

HIDELMAN: This place is "billy-rigged" . . . break downs . . . they jist slap up tar paper . . . leaks in them loose fittings.

STARKEY: I put foam rubber to them "loose fittings" myself.

HIDELMAN: Chemicals is on the floor and lays there. For-ever.

STARKEY: Why don't it show up on no monitor?

HIDELMAN: You git shaky at night? Sit down for dinner sometimes 'n can't hold a fork? That crap kills yer nervous system.

STARKEY: Don't spread rumors, Hidelman.

HIDELMAN: Pipes there drip steam ... acid ... 'n we're used ta it. We don't know anymore.

(*A chime is heard on the public address system.*)

MALE VOICE: Please stand by. Please stand by. Daily announcements.

(*The women pull away from their machines and walk center stage lazily. They sit on chairs or stand next to the small table in the coffee break area.* ELLIS *runs quickly to the washroom and pushes the playpen to prop open the washroom door so she can hear.* ELLIS *strokes the sleeping baby as she listens.*)

HIDELMAN: (*Waves her arms in the air in a slapping gesture*) Another pimp slap.

MRS. STARKEY: (*Mocking the announcement*) Don't smoke outside the washroom.

ELLIS: (*Mocking the announcement*) Make sure all lockers is secure.

HIDELMAN: (*To the P.A. system*) Come on. Pimp slap us.

(*Another chime is heard. A male voice comes over the speaker.*)

MALE VOICE: Good morning. This is Martin Yarde speaking for our General Manager, David Talbert. (*Pause.*) As you know, today is half-day for Department B.

(*The women cheer.*)

MALE VOICE: According to our consent with Negotiations ... see your "Professional Agreement" ... Page 10, Article V ... Management wishes you a pleasant afternoon in the Arcade Room ... where, I am pleased to announce, a new computer blackjack board has just been installed.

(STARKEY *and* HIDELMAN *cheer.*)

MALE VOICE: Mr. Borris, Assistant General Manager, is presently in conference with the "Small Inventory Committee." Floor Supervisors will be investigating small-item loses. (*Pause.*) Speaking for Mr. Talbert, I am hoping production-speed can be increased. Every day brings new customers. This morning, we received a contract for our reactor-parts from Peking. China. (*Pause.*) So I leave you with these words ...

HIDELMAN: Jist leave us!

MALE VOICE: Have a good day.

HIDELMAN: (*Yelling at the P.A. system.*) Coolies is hired for life. They don't git laid off!

BETTY: Yah?

HIDELMAN: Sure. I read that.

(ELLIS *shoves the play-pen back inside the washroom and returns to the work area.*)

ELLIS: I don't hear too good in there. Innythin bout cutbacks?

BETTY: No.

HIDELMAN: You're gonna git us in trouble with that kid.

BETTY: (*Defensive for* ELLIS) She don't take chances.

ELLIS: I give him phenobarbitol ta sleep.

BETTY: It's a good little thang. Out like a light all the time.

ELLIS: (*Proudly. Tenderly*) Got hisself a dingus the size of a eight year old.

MRS. STARKEY: (*Impressed*) Yah?

ELLIS: Big as eight years old.

MRS. STARKEY: That's competition with my "ex."

(STARKEY *winces in pain.*)

BETTY: A real well behaved little boy.

JUBA: (*Defensive for* ELLIS) I don't like chillun who feel they have too much mischief in they head.

BETTY: This here's *Year of the Child,* Hidelman. I heard that to the TV.

HIDELMAN: Hee . . . llll. I got me four kids. Took care of. I don't put people in jeopardy.

ELLIS: We'll git us a nursery. Come 1980. Like Mavis said.

JUBA: (*Strongly defensive for* ELLIS) It ain't abuse she abusing that little one. Is love her lovin him and *keep him* her keepin him, what that is!

(HIDELMAN *glares at* ELLIS.)

MALE VOICE: . . . and please . . . no smoking outside the washroom. Thank you.

(*A shrill bell rings and the women begin working their machines.*)

STARKEY: Hey, new blackjack board.

MRS. STARKEY: (*Disgusted*) Who wants ta play blackjack?

STARKEY: Come on, Mom. Play the new machine.

BETTY: (*To* STARKEY) She don't care ta play 'n no use talk her inta it.

STARKEY: (*To her mother*) Don't you ivver wanna do nothin new?

JUBA: My self cool, but the mouth is dry. (*She slows down in her work.*)

QUASHIE: I got some for if the leg do start hurtin.

MRS. STARKEY: (*Aside. Shaking her head toward* QUASHIE) Centipede city.

JUBA: Nothin bout trouble drink don't fix. (*Pause. To* QUASHIE.) You got *Two Dagger*?

QUASHIE: Woman want *Two Dagger*.

JUBA: You got half a quart of Appleton's?

QUASHIE: Buh!

JUBA: What have you to drink?

QUASHIE: Exactly what I have every Gord day since I been here.

JUBA: You got *Black Seal*?

QUASHIE: This here ain't Nassau the Bahamas.

JUBA: You got South African Sherry, Quashie?

QUASHIE: Don't bawl out my name. Whole room ain't talkin to you.

JUBA: No *Black Seal*?

QUASHIE: Her say that like *Black Seal* and South African Sherry pourin all over, God will come to earth and make everybody happy. I mightn't give you a drink even if I have. (QUASHIE *reluctantly takes a pint bottle out of her pocket and hands it to* JUBA.)

MRS. STARKEY: (*Looking at the bottle. Making a face*) California Port.

STARKEY: Yer not suppose ta drink on the job.

QUASHIE: (*Officious*) Dey don't serve you on crutches in a bar, darlin . . . it be against the law.

JUBA: I give the machine somethin to keep it happy. (JUBA *dabs out a couple of drops from the bottle as if it were perfume and dabs the drops of booze behind a couple of the levers.*)

STARKEY: You'll have "Maintenance" on our back.

JUBA: Only the machine can tell you what it drink and what it ain't drink.

BETTY: What if Elmhurst saw . . .

MRS. STARKEY: Juba, give my machine a snort. Maybe it'll git horny.

STARKEY: (*Embarrassed*) Mom!

MRS. STARKEY: (*Vamping the machine and moving her body against the levers*) Turn on ta me, big thang. Go! (*Pushing the levers.*) Push it all the way. (*The others ignore* MRS. STARKEY.)

JUBA: (*After taking a long drink*) This bottle, girl, it small.

QUASHIE: Who you think you is . . . white? Same bottle I do have every Gord day.

(JUBA *takes a final drink from the bottle savoring it.*)

MRS. STARKEY: (*Turning her backside to the machine lever and trying to move the lever with her rear*) From the back . . . oh . . . come on, you stud. . . . (*After a pause, she turns to face the machine in disgust.*) Know what? You ain't got no technique, buster. (MRS. STARKEY *goes back to working regularly. The others ignore her.*)

JUBA: (*Jiggles the empty bottle*) End of the bottle don't live for the end.

QUASHIE: It dead.

(JUBA *tries drinking from the empty bottle, tapping it.*)

QUASHIE: Won't do you no good, that.

HIDELMAN: You ain't pushin none, Juba.

JUBA: I don't try to beat the machine. I just go long with it. (*Pause.*) Back home, when the blazin hours was pon you, it be too hot for sleep, too hot for work, too hot for "bally-dash." Only thing left to do was *nothin*—and the long cold drink in you mouth.

(*There is a pause.*)

JUBA: (*She takes some corn kernels out of her pocket*) This here grains of corn. 99. Just 99. (JUBA *scatters them on the floor around her machine.*) That there will keep the fire-hags away.

HIDELMAN: Only "hag" ta this place is Mavis.

MRS. STARKEY: (*To* JUBA) Fired-city . . . right out of here.

BETTY: Why 99, Juba?

JUBA: So intent they on finding hundredth grain, they don't bother me.

BETTY: (*Innocently*) Oh.

HIDELMAN: (*Disgusted*) Jeeee . . . us.

(JUBA *goes back to work. There is a silent pause as they all work.*)

ELLIS: Inventory . . . they don't ivver inventory little stuff.

BETTY: Think they been missin thangs?

ELLIS: Maybe new trainees is messed up.

STARKEY: We ain't had new trainees 'n months.

ELLIS: (*Worried*) You hear inny-thang, Betty?

BETTY: Me? I don't go nowhere. I pay fer practical nurse in the day. I can't ford it no more at night.

ELLIS: If ya hear, Betty.

MRS. STARKEY: Maybe Mavis knows.

HIDELMAN: Knows what!

ELLIS: (*Worried*) I don't like management come round sniffin' us out.

HIDELMAN: What-a-ya so hot bout?

ELLIS: Who's hot?

MRS. STARKEY: Hold yer water, everybody.

STARKEY: We're suppose ta have good morale. Half day, member?

MRS. STARKEY: Seems like ever-body always gets worked up on half days.

BETTY: That's not true.

MRS. STARKEY: Last time, Hidelman 'n Mavis got inta it.

HIDELMAN: Woman's not worth shit.

BETTY: She does committee work her own time.

MRS. STARKEY: Why don't you do it, Hidelman?

HIDELMAN: Maybe I will.

MRS. STARKEY: Sure . . . 'n give up moonlightin.

ELLIS: (*Interested*) You sell much Sarah Coventry? Make anythin' offa that?

HIDELMAN: Moonlight—ya git less, but it don't take so much outta ya.

BETTY: We got us a nice coffee area.

HIDELMAN: Sociation wins when the fuckin company wants hit to.

BETTY: Better 'n no Sociation at all.

HIDELMAN: Lighting's bad. We got us shadows. Half the time I don't see me numbers on them gauges tell from shit.

QUASHIE: They is buffalo hours, starvation wages, and that's the way those drums roll, and you can talk and talk till morning come and dawn, I say you can't do no good.

HIDELMAN: Cafeteria ten miles away. Have ta run there 'n back ta make it on time.

BETTY: It's good fer the figure.

HIDELMAN: Shit.

QUASHIE: We is Union workers, but we is still slums of de Company.

HIDELMAN: Bills up ta here . . . takin on my sister now . . . supportin two families . . . (*Looking at* ELLIS.) Billies . . . they have came up here from *Kan*-tucky . . . grab off all the jobs . . .

BETTY: (*To* HIDELMAN) Yer sister find work yit?

HIDELMAN: (*Glaring at* ELLIS) Waitressin . . . Coffee Shop to the Cass Hotel.

BETTY: She lookin fer somethang else?

HIDELMAN: (*Angry*) Yah! (HIDELMAN *stops working and walks away from her area and goes to* ELLIS's *area. She stares at* ELLIS *a couple of seconds as* ELLIS *continues to work*.) Have you ivver waitressed?

ELLIS: I couldn't.

HIDELMAN: (*Mocking*) You couldn't . . . 'n why couldn't you?

ELLIS: Cysts. Ta my ovaries.

MRS. STARKEY: Hidelman, don't you have innythin' better ta do?

STARKEY: Git back ta yer own area, Hidelman.

ELLIS: I couldn't help me cysts. On both of 'em.

HIDELMAN: Sure.

ELLIS: What-a-ya-mean?

STARKEY: Hidelman, you don't fake ovaries.

HIDELMAN: (*She takes a hold of* ELLIS's *uniform and pulls her away from working*.) My sister has lived here in Ill-a-noise all her life.

(ELLIS *is guarded. She has a healthy fear of* HIDELMAN. *After a pause*.)

HIDELMAN: Troy 'n Earlville . . . 'fore she come ta Chicago.

STARKEY: (*Goes to* ELLIS's *area.*) Hidelman, leave her 'lone.

HIDELMAN: How many kids you got?!

ELLIS: (*Weakly*) Six.

HIDELMAN: That's right! (*Pause.*) My sister's got her eight.

MRS. STARKEY: (*To* HIDELMAN) Tell yer sister to use foam.

HIDELMAN: (*Glaring at* ELLIS) She does.

MRS. STARKEY: . . . "industrial strength."

STARKEY: (*Takes* HIDELMAN's *arm*) Go on . . . git back. What if Elmhurst was ta come . . . .

ELLIS: (*Defensive but not hostile*) I trained fer weeks with no pay. When I was started out. Them "white hats" sent me out fer thangs ta Maintenance. So I couldn't watch 'em 'n learn.

BETTY: That was a-ginst rules, Ellis.

ELLIS: You don't find that out till you git round people which already know it. (*Pause.*) I had ta sneak myself looks ta learn. (*Pause.*) I ain't had no hand-outs.

(HIDELMAN *gives a final hostile tug to* ELLIS's *uniform and then goes back to her area. There is a silent pause for a few seconds as they work.*)

QUASHIE: I don't like Elmhurst.

JUBA: When can you like the boss or not? You retired and live pon you mansion?

QUASHIE: *Worker* has got to be defiant. *Boss*—now he must be humble.

JUBA: (*Good natured squabbling*) Shut you mouth, Quashie.

QUASHIE: Who the hell you tellin "shut de mouth," not me? (*Pause.*) Fightin this machine. Fight like the Army. And that (*Points to machine*) . . . it the enemy. My back all bent up like a roll of copper wire.

JUBA: You just don't like the machine cause you can't old-talk with you family while you work.

QUASHIE: Don't speak at me slight, woman.

JUBA: When that Elmhurst calls . . . you answer "yes" back quick and brisk, or it get cold pon you plate till next never.

QUASHIE: I rebuke that.

JUBA: You fight that machine so bad you can't get enough words out of you mouth—even side ways.

QUASHIE: It don't be the work, darlin. This here ain't *real* work. (*Pause.*) I is savin up for Cat Island.

HIDELMAN: Real outdoor work there, Quashie?

QUASHIE: (*To* HIDELMAN) You come there with bags to fill with bay leaves—for bay rum. (*Pause.*) Cat Island don't have no wharf. Water . . . it be so shallow you have to anchor half a mile away. (*Pause.*) Then you git in the surfboat . . . take the short tiller oar . . .

(QUASHIE *stands sideways and holds on to a lever of the machine like an oar with both hands. After a pause to* HIDELMAN.)

QUASHIE: Woman . . . take the oar.

HIDELMAN: I ain't been in no boat before.

QUASHIE: Take the oar!

(HIDELMAN *looks at* QUASHIE *and holds on to the lever with both hands like an oar moving it.*)

JUBA: You both gonna be "oared" outta here.

QUASHIE: . . . then paddle like the dog ears goin: Paddle . . . (*To* HIDEL-MAN) . . . paddle harder, all you do!

(*After a pause,* QUASHIE *stops.* HIDELMAN *stops a little after* QUASHIE. *After a pause, then.*)

QUASHIE: . . . wait for the right wave. And ride like you is on a surf board. Right to a flat rock. Then jump to a speck of red sea-weed underneath . . . your feet in a soft ride of grass . . . breeze comes off the mango tree. . . .

HIDELMAN: (*Dubious. After a pause*) Cat Island. (*Pause.*) Sounds like a whore outfit.

QUASHIE: (*Peevish*) You vex me, woman. I'm from good Jamacian-Nassau family. I is house-proud people. After I was born, my mother, her bury my navel string in the yard so I be a home-girl. If-ing I didn't have the spirit of the Lord in me, I would not old-talk with you at all . . . at all.

(QUASHIE *goes peevishly to working her machine.* HIDELMAN *shrugs like "big deal" and goes back to working. After a pause.*)

ELLIS: Ship thangs all the way ta Peking. How bout that.

HIDELMAN: What's so damn great 'n sell ta Commies?

ELLIS: They pay money jist like inny body else.

HIDELMAN: (*Angrily. To* ELLIS) My old man was ta Service fightin gainst dictators.

ELLIS: Keeps us working.

HIDELMAN: Commies is gonna take over this here country without firin a shot.

JUBA: (*To* HIDELMAN) Devil gonna find something for you to do, you don't stop that talk.

(*The chime is heard over the public address.*)

HIDELMAN: (*Waves her hand at the P.A.*) Pimp-slap time.

(ELLIS *runs to the rest room and puts the play-pen in the half open door and sits there so she can hear.*)

MALE VOICE: Professional growth! Thank you.

MRS. STARKEY: Who's goin? I went last time.

HIDELMAN: (*Goes to the washroom*) *She* goes!

BETTY: Ellis went yis-ter-day.

STARKEY: Hidelman, when you gonna lay off on that?

HIDELMAN: . . . when billies git theirselves shot at ta wars like ever-body else.

ELLIS: I knew me a guy from Nam *give* his wife the clap . . . 'n her pregnant. That there baby it was born blue 'n without no nose.

STARKEY: (*Shocked. In disgust.*) Blue!

ELLIS: (*To* HIDELMAN) I'll go. I ain't 'fraid of no work. (*Pause.* ELLIS *looks to* STARKEY.) Will you look ta the clamp on my play-pen, Starkey? (STARKEY *follows* ELLIS *to the washroom.*)

STARKEY: (*She fiddles with a clamp on the fold of the play-pen*) Jist needs yer "toggle bolt." I kin fix it over lunch. (*Pause.* STARKEY *looks intently at the baby.*) One arm's bigger 'n the other is.

ELLIS: Don't git spare-parts maintenance on a baby, Starkey.

STARKEY: (*Still staring*) . . . jist lies there like a rag-doll.

ELLIS: Don't you ivver want you a baby, Starkey?

STARKEY: I ain't seen me no mother which has took care of a baby like she is took care of a doll back when she was little.

ELLIS: (*Looking at the baby happily*) I was hoping he was twins.

STARKEY: Why?

ELLIS: Take care of one, might's well take care of two.

STARKEY: (*Staring at baby*) Whatta ya feed good ta it?

ELLIS: Nothin. I don't feed nothin good ta ma-self, neither. (*Pause.*) I was ta the fields when I first got married. Husband 'n me didn't git on so good with crops. But I grew me babies even if I didn't grow me much beans 'n stuff.

JUBA: (*Goes to the washroom. Saying to* ELLIS) Last child of mine be pretty old, you know. Look here, let me sing to him and such like.

ELLIS: Thanks, Juba.

(JUBA *rocks the play-pen in the half opened door of the washroom. She begins to speak more to the baby than to the others.*)

JUBA: Used was to take care of the house and little ones for the rich people in Nassau and Kingston. Them people, they say: "Don't break this ... and don't break that." They worry I could smash something. You could poison they children ... but it be gravy-bowls and lamps they worry about and jump up and down for like they catch the spirrid.

QUASHIE: (*To* ELLIS) I go with you, darlin. (QUASHIE *and* ELLIS *exit.*)

MALE VOICE: Please take out your production manual. Review page 284. Thank you.

(*Each person has a manual, phone-book thick, hanging by a hook on the side of the machines, and they go to their machines and lift off the book. As they look through their manuals,* JUBA *sings her song to the baby.*)

JUBA: (*Sings*)
Dey call him Jimmy Rum Bum
Broke de heart of he sweet lovin mum.
Yuh can hear har saay
De live long day:
    "I only a rum bum mum;
    Ah is jus a rum bum mum."

Jimmy ga black beans in he brain
Ga prune seeds in he drain,
Gully roots for he nose
Lime leaves for he toes
Broke de heart of he very own mum.
Yuh can hear har say

De live long day:
   "I only a rum bum mum;
   Ah is jus a rum bum mum."

(*The last verse of the song is sung very softly as the women talk.*)

Jimmy ga soursop for he eyes
Flour sack for he ties,
Cacoa beans for he head
Banana leaves for he bed
Broke de heart of he very own mum.
Yuh can hear har saay
De live long day:
   "I only a rum bum mum;
   Ah is jus a rum bum mum."

(*After* JUBA *finishes her song, she continues to rock the baby. After a pause.*)

BETTY: I don't know why mornings is so long half days.

MRS. STARKEY: This here's the most boring job 'n the world.

BETTY: It's so hot down ta the *repair pit,* cigarette matches start fire in them girls' pockets.

MRS. STARKEY: (*Tired of hearing this*) I know ... I know.

BETTY: Spot welders in the sub-assembly ...

MRS. STARKEY: I'm inner-rested ones got it better.

STARKEY: You'll jist make yer-self sick thinkin like that.

BETTY: We got it good—job off the line.

MRS. STARKEY: Off the line! We're jist the last line.

STARKEY: We got us "Pension Plan."

MRS. STARKEY: God! Nineteen year old droolin over Pension.

BETTY: Before ... people worked till they died.

(ELLIS *comes in wheeling a small serving cart with a big tea brewer on it.* QUASHIE *follows with a tray of tea cups and bread on her head.*)

STARKEY: Take that off you, Quashie. Elmhurst don't like ta see no "Voodoo" here.

QUASHIE: When I was a little girl, I started with one stone on my head. Later it was coconuts ... custard apples ... sage and cabbage, monkey-oranges ... (*Pause.*) Hands, they are not for carrying things—heads are.

HIDELMAN: (*Defensive for* QUASHIE) You're looking at good outside work.

BETTY: (*Looking at* QUASHIE *with head carrying*) Gives me the creeps.

QUASHIE: (*Defiantly takes the tray from her head*) I'll just carry my heart on the inside for a change.

(MRS. STARKEY *takes the manual and puts it on her head. She holds the book with her two hands and walks a few paces.*)

BETTY: That don't count the way you're doin it, Mrs. Starkey.

MRS. STARKEY: One hand, then. (*She proceeds to hold the book with one hand.*) Cause I was to no island in my life. So I'll take me a "handicap." Like bowlin.

BETTY: Sure.

MRS. STARKEY: Pulls the tits up 'n out.

STARKEY: Mom, put that down.

MRS. STARKEY: (*Stops walking*) Juba, you ever screw doin this?

JUBA: Darlin ... my mahn, him come up real nice from behind the stink-pea bush ... this piano on my head ...

HIDELMAN: Piano!

JUBA: ... breathin quick in the back of me. His cane bill movin. That man could pump to a hairy mango so wild like a bush black for me.

(MRS. STARKEY *is living* JUBA's *words, eyes closed.*)

HIDELMAN: (*Dreamily*) Damn. Outdoor work.

MALE VOICE: Please stand by for "Professional Growth." Please stand by for "Professional Growth." Thank you. (*Pause.*) This is Mr. Basenfelder speaking for Mr. Thomas, quality control engineer. (*Pause.*) We have already announced the news that Peking has just submitted specs to us for our reactor-parts. (*Pause.*) So today's professional growth is unleavened bread and ming tea to honor our requisition from Peking. Thank you.

HIDELMAN: (*Drinking from a small Chinese cup*) What the hell's ming tea?

ELLIS: This here. (*Drinks.*) Cups with no handles.

(ELLIS *returns to her baby in the washroom. On her way, she takes some napkins from a holder on the table and stuffs them in her pocket secretly. Nobody sees this.* JUBA *puts the baby back in the play-pen and returns to her area.*)

HIDELMAN: (*Sputtering the tea out*) What the . . .

MRS. STARKEY: Tastes like melted-down Vicks.

BETTY: (*Eating the bread and making a face*) Wait till ya eat unleavened bread.

MRS. STARKEY: (*Eating*) Styrofoam!

HIDELMAN: (*Tasting*) Pig food. What Coolies and Billies eat.

QUASHIE: No red pea soup with dumplings . . . salt beef and paw paw with guava jelly.

STARKEY: What's this stuff?

JUBA: Ain't Jamaician moonbread.

MRS. STARKEY: (*Eating*) Like crackers.

BETTY: I don't think yer yeast's in it.

QUASHIE: Last week, somebody in the cafeteria found a gold tooth in the spareribs.

JUBA: Cannibals!

MRS. STARKEY: *Soul Food* . . . with a little "body" thrown in.

STARKEY: Mavis know bout that?

QUASHIE: If you eat in the Cafeteria, is you look out.

HIDELMAN: (*Disgusted. Looking at the bread*) Professional growth!

STARKEY: The job, Hidelman.

(*There is a pause as they eat for a few seconds.*)

HIDELMAN: We have jist ate Commie food.

STARKEY: We got us a big order from there.

ELLIS: Keeps us working. (*She takes a bite and makes a face.*)

(*After a few seconds of eating, a loud noise is heard. Then a bucket comes rolling across the floor.* MRS. STARKEY *stands in surprise.*)

MRS. STARKEY: It's the Day-Tripper!

(ELLIS *comes out of the washroom to stare. All the women stare. The* DAY-TRIPPER *then comes quickly and loudly across the floor. A short mop is tied to her side with a dust cloth.*)

QUASHIE: (*Saying as the old woman is moving*) Day-Tripper. Her crazy. Her movin sideways cross the floor like some cranky hound pickin up a scent.

JUBA: Hey, you Day-Tripper. Look way you goin now. Slow down a little bit.

QUASHIE: Her run wild like a bush beast.

(*The old woman finally collapses on the floor in a dead stillness by the coffee area table.*)

JUBA: Oh Lorse . . . oh Lorse, what happen?

(*They gather around the old woman.*)

HIDELMAN: She's stoned again.

BETTY: Somebody oughta do something.

JUBA: You need "Coolie Foot" sugar and limes to bring her out of it.

MRS. STARKEY: She's in no pain.

STARKEY: (*Patting the old lady's face gently*) Come on . . . come on . . .

QUASHIE: When will you learn to let a person rest in peace? It takes a little time to get used to the pleasantness on the other side before you take her back to this old place of stupidness.

MRS. STARKEY: Old woman working—at her age.

ELLIS: She gits a free hot lunch for cleaning up, Mrs. Starkey.

STARKEY: It's only one hour a day.

HIDELMAN: Part time work ain't worth shit.

BETTY: She likes doin it.

QUASHIE: Day-Tripper! We had them on Cat Island. Folks who come just for the day—when the hot time takes set.

HIDELMAN: Part time work is shit.

MRS. STARKEY: Where's she get money for a joint? Me . . . all I kin 'ford ta git high on is crunching up aspirin real good in my cigarette.

STARKEY: (*Disapproving*) Aspirin!

HIDELMAN: (*About* DAY-TRIPPER) She don't buy food, that's how. I seen her chow down in the Cafeteria nough for eight people.

MRS. STARKEY: Food to the Cafeteria ain't fit wages for a mule.

DAY-TRIPPER: (*Abruptly sitting up*) I'm all right. Don't tell Elmhurst.

BETTY: Want some coffee?

DAY-TRIPPER: (*Jumping up*) No. No, Betty. I don't want me nothin.

(ELLIS *goes back to the washroom and props open the door with the play-pen.* ELLIS *slips some toilet paper in her pocket, the others don't see. Then* ELLIS *takes the trash can lid and begins poking more holes in it with a large blunt pencil. The* DAY-TRIPPER *takes out a flower from her pocket.)*

DAY-TRIPPER: For the baby. (*She smells it as she walks to the play-pen.*)

JUBA: (*To the* DAY-TRIPPER) Don't smell the flower you give away. That be stealin.

(*The* DAY-TRIPPER *abruptly pulls the flower away from her nose. She then puts it in the play-pen and returns to the others.*)

MRS. STARKEY: Girls in "Floor D" said the *Van* was gonna be out back this afternoon.

DAY-TRIPPER: That's right.

HIDELMAN: You gonna visit the Van, Betty?

MRS. STARKEY: Two young studs out there to the parkin' lot, Betty.

(BETTY *is embarrassed*)

QUASHIE: Look at her tan up like she's short.

ELLIS: Only girls ta "Shipping" gits over-time. Who's got the money?

MRS. STARKEY: I always did like ballin without no fuss.

STARKEY: (*Angry*) You'll git yerself fired, Mom.

MRS. STARKEY: Them poor guys is putting theirselves through DeVries Technical School.

HIDELMAN: (*To* STARKEY) Open up yer heart, kid.

JUBA: It be *legs* they want "open up."

BETTY: (*To* DAY-TRIPPER) Got innythin from the Repair Pit?

DAY-TRIPPER: I come up the back way 'n they give me this. (*She takes a paper napkin out of her pocket. It has a message in lipstick. She gives it to* BETTY.)

BETTY: (*Reads the message. Pause*) They wanna know bout the Van.

MRS. STARKEY: Come on, Day-Tripper. What's the word?

STARKEY: We can't ford us gettin mixed up with no Van.

MRS. STARKEY: Don't listen ta her. (*Pause.*) Come on!

(*The* DAY-TRIPPER *takes out an advertisement from her pocket. It is shiny black and shaped like a jock strap. She gives one to* MRS.

STARKEY.)

MRS. STARKEY: (*Holding out the ad*) This is new, Oh, la ... la. Git me inta one of them.

STARKEY: Mom!

MRS. STARKEY: (*Studying the ad*) ... will ya look at that. They have got theirselves a regular menu now.

HIDELMAN: Yah?

(*The women all crowd around* MRS. STARKEY *who stands aside coldly.*)

MRS. STARKEY: (*Reading*) "Over Easy" ... ten bucks.

ELLIS: I don't have me that kinda money.

MRS. STARKEY: (*Reading*) "Suck of the Day."

HIDELMAN: Goin down on a guy rots yer teeth.

QUASHIE: I'm sick of that parkin lot. They does everythin in that parkin lot—it be no place for good clean people.

DAY TRIPPER: (*Takes out a little shiny black hat with a picture of a red van on it, then she sings*)
Where does all the *come* come from
Come come from
Come come from,
Where does all the *Come* come from?
From the Van, Man!
From the Van, Man!

(*There is then a silence. After a pause.*)

JUBA: How much do you make for all that, darlin?

DAY-TRIPPER: I get me a free one.

HIDELMAN: Jesus!

JUBA: They be good as girls say down in that Repair Pit?

MRS. STARKEY: You gotta have talent in any profession.

DAY-TRIPPER: (*Happily*) It takes a real hunk ta get me outta my support hose.

HIDELMAN: It takes *some* dude get his dick inna marshmallow.

DAY-TRIPPER: (*Offended*) I had all my kids natural. No stitches.

MRS. STARKEY: Don't talk tight-twat ta me at 75.

STARKEY: (*Amazed*) Seventy ... five.

HIDELMAN: Hey, Day-Tripper. Let's see yer jugs.

(*The old lady moves her upper arms. She has a breast tatooed, one on each upper arm.*)

DAY-TRIPPER: Never had innythin up top ta speak of. Even when I was young. Now I got some real good tiddies—drawed there. Turns the men on—more 'n real ones.

(*Everybody laughs good naturedly. The* DAY-TRIPPER *then goes about working, filling the napkin holder and humming as she does so. Then she stops and pauses before her work.*)

DAY-TRIPPER: I member how it was . . . working full time. I put in 30 years to the Cannery till they called me surplus. (*Pause.*) I got it good now. Social Security . . . part time work . . . kids moved away . . . husband dead on me. (*Pause.*) Lotta women . . . they commit marriage a-gin cause of silence. Silence ain't lonely. I make up inny singin . . . jist like I make up what I say. Don't mean a thin' without *me*. None of it.

(*The* DAY-TRIPPER *continues working on the floor and general cleaning, humming as she does this. A horn is sounded. Everybody goes back to their machine to turn it on.* ELLIS *puts the baby inside the washroom again and goes to her work area. They work silently with their levers for several seconds. When the women aren't involved in conversation, they dwell in their own dream world.* DAY-TRIPPER *continues to clean.*)

MRS. STARKEY: My brother outta Rockford called last night, Betty.

BETTY: He ever give back yer money?

MRS. STARKEY: He's got hisself four kids. Sick wife.

BETTY: How kin ya get ta beautician school?

MRS. STARKEY: Come August, he might pay back ten a month.

ELLIS: (*Mostly to herself*) August . . . that's yer bad month . . . gotta buy school clothes for the kids.

STARKEY: Uncle Wes give *inny* of it back?

MRS. STARKEY: All them kids . . . Aunt Emmie with the Bell's Palsy.

STARKEY: I got me over 1,000 to the bank from that part time job last summer.

MRS. STARKEY: I can't take money from my own kid.

STARKEY: Why not?

MRS. STARKEY: I don't wanna answer to no kid of mine.

STARKEY: If you went back ta Daddy . . .

MRS. STARKEY: Don't start on that a-gin.

STARKEY: You told me you'd think on it.

MRS. STARKEY: I never said I was goin back ta him.

STARKEY: You're still married!

MRS. STARKEY: Separated!

STARKEY: That's still married!

MRS. STARKEY: Look . . . I want me somethin better. Ta feel! Yah! Sex in marriage's like wine at Church . . . *there* . . . but ya don't get drunk.

(*Pause.*)

MRS. STARKEY: I never had no excitement. Jist one man that married me at fifteen. What did I know? Not like they do ta-day. My God, we was parked over ta Roosevelt Road . . . him rubbing his prick on me.

STARKEY: (*Tense. Eyes shut painfully*) . . . I don't wanna hear.

MRS. STARKEY: (*Very slowly working the machine*) He begged ta "feel me up." I kept sayin "no." Well, I ended up lettin him, so I might as well said "yes" to begin with. (*Pause.*) . . . then I'm all wet down there. I thought he'd done something. I bawled: "You stuck it in me." (*Pause.*) That's why I got married. (*Pause.*) But he didn't. Not that night. Cause I'd come on myself. I didn't know from nothin. A kid . . . that's all.

(*There is a silent pause.*)

QUASHIE: Make me a gift of the time, Juba.

JUBA: When you gonna learn ta read the clock, woman?

QUASHIE: The *hours* is fine. *Minutes* and *seconds* —those hands is crazy like they be in infancy all day long.

JUBA: (*Studying the clock*) Eight-thirty sharp. No at-home time stupidness.

QUASHIE: (*Disgusted*) These days, you can't rely on the morning to be late.

DAY-TRIPPER: (*Stands up from her working*) Gettin hot in here. (*She fans herself with her dress and a flash of underwear shows.*) I'm glad I got me part time.

MRS. STARKEY: What kinda underwear you got on?

DAY-TRIPPER: (*Holds up her dress to reveal red underwear*) Frederick's Fashions. My niece give 'em to me.

HIDELMAN: God damn!

MRS. STARKEY: Some man'll go for it.

BETTY: (*About* DAY-TRIPPER, *dreamily*) She's so healthy.

MRS. STARKEY: I know me this young guy that got the hots for some old woman. Made people madder 'n hell cause that old lady cheated her last years like that. Well, I'll tell ya, love 'n death don't fit no pattern.

BETTY: (*Softly*) Yah.

HIDELMAN: (*Contemplating*) Young stud 'n old crow, huh?

MRS. STARKEY: Like fuckin in high cotton.

ELLIS: (*After a pause*) You miss havin little ones, Day-Tripper?

DAY-TRIPPER: (*Proudly*) See this? Locket. I won that at the Glass Pitch to our block party. (*She goes to* ELLIS *at her machine.*) Go on. Look to the inside.

(ELLIS *opens it. After a pause,* ELLIS *looks at the* DAY-TRIPPER *puzzled.*)

DAY-TRIPPER: (*Proudly*) That's right. There ain't nobody inside. (*She laughs happily.*) Empty! I got it good. (*She picks up her bucket and walks toward the exit. Pause.*) My friends . . . they are dyin and old. It's like life is jist gathered them up ta-gether in one little knot. (*Pause.*) Not me. Well it rains. . . 'n I don't have trouble with my bunions or my memories. (*Pause.*) I can see me a future for the first time. (*Pause.*) One more floor ta go. (*She exits.*)

BETTY: (*Saying after her*) Funny . . . how a person that don't love life . . . is still loved back by life innyway.

(*There is a pause as they work silently. Then,* ELLIS *looks at the clock.*)

ELLIS: I need 'n give my baby his milk.

(ELLIS *dashes to the washroom and holds the bottle to the baby as it sleeps in the play-pen. After a few seconds, her machine starts to bleep black and red distress lights.* ELLIS *runs frantically to her machine.*)

ELLIS: (*Terrified*) No!

HIDELMAN: The machine's finkin on ya, Ellis.

ELLIS: God! God! (*She hurriedly pushes gauges.*)

HIDELMAN: (*Laughing*) Yer officially behind.

QUASHIE: That's bad . . . nasty bad for truth.

HIDELMAN: Ellis is puttin us in jeopardy.

STARKEY: I'll double the 25-gauge.

(STARKEY *quickly adjusts some gauges and works some levers.*)

JUBA: Ten . . . ten . . . the Bible ten.

QUASHIE: No "Bible ten" can do nothin. What wrong with you.

(*Finally the machine becomes silent. After a few seconds:*)

STARKEY: (*Proudly*) You kin fool a *person*, but ya don't put nothin over on *them*. (*Points to the machines.*)

ELLIS: (*Weakly*) It got ra-corded. That I'm not kept up.

QUASHIE: Outside . . . you are watched by palms, snake-nuts, water . . . everything—without love, hate or put-en.

(ELLIS *continues working, but she is shaken.*)

HIDELMAN: (*To* ELLIS) They got yer number.

STARKEY: It ain't gonna do inny of us no good, Hidelman.

(*There is a silent pause as they work. After a pause,* HIDELMAN *sees* ELLIS *looking in her pockets and fingering clumps of napkins and toilet paper.* HIDELMAN *suddenly springs up like an animal and jumps on* ELLIS. HIDELMAN *knocks her to the floor.* ELLIS *knows she is outstripped and does not fight back.* HIDELMAN *knocks her about and pulls at her hair.*)

HIDELMAN: I seen you was stealin . . . you hairy billy.

MRS. STARKEY: Oh my God!

(HIDELMAN *is making kicking jabs at* ELLIS *on the floor.*)

STARKEY: Hidelman . . . she's got her baby in there. (*Points to the washroom.*)

HIDELMAN: Billy was stealin on us. (*She empties* ELLIS's *pockets.*) Napkins! Toilet paper!

STARKEY: You kin put it back now, Ellis.

HIDELMAN: That cud git us *cut*!

ELLIS: Don't tell 'em . . . please . . . don't tell 'em . . .

STARKEY: This floor don't have a chance something like that gets out.

ELLIS: (*Weakly*) . . . creamers from the Cafeteria, too.

HIDELMAN: Jesus!

ELLIS: . . . soap from the washroom.

HIDELMAN: Even goddamn urinal soap!

ELLIS: ... old uniforms ... cut up fer on his crib. (*Strongly.*) My baby needs him sheets ta the crib.

BETTY: (*Meaning to defend* ELLIS *but it doesn't come out that way.*) Ta the Cresten Factory, why there is so much stealin, they has sewed up all the women's pockets.

MRS. STARKEY: (*To* ELLIS) Go in and wash yer face off, honey.

JUBA: (*To* ELLIS) Let me help you, darlin.

(ELLIS *puts the stolen things on the coffee table. Then* JUBA *and* ELLIS *go to the washroom.* JUBA *helps* ELLIS *wipe her face.*)

STARKEY: Hidelman, you coulda killed her.

HIDELMAN: You couldn't hurt that billy with no two-by-four.

(*There is a pause and then* HIDELMAN, QUASHIE, STARKEY *and* MRS. STARKEY *go back to their machines. After a pause.*)

ELLIS: (*She comes out of the washroom*) You won't tell on me ... (*Weakly.*) ... They sent home a woman last week jist fer puking on a machine.

MRS. STARKEY: Even machines puke.

QUASHIE: I want to cascade....cascade on that machine right now me-self....and work off my mad. (QUASHIE *fake-gags on her machine.*)

(ELLIS *goes to her machine and starts working.*)

HIDELMAN: She'll git us all thrown out.....bringin in her kid... stealin....

QUASHIE: (*To* HIDELMAN) Let dot womahn be.

HIDELMAN: Damn Baptist "Jumper."

MRS. STARKEY: We can't all be Catholics.

BETTY: (*Meekly*) I'm Luthern.

HIDELMAN: (*To* BETTY) ....better 'n "Jumper."

ELLIS: (*Softly*) God don't be only ta Lutherns 'n Catholics.

BETTY: (*Innocently, in defense of* ELLIS) God belongs ta Pagans, too.

HIDELMAN: (*To* ELLIS) Why don't ya go back ta *Kan*-tucky!

(*After a pause,* HIDELMAN *goes to* ELLIS's *machine and jerks off two of the detachable levers.*)

HIDELMAN: You ain't got no right to this work, billy!

(ELLIS *tries to grab them back, but* HIDELMAN *dodges her.*)

STARKEY: (*Angry*) Hidelman...Hidelman...(STARKEY *rages toward* HIDELMAN *with a wrench. Pitch anger.*) I set those...I put them levers on myself! (STARKEY *grabs the levers from* HIDELMAN's *hands.*) You ivver do that a-gin, I'm gonna let yer machine spill on ya. Hear me! All over you good. I'll let it kill ya!

(HIDELMAN *backs away. Then* STARKEY *carefully and lovingly puts the levers back on* ELLIS's *machine.*)

MRS. STARKEY: My kid, the mechanic. She handles "know-how" like a knife—without no love.

(*They all work for a few seconds quietly.*)

ELLIS: (*Looking at the clock*) Elmhurst!

(*They all begin to work their levers more quickly.* ELLIS *runs to the washroom and picks up the baby. She takes the cardboard lid off a large trash can in the washroom, puts the baby in gently, then puts the lid partially on the top. The lid has large round holes punched in it. She hurriedly folds the small play-pen and puts it in a toilet stall in the washroom. Then she returns to the work area where they are quiet and serious.* HIDELMAN *glares at her as she returns to work. After a few seconds,* MR. ELMHURST *comes on stage with a clipboard. He is wearing the work uniform and a white helmet. "ELMHURST" is written on the back of his uniform in large, red letters. He goes promptly to the washroom and bangs on the door.*)

ELMHURST: Washroom check! (ELMHURST *looks at* STARKEY.)

STARKEY: All clear. (*As* ELMHURST *goes into the washroom.*) Hand dryer don't work right.

(ELMHURST *does not react to* STARKEY's *words. He looks around, flushes a toilet by a foot pedal, taps the vanity mirror with his clipboard, looks around, then sees the trash can and straightens the top. He sees he has gotten some grime from the trash lid. He puts his clipboard in his uniform pocket and then washes his hands in the sink. He turns on the hand blower, but it doesn't work. There is no towel dispenser. When he punches the "blower" it makes a beginning roar and instantly dies.*)

ELMHURST: Damn! (*He flaps his hands trying to dry them as he comes out of the washroom.*) Hand dryer don't work right!

ELLIS: Elmhurst, I...

BETTY: Mr. Elmhurst, could we... discuss *pension.*

HIDELMAN: We got us air burns, Elmhurst.

ELMHURST: (*Mock cheerfulness*) Half day. (*Pause.*) There's a ten per cent decrease in production speed. Upstairs is talking "nanoseconds." Know what that means?

HIDELMAN: Yah!

HIDELMAN *and* MRS. STARKEY: (*Together*) One-billionth of a second.

ELMHURST: Yer damn right! (*Now turns to* QUASHIE.) How's the leg, Quashie?

QUASHIE: Wherever you is, you is in life and that's sickness and death.

ELMHURST: Mavis told me.

QUASHIE: That doctor, he don't even "sound me."

(ELMHURST *looks at* QUASHIE *curiously.*)

JUBA: Mr. Gentleman... Quashie means the doctor don't listen to her heart... with that thing. (*She gestures a stethoscope.*)

ELMHURST: (*Disregarding that as usual* "QUASHIE" *talk*) How long on that?

QUASHIE: I make birthday in three weeks, and I make birthday "fine fit."

ELMHURST: (*Matter of fact*) Three weeks in the cast. (*Pause.*) Home accidents can take a person off the job like work accidents. Carry safety home, Quashie.

(ELMHURST *writes this accident down on his clipboard. He is still dealing with wet hands and they smear the ink. He angrily rips the paper off, crumbles it and puts it in his pocket.*)

ELMHURST: (*He writes. Pause*) Ok. Let's turn em off. Starkey!

(STARKEY *takes a special wrench and turns some device on the wall. The machines turn off.*)

ELMHURST: Open all crib doors.

(*They all open a bottom door on their machines.*)

ELLIS: (*Holding out the door*) No damage.

ELMHURST: (*Writing*) Check.

BETTY: I've got a bum one. (*She pulls a small bent wire out of the crib door.*)

ELMHURST: That's the second time.

STARKEY: I told ya, the moulding hole punch is dull. It needs oil.

ELMHURST: (*Irritated*) Ok... ok.

STARKEY: So if you was ta bring me some, I'd fix it.

ELMHURST: Right.

QUASHIE: (*Holding out the crib door*) Nottin.

ELMHURST: Check.

JUBA: Dis here clear.

ELMHURST: Check.

HIDELMAN: Clean.

ELMHURST: Check.

STARKEY: No damage.

ELMHURST: Check.

MRS. STARKEY: (*Holding the door*) Beat up rod. (*She pulls out a twisted rod.*)

ELMHURST: Damn!

STARKEY: Slug marks in the panel. It's pickin up buckles.

ELMHURST: Engineers tell me something different every day. Either they say zero, or everybody tells me something different.

STARKEY: I'll fix it, Elmhurst. I kin keep it out of writing.

ELMHURST: Ok... ok.

(*There is a pause as the women close up the bins.*)

ELMHURST: Let's turn 'em back on!

(STARKEY *turns on the wall device with her wrench.*)

MRS. STARKEY: When we ivver get ta wear real clothes?

ELMHURST: The job, Mrs. Starkey.

BETTY: (*Following* ELMHURST *around with her eyes as she works*) Mr. Elmhurst... Mr. Elmhurst....

ELMHURST: (*Not looking at* BETTY *as he is checking the area*) How's the mother, Betty?

BETTY: Mother 'n law.

ELMHURST: Right. How's the mother-in-law?

BETTY: Doctor has her on Cortisone. Now she has took sick from that ... they have give me pills ta help 'er with the Cortisone. I got me double medicine bills.

HIDELMAN: (*To* BETTY) Git some horse-temperature medicine. Doctors is not worth shit.

ELMHURST: There's no money for increases, Betty.

BETTY: I heard on the TV last night, companies don't put in to the Pension what they should.

ELMHURST: (*Turns to face her*) I belong to the Pension Plan. Would the company do that to me?

(BETTY *goes meekly back to her working and* ELMHURST *continues inspecting.*)

HIDELMAN: We got us air burns, Elmhurst.

ELMHURST: Later.

HIDELMAN: Leaks round the agitator shafts.

STARKEY: I kin put on the "Arkansas patch."

(ELMHURST *hands* STARKEY *some material.* STARKEY *then applies some plastic moulding to* HIDELMAN's *machine.*)

HIDELMAN: Ain't gonna last fer-ever. That's "billy-riggin"...slap up inny old thang.

ELMHURST: Some problems don't have answers, Hidelman. Take yer Tic-Tac-Toe Game. Lotta times nobody wins. Stalemate.

HIDELMAN: I ain't bout ta stale-mate with no machine. What about berylium dust?

ELMHURST: It's controlled.

HIDELMAN: We need the dust regulators.

ELMHURST: For what?

HIDELMAN: Fer our lungs.

ELMHURST: I've been here 12 years, and only one employee was hospitalized with lung spots.

MRS. STARKEY: (*Aside to* HIDELMAN) Pick beans in California, Hidelman.

HIDELMAN: Billy work.

MRS. STARKEY: (*Aside*) Git yerself some good outta those billy-kickers.

HIDELMAN: (*Grumbling*) Inside work.

ELMHURST: (*Routine warning*) Company gets new complicated safety machines, and they'll come with new trained people to work 'em. (*Pause.*) Hidelman, sister of yours find a job?

HIDELMAN: Waitressin. To the Cass Hotel. Nights.

ELMHURST: (*Still checking*) ...tips...good food.

HIDELMAN: She needs her somethin else... ta pay off bills.

ELMHURST: My wife was in Michael Reese Hospital. Just came home. I know bills.

HIDELMAN: ...eight kids.

ELMHURST: ...she's still not back to normal. I eat cold cereal in the morning. By myself.

ELLIS: I've been hearin we was having cutbacks.

ELMHURST: Don't listen to rumors.

HIDELMAN: Gallagher told me. I cashed my check to the Twins last night.

ELMHURST: Cash that check at a bank.

HIDELMAN: They don't cash fer free 'less you got an account there.

ELLIS: Who kin 'ford that?

STARKEY: I kin. (*Looking at her mother with a pleased smile*) Got me account at the Harris Bank.

MRS. STARKEY: Git married...'n you'll be to the Twins with yer check.

HIDELMAN: So what about Gallagher? He don't run off at the mouth.

ELMHURST: This company *does not* run by Gallagher.

HIDELMAN: He was first ta know bout Nadine Sitzes.

ELMHURST: (*Genuinely curious*) Nadine Sitzes. Where did Nadine go?

HIDELMAN: Last I heard, she has went ta the brewery in St. Louis.

ELMHURST: That right?

HIDELMAN: That's what I heard.

ELMHURST: How's she like it?

HIDELMAN: All I know, she has went ta St. Louis 'n found herself somethin at the brewery.

ELMHURST: Nadine Sitzes. (*He shakes his head in interest.*)

HIDELMAN: So if one or more of us is going, I say sooner we know, sooner ta start lookin.

ELLIS: (*Shaken*) Lookin?

ELMHURST: (*Becoming angry at the nagging*) I'm saying ... and I'm saying to all of you. Straight. I've heard there's attitude problems here.

BETTY: We git long fine, Mr. Elmhurst.

ELMHURST: . . . speed down on this floor.

STARKEY: We're working it out, Elmhurst.

ELMHURST: Food and pop in some of the machine cribs. Smoking outside the washroom. Pounding messages all ta hell to the Repair Pit . . . (*Pause.*) One more incident . . . one more.

STARKEY: We're shaped up now.

ELMHURST: This floor has to be! Cause some of management thinks there is waste here. (*Pause. He suddenly turns to mock cheerfulness.*) Not many places have half-days once a month. Recreation on company time. New computer blackjack.

HIDELMAN: (*Sullen*) Strings ta that, too.

ELMHURST: We like employees to participate. To compete. Learn to fight everything that wants us out of business.

ELLIS: (*Nervously*) Elmhurst, I was . . . I was wondering bout inventory thang we heard in announcements. (*Pause.*) Maybe new trainees is messed up?

ELMHURST: No new trainees anymore. You know that.

ELLIS: (*Meekly*) About the day nursery . . .

(ELMHURST *is busy with last minute inspections on the machines. He walks around* JUBA's *machine and steps on some corn kernels in his paper scuffs.*)

ELMHURST: God damn! (*He picks corn kernels painfully from his scuffs.*) What the hell's that!

JUBA: My "ju ju" workin.

ELMHURST: Get that "third world crap" off the floor, Juba. (*Pause.*) And whose safety mask is this? (*He picks it up . . . then looks for a blank space on the machines to see where it goes.*) I scream upstairs six months to get you women these, 'n nobody wears them. (*He replaces* HIDELMAN's *mask on her machine. Pause. Still groaning over his feet.*) Tarpaulin is not authorized. I told you that last week. I want it off. Tomorrow! (*He kicks at the floor. Does one final look around the area. After a pause.*) Starkey, over here for a minute.

(STARKEY *and* ELMHURST *go near the washroom to talk privately.*)

ELMHURST: I need some advice.

STARKEY: It jist wants fer oil.

ELMHURST: Not that. (*Pause.*) Doris . . . well . . . she's been home from
the hospital. A month now.

STARKEY: (*Pleased*) A month already?

ELMHURST: . . . she don't . . . well . . . you know . . . she don't . . .

STARKEY: . . . have her strength back.

ELMHURST: (*Eagerly*) That's right. (*Pause.*) She . . . cries all the time.
All the time. She says she came home without a baby . . . the first
time she came home from the hospital without a baby.

STARKEY: Jist tired. Organs that is left, Elmhurst, are doubled up.

ELMHURST: I . . . I don't know who else ta ask. I can't just go up to
Doris's mother. Or the doctor. Christ, the doctor's a woman.

STARKEY: Even when it's a woman, they're used ta it.

ELMHURST: You're young. The swinging generation
. . . acid . . . disco. Tell me . . . (*Pause.*) A total hysterectomy,
Starkey. You know what that means? (*Pause.*) We used to lay in
bed at night . . . and talk about the kids . . . how we loved each
other . . . touching . . . (*Pause.*) Now we lay in bed at night . . . . and
Doris tells me all the things the doctor took out. She knows the
medical names of everything. (*Pause.*) What's *fibroids*?

STARKEY: (*After a pause*) It all come out?

ELMHURST: Cause that's what I wanna know. (*Pause.*) She looks the
same. I can't tell the difference. (*Pause. Softly.*) The woman's only
45. She won't put a hand on me.

STARKEY: Forty-five! (*Pause.*) She . . . was . . . born in the . . . thirties.

ELMHURST: Is it all sewed up?

STARKEY: (*She looks at him blankly*) Elmhurst . . . I . . . I can't leave
my machine no longer . . . .

ELMHURST: (*Weakly*) Who else am I gonna ask, for Christsakes?

(ELLIS *goes back to her machine. After a pause, the hand blower is
heard coming on.* ELMHURST *listens, then reverts back to his business-
like composure and goes in the washroom. Inside he jiggles the
machine. It dies. He jiggles it some more and it sputters and then dies
again. Angry, he writes something on his clipboard. Then he looks
around for a final check, pats the trash can with his clipboard and is
about to leave when he sees something on the floor. He picks up a*

small baby bottle. He comes angrily out of the washroom holding the bottle.)

ELMHURST: Baby bottle!

HIDELMAN: It ain't mine.

(ELLIS *is white with fear.*)

ELMHURST: One of you women got a baby to . . .

ELLIS: It don't mean nothin.

ELMHURST: . . . to the parkin lot again?

HIDELMAN: (*Looking at* ELLIS) Mine is took care of. By sitters.

ELMHURST: That's all we need here. My God, I'm trying to hold on to this floor. I'm trying to keep all of you working.

(*There is a pause as he looks around at the working women.*)

ELMHURST: And requisition a new cover for the trash container in the washroom. (*After a pause. With a martyr attitude.*) Last foreman on this floor sold cars on the side. Buy a car from him—and he saw to it you girls worked yer fannies off to the factory for the next hundred years to pay it off. Do I do that? Do I take advantage? (*Pause. In desperation.*) What the hell do you women want?

HIDELMAN: (*After a pause*) I'd as soon be cold now, Elmhurst, than a lot colder tomorrow.

(ELMHURST *stares at her silently and then walks off the stage. After a pause.*)

HIDELMAN: (*To* ELLIS) You've done it now, billy! (ELLIS *runs to the washroom—puts the baby back in the play-pen.*)

STARKEY: Shut up, Hidelman. He don't know.

HIDELMAN: Mavis is gonna come through here now 'n take this floor apart . . . shake that kid outta us. We'll git throwed out on our ass.

BETTY: Mavis wouldn't do that.

HIDELMAN: (*She dramatically crosses her two fingers*) Mavis 'n the company are jist like *that . . .* 'at's Mavis on the bottom.

MRS. STARKEY: Nobody's seen them nothin'.

JUBA: (*Angry. To* HIDELMAN) You too damn gypsy, woman.

(ELLIS *returns frantically to her machine. They all work quietly for a few seconds. Curtain.*)

ACT II

Time: *Break time*
Later in the morning

At Rise: HIDELMAN *is checking out a fire-extinguisher to one side of the area.* STARKEY *is working on a machine.* ELLIS *is standing near the play-pen with the cardboard lid of the trash can punching in more holes as* BETTY, MRS. STARKEY, QUASHIE, *and* JUBA *stand near her in the washroom.*

ELLIS: (*Punching holes*) I'll jist git more holes to this 'n put him down deeper ta the trash can.

BETTY: That ain't the best place in the world fer baby, Ellis.

ELLIS: (*Defensive*) Not that much different 'n stale timothy hay 'n cow beddin to a barn.

MRS. STARKEY: We'll jist have ta requisition us new cover . . .

ELLIS: I kin make smaller holes so they don't see . . .

JUBA: (*Warning*) My old grandmother "dreamed me" last night, and say be careful of the mash-mouth white lady.

ELLIS: Mavis ain't gonna find him. (*Pause. Looking at them pleadingly.*) I know me this old lady ta down home . . . 'n she were like touched in the head 'n all . . . 'n people, they is criticized her cause she had this parakeet bird in a tiny bitty box and it couldn't even spread its wings.

QUASHIE: Poor little thing.

ELLIS: Oh, no. It was took real good care of.

MRS. STARKEY: (*Looking at the baby*) Yer mama know bout this?

BETTY: It can't be wrong, Mrs. Starkey, else Ellis would feel bad doin it.

ELLIS: I'm gonna keep him hid better.

(BETTY *and* MRS. STARKEY *and* JUBA *and* QUASHIE *look at* ELLIS *doubiously. Then they go to the mirror of the washroom to primp and chatter.* ELLIS *remains by the crib punching holes in the lid.*)

HIDELMAN: (*Holding an extinguisher*) Wheel-dry chemical extinguisher and the nozzle is broke off at the bottle.

STARKEY: It's on order.

HIDELMAN: We jist got us B and C extinguishers. What if yer type A fire starts?

STARKEY: The scram-alarm, Hidelman.

HIDELMAN: Heee . . . lllll. It's cheaper for them ta risk compensation payments ta the dead 'n beat up 'n buy decent equipment.

(*She slams the extinguisher angrily against the wall and goes inside the washroom.* STARKEY *remains working on the machines.* MRS. STARKEY *comes out of the washroom. She sits in the coffee area and calmly and defiantly smokes a cigarette. After a few seconds, the smoke alarm goes on.* STARKEY *runs to her mother, the others are used to this incident and go about their chatter.*)

STARKEY: Mom! The smoke alarm.

MRS. STARKEY: Ok . . . ok. (*She calmly waves the smoke away and puts the cigarette out in a kleenex in her pocket. After a few seconds, the alarm goes off.* MRS. STARKEY *takes out a plastic rain scarf and puts it on her head. Then some misty rain falls from a ceiling sprinkler for a few seconds as she lights up another cigarette.* STARKEY *goes to an inter-com phone on the wall.*)

STARKEY: (*Into the phone*) Floor B. False alarm.

(STARKEY *hangs up. Her mother takes off the rain scarf and lights up another cigarette, keeping it held way down from her near the floor.*)

MRS. STARKEY: "Break" is late ta-day.

STARKEY: We was early last week. (*Pause.*) Yer suppose to do that inside.

MRS. STARKEY: You have aspirin? Feels like my skull is splitting open.

STARKEY: (*Suspicious*) Oh, no!

MRS. STARKEY: Yer not too old ta be slapped. (*She yanks at* STARKEY's *arm.* STARKEY *winces in pain and then goes to the first aid box on the wall and gets a tin of aspirin and thrusts her hand out to her mother.*) I ain't gonna main-line it. (*Pause. Seeing her daughter doesn't believe her.*) Wanna put it on my tongue?

STARKEY: You'll ruin the health what you got, mama.

MRS. STARKEY: (*Holding out an aspirin*) Nice little harmless "toke" like that?

STARKEY: (*Trying to scare her*) I seen me this old man once . . . 'n he didn't have him no more room to his arms . . . he was shooting up ta the veins in his head.

MRS. STARKEY: Aspirin! Shootin stuff's a hassle . . . keeps ya runnin ever minute . . . so ya ain't got time fer nothin else. (*Pause.*) Between me 'n the rent 'n a few good-lookin dudes, the money don't last.

STARKEY: (*Determined but with a pleading tone*) I was down ta Halstead Street and here you come . . . old wig on yer head, wrinkled up clothes . . . drunk. (*Pause.*) I don't want my mama down on Halstead drinking 'n dropping pills jist like everything else I see ta the street on Friday night.

(*There is a pause.* STARKEY *just glares at her mother.* MRS. STARKEY *puts the aspirin dramatically on her tongue.*)

MRS. STARKEY: There!

STARKEY: (*Going to the cooler for a glass of water*) It kin burn yer stomach dry like that.

(MRS. STARKEY *makes a gulping motion. Then she takes a long sensuous drag from her cigarette.* STARKEY *hands her the water, and* MRS. STARKEY *suddenly begins to shake.*)

MRS. STARKEY: Ahhhhhh . . . Turnin on! Gettin me "Bliss" . . . I got sin . . . from Buff—a—rin!

(MRS. STARKEY *waves the glass of water in the air and then stands up on her chair yelping.*)

STARKEY: (*Truly concerned*) Mom . . . you come down . . . you come down from there. (STARKEY *runs to the washroom and calls to the others. Desperate.*) You gotta help me with my mother. She is took sick.

(*Everybody comes to the door of the washroom, stamping out their cigarettes before they come out.*)

HIDELMAN: What the hell!

(MRS. STARKEY *abruptly stops and gets off the chair.*)

MRS. STARKEY: My kid jist give me some bad stuff.

STARKEY: (*Relieved*) Don't scare me like that, Mom. It ain't funny!

(*The others shrug, used to* MRS. STARKEY's *madness.* STARKEY *begins cleaning up the broken glass from her mother.* HIDELMAN *and* ELLIS *return to the washroom.* HIDELMAN *massages her scalp and smokes and stares in the mirror as she does this.* ELLIS *is sitting on the floor next to the play-pen punching more holes in the trash-lid.* QUASHIE *and* JUBA *go to their lockers and get out their mesh bags of coconuts. They take them to the coffee area table where they sit and paint blue circles on the tops of the coconuts.* BETTY *watches.* STARKEY *goes to the pay phone in the coffee area and* MRS. STARKEY *follows.*)

STARKEY: I'm calling Daddy.

MRS. STARKEY: What for?

STARKEY: You're gonna talk ta him! (*She puts money in and dials.*)

MRS. STARKEY: Like hell.

STARKEY: It's busy. (*She hangs up.*) You said you was willin ta talk. (*Weakly.*) I . . . I want us family again.

MRS. STARKEY: You wanna be a hot-shot mechanic. Well a family don't know inny-thing. It don't pass on no information to what you need with *them.*(*Points to the machine. Pause. Not harshly.*) I'll smoke to the washroom if it makes you so damn almighty happy.

(MRS. STARKEY *walks to the washroom where she goes to comb her hair and primp while smoking.* STARKEY *follows her.*)

JUBA: (*To* BETTY) You want to buy a nice coconut, darlin?

BETTY: I can't eat 'em. I got me "floating plates." (*She moves her mouth awkwardly.*)

JUBA: These come from my cousin. Right on Air Jamaica.

BETTY: Why ya paintin that there on it?

JUBA: So the rats won't eat them.

QUASHIE: We sell these by the lake-front on Sunday. Juba and me was higglers back home when little girls in "Bessie-My-Nanny Gap." (*Pause. Wistfully.*) I had this old house there . . . with a back porch to the ocean . . . broken down old house that did sing just from its water-side.

(*There is a silent pause.* BETTY *watches intently as they work and talk.*)

JUBA: I hear Adassa wants to marry the new overseer at Half-Way-Tree. That overseer, him a jackass.

QUASHIE: That's just gossip.

JUBA: It's gossip whether I say it or not. (*Pause.*) You know, Ismay got she-self engaged to Gobin.

QUASHIE: That Gobin . . . he brave in he front-porch way.

JUBA: He has over three thousand in the Barclay's Bank.

QUASHIE: You hear somebody theif Man-Boy's wallet? They found it empty in the shallow water top-side the market.

JUBA: My Lor's. My Lor's.

QUASHIE: My aunt just come from Kingston. Cleaning work's scarce and is three weeks now she ain't workin.

(MRS. STARKEY *comes out of the washroom.*)

MRS. STARKEY: I got something ta show you, Betty. (*Hands her a small snap shot from her pocket.*) See this?

BETTY: (*A pause as she stares at the picture blankly.*)

MRS. STARKEY: Look long enough, you kin see the face of Jesus.

BETTY: Nothin here but wavy lines.

MRS. STARKEY: It's a picture of the ocean. Took by a sailor from Moline in a typhoon. (*Pause as* BETTY *studies the picture.*)

BETTY: I can't see nothin.

MRS. STARKEY: You jist keep it till ya do. Took me two hours. Then I seen the beard 'n right way my brother calls ta tell me he could maybe pay back ten a month come August.

(*There is a pause.* BETTY *stares at the picture and then passes it around to* QUASHIE *and* JUBA. *They look at it blankly and finally return it to* BETTY.)

BETTY: When I married Al, the old lady was up ta Peoria, Ill-a-noise. Maybe we seen her twice a year. That's all. (*Pause.*) I never had me no kids. We tried. (*Pause.*) Some people said we was lucky. Come 'n go like at when we wanted. I could keep thangs one with kids couldn't . . . white throw rugs . . . (*Pause.*) Then Al died. Old lady took sick.

MRS. STARKEY: Nothin ivver works out like ya want it to. I had me five hundred dollars. Could-of been through beauty school by now.

BETTY: ... a friend from down-home come to visit last week. Ta spell me from the old lady. Know what I did? (*Pause.*) I called Leota cross the street. Leota, I says over the phone, Leota—I'm coming over ta-night. I got somebody here with Mom. I don't care ya got plans or not. If yer taking off somewheres, I'll stay anyway ... by myself ... to yer living room. (*Pause.*) And I did. (*Pause.*) Sometimes I get scared. Scared of bein lone with her. I see her lay there ... eyes closed ... 'n think she's dead. I don't hear no breathin. I go up ... touch her mouth 'n sometimes even then it don't move. But the stomach twitches ... jist a little ...'n ...

MRS. STARKEY: (*Trying to be cheerful*) Come on, Betty. I got us a hor-ror-scope.

(MRS. STARKEY *takes a page of a newspaper from her pocket.*)

MRS. STARKEY: What's yer sign?

BETTY: Tarus.

MRS. STARKEY: Leo.

(MRS. STARKEY *and* BETTY *sit close together and look at the paper.*)

BETTY: This here is last week's.

MRS. STARKEY: I know.

BETTY: What good's last week's horra-scope?

MRS. STARKEY: So I kin tell what has came true.

BETTY: Oh.

(BETTY *and* MRS. STARKEY *look together at the article and converse quietly.* HIDELMAN *is still in the washroom. She goes to* ELLIS *and stands over the play-pen.*)

HIDELMAN: (*Looking at the baby*) Think I wouldn't like one of *mine* here.

ELLIS: (*Anxious*) Yers is older, Hidelman.

HIDELMAN: (*Rattles the play-pen side where the bolt is loose*) Where'd ya git this?

ELLIS: (*Proudly*) It was little Donny's ... 'n give ta me by my sister over ta Romeoville.

HIDELMAN: You get it from the "Sally"?

ELLIS: I don't buy me innythin to the Salvation Army ... cause of one give Sue Ellen lead poisoning.

HIDELMAN: You got you "Sally" clothes, 'n "Sally" furniture ... n' ...

STARKEY: (*Annoyed with* HIDELMAN's *taunting*) Hidelman!

HIDELMAN: Go ta Ellis' house 'n see yerself No. 10 cans of beans 'n corn ta the table.

STARKEY: You are wasting "break." Let's git us a pop.

HIDELMAN: (*To* ELLIS) Don't ivver come outta here ... you too good, Billy, 'n talk ta the rest of us?

ELLIS: Down home ... you has knew people since you was born 'n they know if you sucked yer thumb or if you're shy or got the hives. Saves a lotta talkin. (*Pause.*) I'm jist not used ta it, Hidelman.

HIDELMAN: Hee...llll. (*Pause. Looking at the baby.*) Don't git us "dumped on" cause of that kid.

STARKEY: Hidelman ... come on ... you said I could see what ya got yer cousin fer wedding gift.

(HIDELMAN *comes out of the washroom with* STARKEY. HIDELMAN *gets a package from her locker.*)

HIDELMAN: I got these ordered outta Rockford. For her weddin night. (*Holds them out. Pause*) Six pair of purple pants with no crotch in 'em.

(STARKEY *is embarrased.*)

MRS. STARKEY: What's that you got, Hidelman?

STARKEY: (*Embarrassed*) Jist *purple,* Mom.

MRS. STARKEY: (*Laughing lewdly while looking at them*) He's gonna lose it all over hisself.

HIDELMAN: (*Taking this as a criticism*) She ain't hitchin up with no one-shot-a-night.

MRS. STARKEY: That's what they all say.

(STARKEY *looks at her mother embarrassedly and then goes to the pop machine.*)

MRS. STARKEY: (*After a pause*) Let me buy one offa you?

HIDELMAN: No way! These was on back order for two months so many people has bought them!

BETTY: (*Innocently*) Those wouldn't fit you, Mrs. Starkey.

MRS. STARKEY: It's what *fits* the man, Betty. I got me a "tight little box."

STARKEY: (*Embarrassed. Drawing attention from her mother, she stands at the pop machine. To* HIDELMAN:) You got change for five?

HIDELMAN: It's been so long since I had *five* on a Thursday, Hee . . . lllll, I don't member last time I did. (*Puts her money in and takes out a cup from the machine.*) Looka that. Coke with no ice. (*She puts the cup back in the machine and pounds on it. The machine now "sprays" out coke all over* HIDELMAN's *feet.*) Shit!

MRS. STARKEY: (*Not even looking up from her paper*) Machine pee-in' on you again, Hidelman?

HIDELMAN: (*Looking down at her feet*) I've been pissed on so much by this damn place my feet is yellow. (*Takes out the cup and shakes it. Angry.*) Putrid!

BETTY: You don't have ta drink it, Hidelman.

HIDELMAN: (*Suffering as she drinks*) I paid for *this*. (*Finally drinks it all down as if it were medicine and angrily crumbles the cup and throws it in the trash. She reaches for the napkin holder to get a napkin, but the napkins are so tightly packed they won't come out.*) Damnit ta hell. (*Holds the container by the inside napkin, dangling the container in the air.*) How ya 'spose ta git one?

BETTY: Maintenance does that so they don't come out too many.

(HIDELMAN *puts the container on the floor, puts her feet around both sides, yanks. A clump comes out. She wipes her hands and puts the container back. As she is doing this,:*)

HIDELMAN: You mean so the billy don't steal 'em.

STARKEY: Forget that, Hidelman. If Elmhurst . . .

HIDELMAN: Fuck Elmhurst.

BETTY: Elmhurst has ta push 'n nobody likes a pusher.

STARKEY: He don't, somebody else does.

JUBA: I accept the boss if he don't hag me or slap me on the back with a knife.

QUASHIE: Used ta be if you wanted something bad, you could dip in Tilla's conch chowder back home.

BETTY: Want to look to this picture, Starkey, 'n hunt for the face of Jesus?

STARKEY: I seen that 'n there ain't nothin on it.

BETTY: (*In mild rebuke*) If you died, Starkey, if you was to pass-away now . . . where would you spend eternity?

STARKEY: (*Assured. Sassy*) Down there! (*Points to the floor.*) It's gonna be all done up real good with thermostats 'n dials 'n stuff. It ain't like yer old hell.

BETTY: (*Shaking her head in disapproval at* STARKEY. *To* JUBA) Juba, play me sum checkers?

JUBA: All right with me, yes. But I'll win again, darlin. (*Pause.*) Quashie, put these coconuts back. Work be starting soon.

(*Suddenly a strong glare of light comes through the blackened panes of the large factory window.*)

MRS. STARKEY: Look . . . the wind-das is lit up.

QUASHIE: Sun's out.

(*All the women go to the window, crowd around it, and find a blackened panel to spread their hands against a blackened pane. Except for* STARKEY. STARKEY *just watches them.*)

QUASHIE: I need to see the sky.

STARKEY: Why?

QUASHIE: It is big and empty like the sea.

BETTY: I like me the Chicago River. Funny bout a river . . . it's always changing . . . it ain't like yer ocean, Quashie . . . you jist don't know what it'll do . . . what's gonna be round that next bend.

QUASHIE: Work . . . work . . . and I can't feel the air.

BETTY: Look the way these wind-da frames is cracked . . . little veins ivver which way . . . jist like the outside is strikin back at "in here."

HIDELMAN: Quashie, some day I'm gonna buy me a house with its back ta Chicago . . . an empty lot next ta it. And I'll have open space ta the side. Like country.

MRS. STARKEY: It would be nice if factories lived like people . . . maybe 60 . . . 70 years. Then died. But damn it, they kin go on 'n on. This joint ain't ivver gonna check-out.

(*Suddenly* QUASHIE *bashes in one of the window panes with a coconut she is still holding.*)

QUASHIE: (*Breaking one of the window panes*) Kai-so . . . ai-o . . . kai-so.

(ELLIS *comes out of the washroom to stare.*)

JUBA: (*Goes to her and pulls* QUASHIE *from the window*) What you at, woman? How you do!

QUASHIE: I'll get all of them!

(QUASHIE *tries to break the other window panes. The women move around her to restrain her.*)

JUBA: What is this at all!

QUASHIE: (*Gently breaks away from restraint. She slowly puts one hand through the broken pane*) Humming birds are so tame, they sip the flowers right in your fingers.

STARKEY: (*Alarmed*) Look what you've did, Quashie!

QUASHIE: (*Goes to her machine*) That machine . . . it don't go crazy. (*She calls to the machine.*) You can do anything . . . but you don't go crazy.

JUBA: (*Going to her. Tenderly*) What you don't have, you not meant to get.

QUASHIE: I got blood in me of Gold Coast Slaves.

STARKEY: (*Nervous*) Quashie, you heard what Elmhurst said . . .

HIDELMAN: (*Defensive for* QUASHIE) I know what it's like ta want outside.

MRS. STARKEY: (*Aside*) Floor's carryin loons.

QUASHIE: (*Points to machine*) It will kill the light in my eyes!

JUBA: (*Firmly but tenderly*) If you do this another time, I hope the sperrids drag you away and don't let you come back.

QUASHIE: Folks here . . . they don't fear lightning or thunder or the wind. Nothin from outside. They don't love it, either.

JUBA: Woman, yuh relax 'n jes hold strain . . . jes hold strain.

(ELLIS *goes back in the washroom.*)

HIDELMAN: (*Standing by the broken window pane*) I'll put the safety poster over this. So nobody sees.

MRS. STARKEY: Damn . . . "break's" almost over.

(*The women go back to the area.* QUASHIE *begins gathering up the coconuts in a sack.* BETTY *sets up a checker game on a stool in the coffee area—intermittently looking at her photo of the ocean.* STARKEY *goes to the machine area to give them a look over.* HIDELMAN *takes a safety poster from the coffee area and tacks it over the broken window pane.* MRS. STARKEY *goes back to reading her horoscope.*)

QUASHIE: Folks on Cat Island . . . right now, sitting in they door-mouth old-talking . . . lazin in the shade.

(*There is a silence for several seconds.*)

QUASHIE: I hunt turtle . . . put that turtle on his back, feet out, neck bent. Slit the belly with my knife, then stick my hand inside. I get the heart ... flip it on the ground. That turtle-heart jumps round hard, then it goes soft and beats nice and quiet by itself in the dust. Turtle ... he be so strong he'll live even with his heart gone. Even with he heart there next to he on the dirt.

JUBA: Quashie, you is in Chicago!

QUASHIE: (*Angry*) Plantin machines all over like they're posting they flag of conquest.

JUBA: This here is Chicago and it be the only work we have.

QUASHIE: Cat Island is where you can hold up your head. Cat Island is your peace of mind.

(JUBA *goes to* QUASHIE *and puts* QUASHIE'*s hands firmly to the levers.*)

JUBA: This is where you is and where all you pickney is in and nobody is taking off for Cat Island. We is staying here, all we do.

(*There is a pause. Then the horn sounds.* ELLIS *shoves the play-pen inside the washroom and returns to work.* BETTY *has the picture up against a ledge on her machine. She has put the checkers game on a stool near her machine. The women all work silently at their machines for several seconds.*)

ELLIS: (*Defiant. To* HIDELMAN) We was kids, winter, it was hell. Ten of us ... packed inta three room. Summer—least we was all ta the outside ... workin the bean fields. Not yer eight hours. It was 12 ... 14 hours.

HIDELMAN: Billies like "stoop" work.

ELLIS: (*In defiance to* HIDELMAN) Least ya had yer folks right next ta you. (*Pause.*) We come up hard. I had dogs git sick all over me ... a one-arm-man behind me pickin beans 'n pushin hard ta my back. We is like ate boiled caribou 'n had ta pick the deer hairs off forewe chewed on it even ... worked like damn dogs make it pay off.

HIDELMAN: No billy I ivver saw worked like a damn dog.

STARKEY: Bug off, Hidelman.

ELLIS: ... nights ... I'd git so chilled jist drunk me the juice from a bottle of hot peppers 'n sweated ta keep warm.

BETTY: (*To* JUBA) Yer first this time, Juba.

(JUBA *moves a checker.* BETTY *and* JUBA *play checkers in between moving their machine levers.*)

ELLIS: (*Looking at the clock*) Mavis!

(ELLIS *runs in the washroom, puts the baby in the trash can and hides the play-pen and returns to her machines seconds before* MAVIS *arrives. They all work silently. After a few seconds,* MRS. STARKEY *takes out a cigarette from her purse and smokes it by the machine guardedly.)*

BETTY: *(Hesitating)* Mrs. Starkey . . . yer . . . not sa-pose ta smoke outside the washroom.

(MRS. STARKEY *ignores this and continues smoking.)*

STARKEY: *(She shoves her levers in anger as she looks at her mom.)*

(There is a few seconds of silence and then MAVIS *comes on stage wearing the same uniform as the others.* MRS. STARKEY *hurriedly puts out her cigarette on the floor with her foot.* MAVIS *sniffs the air and then goes to* MRS. STARKEY.*)*

MAVIS: *(To* MRS. STARKEY*)* I don't ivver wanna see you grind out a cigarette cause ya seen me. Thangs go good, jist sneak one by the area. Thangs is behind, I wanna see you snuff out that cigarette 'n jump in 'n git the job done. *(Pause.)* Ok?

MRS. STARKEY: *(Sullen)* Ok.

MAVIS: Now that don't mean Elmhurst.

(MAVIS *goes to the bulletin board to start to pin a notice on it. Then she sees something, takes it off the board and goes to* MRS. STARKEY *in an officious manner.)*

MAVIS: *(Matter of fact and used to this kind of thing)* Rubber-penis don't belong ta a company bulletin board. (MAVIS *lets out the air and hands it to* MRS. STARKEY *and then returns to pin her notice to the board.* MRS. STARKEY *puts the object in her pocket without reacting.)*

HIDELMAN: *(Snickering)* You knock ta Mrs. Starkey's door . . . 'n you'll hear this . . . blllllllllll *(She makes a noise of air coming out of a balloon)* . . . in there makin it with her "Ken doll" . . .

STARKEY: *(Angry)* Hidelman!

MAVIS: *(She is used to all this chatter. Coming from the bulletin board, matter of fact)* All personnel required ta read the Company Bulletin Board before each work day terminates. *(Pause.)* Quashie, leg holding up? I don't want you behind.

QUASHIE: *(Defensive)* You know is one thing I never do.

MAVIS: I see that. But soon as I tell a woman she's doin good, sure as hell the next day her work is shit.

STARKEY: Quashie is kept up, Mavis.

MAVIS: I don't wanna see this here floor charged with "lost-time-acci-dent."

BETTY: Mavis . . .

MAVIS: One at the time. One at *the* time.

BETTY: Mavis, when kin we get in-fermation bout pension?

MAVIS: What kind of in-fermation?

BETTY: I hear we put in our share, but the Company don't match it.

MAVIS: I'm on the same pension. You think I'd calmly stand here if Pension was in arrears?

BETTY: . . . if I could go over what I got . . .

MAVIS: (*Takes out a little book*) We got us a job with good gravity. Look, says right here in "Professional Agreement." Says here: "Company oblighed ta match contributions of its 'sociates." (*Pause.*) How's the mother?

BETTY: Mother-n-law.

MAVIS: Mother-n-law.

BETTY: I think by the smell she has her the cancer. (*Pause.*) I got me double medicine bills.

HIDELMAN: Mavis, we hear talk of cutbacks.

MAVIS: Where'd ya hear that?

HIDELMAN: To the Twins. Gallagher.

MAVIS: (*Points to her union book*) Company gives all sociates prior warning from 20 days not to 'ceed 30 of inny cutbacks, be it machine or person.

ELLIS: Did the Sociation hear inny-thing?

MAVIS: I was to the meeting last night. There was no mention of cut-backs.

HIDELMAN: Gallagher told me.

MAVIS: Gallagher don't know.

BETTY: (*More to herself than to the others*) Holdin on ta a job, that's half of it.

ELLIS: (*Nervous*) If ya hear . . .

HIDELMAN: I say sooner we know . . . sooner ta start lookin.

ELLIS: (*Shaken*) Lookin?

HIDELMAN: Yah. Lookin.

BETTY: I got me seniority.

HIDELMAN: Seniority don't mean shit ta the 'sociation.

MAVIS: You give a woman seniority, 'Hidelman, 'n you make her scared ta move. You turn a job right inta the *grave*.

(HIDELMAN *glares at* MAVIS *and then holds out one hand to* MAVIS *in defiance.*)

HIDELMAN: (*Still working but with one hand out*) Whatta ya see, Mavis?

(MAVIS *looks blankly.*)

HIDELMAN: The fingernails!

MAVIS: They're dirty.

HIDELMAN: Look a-gin. That ain't dirt.

(*There is a pause.*)

HIDELMAN: Skin under there's dark blue. From s'posure ta aldrin spills.

MAVIS: (*Firm*) You show me *one* monitor that has registered *spills*!

HIDELMAN: (*Shaking her hand*) Don't tell me!

MAVIS: I got us promised safety showers, Hidelman.

HIDELMAN: That crap goes through unbroken skin.

MAVIS: I do eight hours here ... nother full time job 'n do fer my family at home. Then the sociation.

BETTY: (*Defensive*) Mavis got us air vents.

MAVIS: You kin win a thousand thangs, lose one, yer no good bitch.

HIDELMAN: Sociation don't win less the Company wants it to.

QUASHIE: Hay-men. Hay-men.

MAVIS: I'm responsible for this here table ... coffee and pop machine. We have the decent area fer rest periods.

HIDELMAN: You know what you kin do with benefits.

MAVIS: I got you off Good Friday. Noon ta three.

HIDELMAN: We shoulda had us off *all* day.

ELLIS: Jesus hanged to the cross from twelve ta three.

HIDELMAN: Yah? Is that "Jumper" time?

MAVIS: Who the hell cares when he was on the cross. I got all you off three full hours.

(HIDELMAN *picks up the table and throws it across the room. After the table lands,*)

QUASHIE: Just like lightning strike the house and kill the dog under de porch, what har do that for?

(*There is a pause of silence as the others look on anxiously.* HIDELMAN *stands fiercely by the table. After a pause,* STARKEY *goes to the table and examines it.*)

STARKEY: Couple cracks in the leg. I kin fix it. (*She goes back to her machine.*)

HIDELMAN: I'm tired of losin ... raises, my color TV, snow tires! I want me money—not tables.

MAVIS: On yer 40 cent raise, I git you 20 cents on benefits 'n 20 cents on yer check. (*Angry.*) Floor here is talked about. Floor B has attitude problems.

(HIDELMAN *then carries the table back to where it was. She takes a broom from the side of the area and runs the broom defiantly over the top of the table.*)

MRS. STARKEY: (*Indignant*) I eat offa that.

(HIDELMAN *ignores* MRS. STARKEY's *comment and returns to her machine.*)

HIDELMAN: Ain't nobody lookin backwards. People has went up in 'sociation 'n fergot all the worst places ... where women is bustin their asses off.

MAVIS: I *learned* Elmhurst. Remember! I learned him 'n then watched him go up 'n git more money 'n better job. You think I liked that? (*Pause.*) I'm the only one here that worked to the Repair Pit. (*Holds out her right hand.*) I lost these on the Grinder down there. When my two best fingers was bein ate up, I was screamin my head off fer hours. Only nobody could hear me down there with the noise. Nobody could hear! And don't you forget that!

(*There is a pause as all but* HIDELMAN *act remorseful.*)

HIDELMAN: Like I said, Mavis, you ain't lookin backwards. You got you somethin good in "Shippin."

MAVIS: I got bills up one side 'n down the other. Station wagon last month with broken transmission. Kid in braces. I don't git management pay.

BETTY: Do what you kin, Mavis.

MAVIS: (*Calming down*) I'll bring up kin-cern bout cutbacks to the Sociation next Thursday.

ELLIS: What bout the day nursery? For our kids?

MAVIS: (*Helpless*) Every time I brung that up, I was "out of order." It's always "out of order."

ELLIS: My little Donny, Dwane, Sue Ellen an' Janice has ta stand outside in the rain till school opens every morning. Dwane has took sick from the bronchitis. . . .

MAVIS: (*Helpless*) I got me a whole set of minutes wrote up fer a meetin on "day nursery" which ain't never took place.

JUBA: Children need care, Mavis.

MAVIS: I'm doin what I kin. Cause 'sociation kin git me fired jist as fast as the Company.

(*After a pause.*)

MAVIS: Now I'm jist gonna have me a "look see" ta the washroom . . . 'n out ta the parkin lot.

ELLIS: (*Frightened*) Why?

MAVIS: Elmhurst is . . .

ELLIS: He ain't found him nothin!

MAVIS: (*After a pause of looking at the women*) This floor got them somethin hid?

(*After a pause,* MAVIS *walks to the washroom.* ELLIS, *frightened, follows her.*)

STARKEY: Ellis, machine is gonna "fink" on you agin.

(MAVIS *looks around for a few seconds and then sees the trash can. She holds up the lid with the holes in it.*)

MAVIS: This some kinda game!

ELLIS: (*Pleading*) Mavis . . .

(MAVIS *puts the lid with the holes up against the wall. She picks up an old patch of boarding against the wall and puts it on the trash can.*)

ELLIS: (*Screeching*) No! (*She pulls the boarding off.*)

MAVIS: That's what I thought. (*Pause. Looking at* ELLIS.) I don't know what is hid in there . . . dog . . . cat . . . I don't wanna know . . . but you git it gone ta-morrow.

ELLIS: (*Wimpering*) Mavis . . . you is put little Royce ta yer car in the parkin lot ... when he had hisself a cold 'n couldn't go ta school.

MAVIS: (*Defensive*) Once ... that was a long time ago, Ellis.

ELLIS: (*Weakly, muttering*) ... my little Donny, he is good ta baseball. Why he is hitting from both sides of the plate. But I ain't saw me none of the games ... 'n I couldn't 'ford 'n buy him a baseball glove so I jist stuffed rags inna old sock ...

MAVIS: (*Pause. Not harshly*) Ellis ... tomorrow. Ok? Now I ain't seen me nothin. Ok? (*Pause.*) You git yerself back ta work.

(MAVIS *puts the lid with the holes back on the trash can. When* ELLIS *sees this, she goes back to her machine.* MAVIS *comes out of the washroom. She checks a list.*)

MAVIS: Ok ... who is had them nosebleeds?

(*Silence. There is no answer.*)

MAVIS: (*After a pause. Aggravated*) Well ... suit yerself. I'd bring on in a nasal smear, that's what I'd do. (*Pause.*) 'Sociation gets us free contamination checks. Yer benefit. (*Pause.*) Now, who had them their "period" all messed up?

ELLIS: I'm bleedin heavy...twice a month.

MAVIS: (*Officious*) Urine sample, Ellis. 'Fore next Tuesday. (MAVIS *looks around the room for a final check.*) What the hell's that? (MAVIS *shakes her head in irritation as* JUBA *looks down guiltily.*) Juba, keep "jig-a-boo" off the floor. Elmhurst don't like it. (*After a pause.*) And Hidelman... (*Kicking at the floor covering*)...this don't meet with approval. I told you that last week.

(MAVIS *then goes to the table and turns it around so the cracked leg won't show. She adjusts and pats the table protectively. Then she exits. As soon as* MAVIS *exits,* ELLIS *gets her baby from the trash can and puts him in the play-pen and returns to work. They work silently for a few seconds. Then* HIDELMAN *begins to laugh.*)

HIDELMAN: Well ... billy, looks like the kid is *movin out....*

MRS. STARKEY: I'm glad somebody is. (*After a pause,* MRS. STARKEY *stops working. She puts her hands down on the floor.*) No vibration from downstairs. They have shut off fer "break." (MRS. STARKEY *takes a wrench near her machine and then thumps the floor.*)

STARKEY: Mom, don't do that.

MRS. STARKEY: (*Still pounding*) Come on... come on.... (MRS. STARKEY *stops. After a few seconds, a thumping sound is heard back.*)

BETTY: (*In awe*) The repair pit. When yer underground like that, you'd better be sisters.

MRS. STARKEY: They want prices from the Van.

BETTY: You jist got the *same* in the Van, Mrs. Starkey.

HIDELMAN: Yah. Like home. Vanilla.

MRS. STARKEY: Gonna be "French" vanilla this time. (STARKEY *glares angrily at her mother.* MRS. STARKEY *thumps back a "ten" and then* STARKEY *goes to her and takes the wrench back.*)

STARKEY: (*To her mother*) You want *cut?*

(*They all go back to working. After a pause:*)

BETTY: We don't ivver go ta other departments like we done . . . in the beginnin . . . .

MRS. STARKEY: So what?

BETTY: Sometimes . . . it'd be fun ta . . . you know . . . work some other area for while.

HIDELMAN: (*Stops*) Who wants ta change with me?

STARKEY: Come on, Hidelman, not that again.

HIDELMAN: Somebody trade machines with me.

BETTY: We're not suppose ta 'n you know it.

JUBA: What's wrong with you?

STARKEY: We stay to our own machines, Hidelman. You know that.

HIDELMAN: Ellis, come on. Swap!

ELLIS: (*Nervous*) I . . . I . . .

HIDELMAN: Come on!

ELLIS: (*Meekly*) I don't know, Hidelman.

HIDELMAN: (*Goes to* ELLIS'S *area*) Go on! You ain't fraid 'n steal . . . damnit, you ain't fraid ta "trade."

(HIDELMAN *and* ELLIS *trade machines. There is a pause and they work the other person's machine.*)

HIDELMAN: Nothin to it! (*Happily.*) Piece of cake!

ELLIS: Not too long . . . ok?

HIDELMAN: Git yerself new outlook from nother area.

STARKEY: Come on, Hidelman!

HIDELMAN: Git me some variety round here.

(*Pause of a few seconds.*)

STARKEY: Ok, Hidelman...nough!

(HIDELMAN *gives* ELLIS *a look of contempt and then they both switch back to their own machines. After a pause:*)

JUBA: (*Moving a checker to jump one of* BETTY'*s*) Buh, how a person catch her royal when she don't watch me-self.

BETTY: I didn't see that.

HIDELMAN: Like hell. Why ya let her win all the time?

BETTY: Juba likes winnin. Me... I play cause the "clock is fighting."

MRS. STARKEY: (*Stroking a lever. To* QUASHIE) Your Darlton inny good, Quashie?

QUASHIE: His face all Carib buck. (*Laughing.*) Him suck from a Carib womahn, aw-right.

MRS. STARKEY: My "ex" has a dick so small even the whores on Ogden Avenue don't charge him list price.

STARKEY: Mom! (*She winces painfully.*)

BETTY: Companionship's more important.

MRS. STARKEY: The hell it is! Good screw's like... bowlin a perfect game.

HIDELMAN: I found me these "rubbers" in my old man's glove compartment.

MRS. STARKEY: Yah?

HIDELMAN: Colored ones... red ... yellow ... blue ...*real* fancy.

MRS. STARKEY: Yah?

HIDELMAN: .....'n I jis took a pin 'n I put a hole in all of 'em! Cause that ass-hole is gonna knock up ever bimbo he screws.

(MRS. STARKEY *laughs appreciatively.*)

HIDELMAN: Then I beat up on him.

BETTY: Yer own husband?

HIDELMAN: Ever since my shoe-size went two-digits, I know I didn't have ta take no shit offa nobody.

BETTY: Yer own husband?

HIDELMAN: I like ta pound his ass when he's driving. That way I know

I'm gonna win fast.

JUBA: My Marse Bob from Breadfruit Alley, oh mahn, he be somet'ing. Him wears bossa nova shirt, tall trousers, and hot tie. He say: "Lissen, baby, ah luv yuh." Ah say: "My name is no baby. Yuh rude and I clip you wings fer'yuh, male chauvinst."

BETTY: Did ya, Juba?

JUBA: He just grab my waist an kiss me. Is funny thing how sometimes not able to stop any damn stupidness. (*Pause.*) Ah, Christ, if yuh not careful dese days yuh is a disgrace.

QUASHIE: (*Proudly*) I wuz married in the Church of the Castor Oil Dead. On Cat Island.

HIDELMAN: Mrs. Starkey, let's *relay*.

STARKEY: Oh, no, Hidelman!

HIDELMAN: Guys ta "Arnie's Packing House" 'n Rockford do it all the time.

STARKEY: They git theirselves on "report," too.

HIDELMAN: Wanna "double up." Mrs. Starkey?

MRS. STARKEY: Sure.

HIDELMAN: 5 minutes on . . . 5 minutes off.

STARKEY: Mom, "doubling up" ain't authorized . . .'cept for "E-break."

MRS. STARKEY: This here *is* Emergency Break. I'm dyin of fuckin boredom.

STARKEY: It ain't authorized.

HIDELMAN: Bunch of pussies on this floor. Guys do it all the time!

MRS. STARKEY: You first, Hidelman. I wanna call Donna in Shippin. She jist got herself a "book" ta the Arlington Race Track.

(MRS. STARKEY *walks away from her machine and* HIDELMAN *"relays" by running back and forth to work both machines at the same time.*)

STARKEY: You ain't gonna bet agin, Mom?

MRS. STARKEY: It's *my* money, kid. (*She goes to the pay phone.*)

BETTY: You could git us all in trouble, Hidelman.

HIDELMAN: (*As she is working both machines*) You got you a job movin a brick from one table ta another table. Right? Yer gonna git the same money if ya bust yer ass 'n carry *two* bricks ta the next table fer five minutes 'n yer buddy rests...then let her take over 'n you rest. That way, ya wanna git a pop or call home, ya got the time.

MRS. STARKEY: (*On the phone*) Number six, seven, eight fer 20 cents in both races. (*Pause.*) ...four, four, one in the box fer ten. (*Pause.*) Honey, I know I'm due fer a big hit ta-day.

HIDELMAN: (*After a pause,* HIDELMAN *suddenly stops and holds her nose*) Aw....

BETTY: Hidelman's got the nosebleed.

ELLIS: Pinch the side.

HIDELMAN: I am! (*Pause.*) Dust from the fuckin metaphosphate. (*Pause.* HIDELMAN *goes to her own machine working it with one hand and tending to her nose with the other.*) I can't "double" no more, Mrs. Starkey.

(MRS. STARKEY *goes to her own machine to work it.*)

HIDELMAN: (*Still trying to control her nose bleed*) You owe me "two minutes," Mrs. Starkey!

MRS. STARKEY: (*Aggravated*) Ok. My god, I ain't gonna jip ya outta lousy "two minutes."

HIDELMAN: Ta-morrow!

BETTY: Company doctor oughta see yer nose.

HIDELMAN: They jist give out nose drops.

BETTY: Least ya don't have ta pay for it.

HIDELMAN: All that dye sprayed on the casings.

STARKEY: Jist got you the sensitive nose.

HIDELMAN: (*Caustic*) Sure. (*Pause.*) We need us dust respirators.

STARKEY: Don't start that 'gin.

HIDELMAN: I come home from work yisterday... my neck turned black on me. That crap works up outta the pores of yer skin.

STARKEY: Don't start rumors, Hidelman.

HIDELMAN: Stopped! (*She takes her hand away from her nose and works as usual.*)

(*There is a pause as the women work silently.*)

STARKEY: (*Pause. Coaxing*) You take innythin out fer dinner ta-night?

MRS. STARKEY: Why?

STARKEY: I thought if you wasn't plannin nothin, we could git us chicken 'n fries at *Charlie's*—where Daddy eats.

MRS. STARKEY: Don't force him on me.

STARKEY: Six o'clock. I'm buying.

MRS. STARKEY: I don't know.

BETTY: I haven't had a night out since . . .

STARKEY: I gotta know.

MRS. STARKEY: Don't push me.

BETTY: I was a girl . . . we kept our own chickens . . . 'n I kilt 'n cleaned 'em with the feet on. You kin flip 'em so nice in the batter that way.

STARKEY: They got beer on draft.

MRS. STARKEY: Good stuff?

STARKEY: Sure.

MRS. STARKEY: Budweiser?

STARKEY: Sure.

BETTY: (*Staring at the machine*) I stand here 'n look at the same old machine. And I go home 'n look at the same old lady. Day after day. It don't change on me neither place.

MRS. STARKEY: Gotta wash my hair ta-night.

STARKEY: I'm buying.

BETTY: I call out fer Chinese food sometimes on Saturday night. Rice . . . them little pouches of soy sauce.

MRS. STARKEY: I don't know.

STARKEY: Eat nice 'n slow. Air conditioning.

MRS. STARKEY: My hair's a mess.

STARKEY: Her hair look all right, Betty?

BETTY: Oh, yes.

MRS. STARKEY: I don't know . . .

BETTY: (*Says as everyone ignores her*) Somewhere in my head black thoughts is mean ta her.

MRS. STARKEY: Oh . . .

(*A loud horn is heard. The lights on the machines go out. The machines are dead.*)

MALE VOICE: Shut down. Stand by. Shut down. Do not leave your work area!

HIDELMAN: Second time this week damn thang has went broke.

JUBA: I know sumt'ing like dis happen. Trouble.

STARKEY: Low amperage. Loose anode clamps.

MRS. STARKEY: Let 'em break down.

BETTY: They're down too long 'n we got ourselfs un-ployment.

ELLIS: We had us *down time* two days this week.

HIDELMAN: Them idiots in Central Maintenance, they don't keep "shut down" long nough ta fix it good.

STARKEY: Let me at that job. I'd fix 'em all right!

(MRS. STARKEY *walks over to the coffee area.*)

STARKEY: Yer not suppose ta leave work area, Mom.

MRS. STARKEY: (*Taunting*) You gonna report me?

BETTY: You cud git us all in trouble, Mrs. Starkey.

(MRS. STARKEY *goes to a side door by the coffee area and opens it. She sits on a chair near the door for air.* HIDELMAN *leaves the area to go to the bulletin board.*)

STARKEY: Hidelman!

HIDELMAN: (*Halfway to the bulletin board*) I kin read Company Bulletin Board durin shut-down. You know that. (HIDELMAN *reads the notice* MAVIS *has put up.*)

QUASHIE: (*After a pause. To* MRS. STARKEY) Yuh feel anyt'ing, darlin?

MRS. STARKEY: Little bity breeze.

QUASHIE: On Cat Island, we call de breeze, "doctuh."

MRS. STARKEY: (*She unbuttons her lab coat and pulls out her breasts, laughing*) Doctor me...oh, doctor me....

STARKEY: Mom! (*She closes her eyes tightly so she can't see.*)

MRS. STARKEY: (*There is a pause. Then she leans back in her chair, dreamily*) I was a kid... I walked these two big dogs fer old lady. Legs went on her, 'n she give me a nice piece of change run 'em to the park. (*Pause.*) They was pals, them two dogs. Brang up tagether from pups. (*Pause.*) Bitch come on by, they'd be in heat... well, their peckers would start ta grow... slow 'n lazy like. Bigger. Bigger. I swear ta God, they both swelled up big exactly tagether. (*After a pause.*) I can't ferget it. (*Pause.*) I'd like me somebody ta my side who'd feel all the heat I was feelin...jist when I was feelin it.

HIDELMAN: (*Standing by the bulletin board looking at the notice* MAVIS *put up*) Jeee ... us. (*Pause.*) Jee ... us! (HIDELMAN *turns to face* ELLIS.)

BETTY: What's wrong, Hidelman?

HIDELMAN: They put them out "A-Notice."

MRS. STARKEY: "Alert?"

HIDELMAN: (*Softly*) Yah. (*Pause.*) Stuff is stole from here is..."hot."

ELLIS: (*Anxious*) Whattaya mean?

HIDELMAN: Tainted. Low-level contamination.

STARKEY: That there's jist a warnin.

HIDELMAN: (*In awe*) No wonder that kid in there (*Points to the washroom*) ...ain't kickin'.

ELLIS: He is on phenobarbital!

HIDELMAN: (*Slowly*) ...gettin ate up by crap... from them uniforms you wraps him up in...from soap rubbed on his skin....

STARKEY: Don't listen ta her, Ellis. You know nothin shows up on them "readings" took by the 'sociation. We git us checked ever month.

MRS. STARKEY: (*To* ELLIS) It's the old scare trick ... so they don't git them thangs stole.

HIDELMAN: (*Staring at* ELLIS *softly*) You...You give that kid inny of the "creamers" took from the Cafeteria?

ELLIS: He is jist on pheno! (*There is a pause.* HIDELMAN *stares at* ELLIS. *Then a fire engine is heard through the opened door.* ELLIS *tenses in fear.*)

JUBA: (*To* ELLIS) Don't mean it be goin to your house.

ELLIS: I hear one of them, Juba, 'n I think on that song I skipped rope to... when I was little. (*Pause.*) "Lady bug, Lady bug, fly away home...yer kids is on fire...(*She holds her ears against the sound of the fire engines*)...yer kids is on fire....."

(*The fire engine sound disappears.* JUBA *soothes her. After a pause:*)

QUASHIE: A "swamp place"—that's what this floor is. Folks back home call *this* a "fever hole"...white man's grave.

MRS. STARKEY: (*Fanning herself*) Sweat box city.

BETTY: Least we work off the line.

MRS. STARKEY: Hell, we're just the last line.

(*After a pause, the horn is sounded.*)

MALE VOICE: Machines operable. Machines operable.

(MRS. STARKEY *puts her clothing together and returns to the machine after closing the door.* HIDELMAN *gets a mini-transistor radio out of her pocket and turns it on.*)

STARKEY: You ain't sa-pose ta play that.

HIDELMAN: Ok . . . ok . . . .

MRS. STARKEY: (*To* HIDELMAN) Radio's on . . . but you ain't.

STARKEY: (*After a pause. To* MRS. STARKEY) I like couple three drinks fore supper.

MRS. STARKEY: I'm thinking . . . I'm thinking.

BETTY: (*Holding a checker mid-air before playing*) . . . X-ray man, he says: "Don't breathe" . . . 'n takes a picture of my mother-in-law's chest . . . then he says: "Now you go on a-gin." (*Pause.*) Someday, he is gonna ferget ta tell her . . . *breathe.*

MRS. STARKEY: (*After a pause. To* STARKEY) I don't want him back!

BETTY: (*Now back at her machine*) My own mama . . . she died young. From the flu. In them days, they was hanging up goats ta catch the fever from the air . . . 'n all the skin 'n meat fell right off them goat bones 'fore noon. People they was dying right 'n left. They was took out the bedroom window so as not ta have 'em brung through the rest of the house 'n infect people . . . took right out the window . . . .

STARKEY: (*After a pause*) You like white or dark meat?

MRS. STARKEY: Legs.

STARKEY: Fine by me. I like white.

(QUASHIE *begins to stamp after something on the floor by her machine.*)

JUBA: What are you doing, woman?

QUASHIE: (*Trying to stamp it*) Get this bug.

JUBA: (*Goes to* QUASHIE *in order to stop her*) That could be a "fire hag." You let the bug go about its own thing.

QUASHIE: Witchcraft is crazy, for truth. (*She squashes the bug.*)

JUBA: Witchcraft is a woman's business.

(JUBA *shakes her head in resignation as they both stare down at the dead bug. Then they go back to working their machines and dreaming.*)

ELLIS: (*In defiance to* HIDELMAN) I took my little Donny, Dwane, Sue Ellen, Janice 'n the babies ta Brookfield Zoo ... 'n we seen these porpoises jump through them rings put up high. Well, ones id jump up there 'n make it, they was give a fish. Course those couldn't git high nough, well, they was throwed nothin. It was real pit-eeee-ful. (*Pause.*) I'd give 'em all fish ... even them which didn't make it ta the ring.

STARKEY: (*To* ELLIS) You'd ruin the show that way, Ellis.

(*There is a pause as they work silently for a few seconds.*)

STARKEY: (*Staring at her mother coldly*) The Van don't satisfy.

MRS. STARKEY: It's *professional*.

STARKEY: Damn it, Mom, whatta I have ta do make you see straight? (STARKEY *walks to* MRS. STARKEY'*s area and stands in front of her firmly. She takes a check from her pocket, saying weakly.*) This here's a check. Wrote out ta you. But it goes with Daddy. (*Breaking.*) I want my daddy back. (STARKEY *goes to her mother and buries herself in her mother's arms, crying.*)

MRS. STARKEY: (*Touched*) Hey, don't cry over it.

STARKEY: (*Quietly crying*) I was eight...'n you made me that gypsy dress for Halloween....

MRS. STARKEY: (*Softening*) Why are you crying, baby?

STARKEY: ...I had that beautiful red dress ... all yer rhinestones... pink satin mask round my eyes. (*Pause.*) This old man, he told me ta come up on the porch...'n he promised me little chocolates with the jelly inside...'n...'n he set me on his lap... I felt his "thing" on me ... in the dark....

MRS. STARKEY: You never told me that, baby.

STARKEY: ...it was Halloween, momma....

MRS. STARKEY: Oh, honey...honey... little girls, they are molested all the time... every day...it ain't nothin...(*Softly.*)...every day....

STARKEY: Men is "spills"...killers. I hate 'em. All of em! But

Daddy.

(MRS. STARKEY *holds her and rocks her in her arms.*)

STARKEY: (*Softly*) Please... take it... (MRS. STARKEY *takes the check and puts it in her pocket.* BETTY *is absorbed in her own thoughts and suddenly picks up the picture.*)

BETTY: (*Staring at the picture*) I see it! I see it! Eyes!

MRS. STARKEY: (*To* BETTY) I knew ya would, Betty.

HIDELMAN: (*Turns off the radio. To* BETTY) There ain't nothin on that but *ocean*.

BETTY: I'm gonna git me some good luck now.

JUBA: (*To* BETTY) Is your turn now.

BETTY: (*Happily*) Did you "jump" me?

JUBA: (*Proudly. Holds up a checker*) Is I-self done that with this.

STARKEY: (*To her mother*) Money is left over—'n what I give you. Go to Wig World 'n buy that switch you like so much.

MRS. STARKEY: (*Looking at her daughter*) We're all gonna git us some good luck—come the nineteen-eighties. (*Smiles at her daughter.*)

HIDELMAN: 80's gotta be better. What the hell good is happen up ta now.

STARKEY: We went ta the moon!

HIDELMAN: They've been goin up there 'n space 'n haven't seen nothin yit.

QUASHIE: They go to the moon—that is "duncy-no-good" cause then we lost this earth.

(*After a pause, the inter-com phone lights up and rings. They all look anxiously.* HIDELMAN *turns off her radio.* STARKEY *pauses, apprehensively, and then goes to the inter-com phone.*)

STARKEY: Floor B. (*Pause.*) Yes...yes!!!! (*There is a long pause and then she slowly hangs up the phone.*)

STARKEY: Betty... sitter to yer house called the office. (*Pause.*) She thought yer mother was asleep....

BETTY: Mother-in-law.

STARKEY: ...she is passed away.

MRS. STARKEY: (*Goes to* BETTY *and puts an arm around her*) It's fer the best, Betty.

STARKEY: (*Still standing by the phone*)...They found them lotta blood in her throat... doctor... he is said she was choked ta death. (*Pause.*) Kilt.

MRS. STARKEY: Oh my God.

STARKEY: (*Weakly*) Elmhurst is coming... ta take you....

BETTY: (*Softly*) Take me where?

STARKEY: Police.

QUASHIE: Funny how a person do stay good wid everybody, do find one who turn her bad.

MRS. STARKEY: (*To* BETTY) Honey, you stop working now and go on 'n finish the game...'fore Elmhurst gits here.

(BETTY *stands before the checker game, pauses, then puts a checker carefully in place.*)

BETTY: I got it fixed up fer you, Juba.

JUBA: Ah doan have the heart ta win no more. Hit jus big carry on.

(JUBA *puts all the pieces, black and red, in* BETTY's *pockets.* ELMHURST *comes to the door.*)

ELMHURST: (*At the door. Softly*) Betty...

BETTY: (*Holding out the photo to* MRS. STARKEY) Here, Mrs. Starkey.

MRS. STARKEY: No, honey. You keep it. Till you see the rest.

ELMHURST: Betty...

BETTY: Is she kilt?

ELMHURST: Yes.

BETTY: No matter how far I let myself go 'n dream...some wall was always there.

HIDELMAN: You see she gits cleaned off, Elmhurst. You see ivver-thang's off her skin.

(ELMHURST *does not react.* ELMHURST *and* BETTY *leave. After a pause,* JUBA *looks down at the bare checker board.*)

JUBA: (*Softly and appreciatively*) That's one rash woman...one rash woman.

(*There is a silence as the women work a few seconds. Then* HIDELMAN *begins to sing defiantly.*)

HIDELMAN: (*Singing in anger in a jerky rhythm with working the machine*)

I wanna be a trucker's sweetheart,
I wanna learn ta gearjam drive,
'n love inside the "sleeper cab"
'n see my soul alive.

(MRS. STARKEY *joins in the next verse with the same defiance.*)

HIDELMAN and MRS. STARKEY: (*Singing. In anger*)
I wanna double-clutch me kisses,
I wanna diesel-fuel me sighs,
'n drink a hundred coffees
without no last good-bys.

(*Now* ELLIS *joins in on the third verse.*)

HIDELMAN, MRS. STARKEY, ELLIS: (*Strongly—as a freedom song*)
I wanna be a trucker's sweetheart,
I wanna learn ta long-haul loads,
'n have the windows open
Jist air 'n sky 'n roads....
(*Softly.*)... air ...'n sky ...'n roads....

(STARKEY *does not sing. She does not react to the song but just works the machine without emotion. After working the machines for a few seconds silently.*)

STARKEY: She'll be all right, won't she? (*Pause.*) Won't she?

MRS. STARKEY: I don't know, honey.

JUBA: I ain't think so.

ELLIS: Poor thang.

(*There is a pause as they work silently. Then:*)

HIDELMAN: Ahhhhhhhhh! (*She stoops over the floor in front of her machine.*) My... back ... is locked on me a-gin! Hell! (*Pause. In pain.*) God damn them Bohunk machines...'n Polock mechanics...'n Wop foremen...Spick maintenance ...

ELLIS: (*Kindly*) Least yer democratic, Hidelman.

MRS. STARKEY: ...you don't leave innybody out, all right.

(*After a pause,* ELLIS *goes to* HIDELMAN.)

ELLIS: (*Squats down next to* HIDELMAN. *Grinning*) You know, Hidelman, right now you look like woman is pickin beans. I think you really want you "billy" work.

(*There is a pause. Then* HIDELMAN *slowly begins to laugh even though her back hurts.*)

HIDELMAN: (*Laughing*) Damn . . . Oh, God. . . .

(ELLIS *gives* HIDELMAN *a hand and helps her up. Slowly,* HIDELMAN *gets back to her machine. After a pause:*)

HIDELMAN: Ellis. . .you go home ta-night 'n burn all them old uniforms you have took. Hear me! You git them off that kid. . . .'n don't feed him no more creamers from the Cafeteria.

(*There is a pause.* ELLIS *doesn't answer.*)

HIDELMAN: (*Softly. Almost to herself*) I had me lotta thangs took back. . .but I ain't ivver lost my own baby. (*Pause.*) Ellis! You don't . . . I'm comin over there 'n burn 'em myself!!

(*There is a pause as the women work silently.*)

HIDELMAN: I'm goin down ta the Station 'n see Betty over lunch. You kin bet yer ass it'll be two weeks 'fore the 'sociation makes it.

MRS. STARKEY: We'll all go.

JUBA: Dat's fine with me.

ELLIS: (*Hesitantly*) Even my baby?

HIDELMAN: Sure.

(*There is a pause as the women work.*)

ELLIS: They'll treat her decent, won't they?

HIDELMAN: (*Caustic*) Pigs is gonna treat her great.

STARKEY: (*Firmly*) There is police who is Catholics.

MRS. STARKEY: (*Mocking*) Sure.

STARKEY: No Catholic I ivver known hurt no woman.

HIDELMAN: Well, there is Pigs which is Protestant!

MRS. STARKEY: This is one hell of a half day.

JUBA: This morning is a "haunting dream". . .a real "haunting dream" cause I can touch myself for truth.

(*After a pause, the "after work" whistle blows.* ELLIS *goes to the washroom immediately.* JUBA *follows. The others go to their lockers to dress.*)

JUBA: (*Following* ELLIS) I'll help you with the baby.

(*After she dresses,* QUASHIE *goes to the washroom.*)

QUASHIE: (*Takes* ELLIS *by the arm*) You bring him on out in de open, darlin.

(*After* ELLIS *and the baby are out of the washroom,* HIDELMAN *takes* ELLIS *firmly by the arm even though the others try to prevent her from doing this.* HIDELMAN *gently leads* ELLIS *to a chair in the coffee area.*)

HIDELMAN: Ellis, you sit here. You jist sit here 'n rest.

MRS. STARKEY: Hidelman...

HIDELMAN: (*To* MRS. STARKEY) Let me alone! (*To* ELLIS.) Jist sit, Ellis. (HIDELMAN *gets her billy kickers. She puts them on. Then she goes to* ELLIS's *machine and kicks it over and over as* ELLIS *watches passively.*)

STARKEY: Hidelman!

HIDELMAN: Don't stop me, Starkey. This floor's done fer innyway.

(MRS. STARKEY *goes to* STARKEY *and holds her back from* HIDELMAN.)

STARKEY: (*In anguish*) Ma ... ma ...

MRS. STARKEY: We'll git us some wine, too, at *Charlie's*. Boone's Farm Apple. Couple Budweisers 'n some Boone's Farm Apple.

(*After kicking* ELLIS's *machine,* HIDELMAN *takes a parting swat at* BETTY's *machine and then takes off her shoes and throws them at the machines. She tugs on the floor covering and heaves it against the machines.*)

MRS. STARKEY: Let's git outta this dump.

(*The women finish dressing quickly and quietly.* ELLIS *still sits passively on the chair staring at her baby and rocking him.* QUASHIE *brings* ELLIS's *clothes to her.* JUBA *slowly folds up the play-pen and stands beside* ELLIS.)

QUASHIE: (*Helps* ELLIS *up slowly and puts some of* ELLIS's *clothes around her*) Darlin, you jist think about everything outside on the ground pushing up—flowers and grass—gettin theyselves born hard and hurtin, like all life.

(*A slight pause. Suddenly the low whining sound of the hand-blower is heard.*)

STARKEY: (*Weakly*) Hand-blower is workin a-gin. (*It groans for a few seconds and dies. They pause to listen. Then they slowly exit,* HIDELMAN *barefoot. Curtain.*)

End

Separate Ceremonies

Phyllis Purscell

Characters

CARRIE
FRITZ
JOHN
ADDIE
LAUREN
GRACE

Separate Ceremonies was given a rehearsed reading by The Women's Project on January 15, 1979, directed by Geraldine Court, with the following cast:

CARRIE . . . . Elizabeth Hubbard
FRITZ . . . . Tom Toner
JOHN . . . . David O'Brien
ADDIE . . . . Margaret Warncke
LAUREN . . . . Janet Pennybacker
GRACE . . . . Katherine Squire

It was given a staged reading on April 23, 1979, directed by B.J. Whiting, with the following cast:

CARRIE . . . . Beryl Towbin
FRITZ . . . . Nicholas Saunders
JOHN . . . . Conard Fowkes
ADDIE . . . . Kristin Griffith
LAUREN . . . . Janet Pennybacker
GRACE . . . . Dortha Duckworth

ACT I

Setting: *The livingroom of a small house in the mid-west. Stage right there is an opening that leads to an entry hall offstage. There are two doors stage left: one up stage leading to the bedrooms and one down stage leading to the kitchen. This was the house of an elderly, bookish man. It is comfortable and well organized, but there is a lifetime collection of the things that interested him most. These might include old maps, a model of the Globe Theatre, one or two pieces of furniture from another time in his life — his desk being one of these.*

Time: *Close to midnight. Late spring.*

At Rise: *The stage is dark. There is the sound of a key in a lock from the hall, and then a light comes on from the door stage right.* CARRIE, *an attractive woman in her early forties, comes into the room.* JOHN, *who has been seated stage left, stands.* JOHN *is forty-one, a tall man whose face still shows a boyish quality from time to time. Before either has a chance to speak, we hear the voice of* FRITZ *from offstage.*

FRITZ: That lock always sticks — And now I can't get the damned thing to close properly . . . Oh, well, I'll get it later. (*In a louder voice.*) I'm going back to get your other bag, Carrie.

(CARRIE *walks into the room, and* JOHN, *whom she has not yet seen, walks toward her.*)

JOHN: (*Softly*) Carrie . . .

CARRIE: (*Starts*) Oh, my God! . . . John — is that you? (JOHN *turns on a lamp close by, walks up to* CARRIE *and embraces her. She gives him a hug and then takes a step back.*) What a start you gave me! I

thought ... (*She gives a gasping kind of laugh.*) I thought it was
him.

FRITZ: (*Entering stage right with two suitcases.* FRITZ *is seventy-six.
He will be old soon, but he isn't yet.*) Which room are you going to
use, honey? (*Sees* JOHN *and puts down the suitcases.*) Johnny.
(*They embrace.*) I didn't see your car.

JOHN: I pulled around to the back, Fritz ... I guess I gave Carrie a
start. (*To* CARRIE.) I'm sorry I scared you.

CARRIE: It was just so strange. I thought you were Dad. And I just
saw ...

FRITZ: (*Picking up the suitcases. Overlapping from "And I"*) Where do
you want these, Carrie?

CARRIE: Here, let me take those.

FRITZ: Just tell me where you want 'em.

CARRIE: (*Indicating a corner of the room*) Put them over there for
now, Fritz ... Come on, John. Sit down. (*She sits on the sofa.*) Oh,
Lord — what a day. Uh — what's next? (JOHN *sits next to her on the
sofa.*) I can't think what we do now.

FRITZ: I make us a drink. You've no objection to that, have you?

CARRIE: No.

(FRITZ *exits into the kitchen.*)

JOHN: Are you sure you want to stay here?

CARRIE: I'll be all right. What about you?

JOHN: I don't know. I was thinking maybe I'd ...

FRITZ: (*Sticking his head into the livingroom*) Your father had some
bourbon and I'll find it ... It's in a logical place — he was a
methodical man — the only problem is his methods weren't like
other people's.

(CARRIE *smiles and nods.* FRITZ *withdraws.*)

JOHN: When does Addie's plane get in?

CARRIE: (*Looking at her watch*) Soon, I think. She wasn't sure when I
talked to her last. She's renting a car and driving out from Des
Moines. She insisted — and when we talked last I was in no shape
to argue about that.

FRITZ: (*Coming in with three glasses and a bottle of whiskey*) I found
it. He kept it in the refrigerator so it wouldn't melt the ice so fast.

He told me that once, but I forgot. (*He puts the glasses down on the coffee table, pours them each a liberal drink, and passes them around. Then — to* CARRIE.) Are you all right, girl?

CARRIE: Yes. I am . . . I don't know why — but I am. What about you?

FRITZ: (*Taking a sip of his whiskey*) I've known it was coming . . . And, then, when you're my age you begin to lose people. (*A change of tone — less heavily.*) They die on you — leave you to go it alone — to figure it out for yourself. (*Still lighter.*) I thought your father and I would figure it all out before he quit on me.

CARRIE: (*Smiling at him*) You spent enough time at it.

FRITZ: (*Keeping it light*) Well, we would have gotten it done except that about every five years he'd get very wrong-headed on some point, and it would set us back by months . . . For a younger brother he was curiously resistant to my influence . . . I figure if he'd given me another decade . . . (*Silence, and then, lighter again.*) Well, he'd have been a miserable invalid. Crotchety would only have been the beginning of it!

JOHN: (*To* CARRIE) You were with him when he died?

CARRIE: Yes. He just — went, John.

JOHN: Had he been conscious at all, before that?

CARRIE: By the time Fritz called me and I made the drive from home to the hospital, and that's — what? About an hour and a half? He was pretty much gone. Now and then — some little glimmer — but nothing, really.

JOHN: I wish I'd been there.

FRITZ: I understand how you feel, Johnny. I was with my mother when she died . . . but my old man quit us one summer when I was in Monmouth County haying. I just got home in time for the funeral. It is harder to accept that way. It helps if you see them go.(JOHN *nods, grateful for the understanding.*)\Your dad called me early this afternoon and said he was feeling pretty bad. He'd taken his medication but it hadn't really helped . . . We talked it over and decided that if he wasn't feeling a whole lot better in an hour or so he'd better go back into the hospital . . . I called Carrie at that point, and she decided to come on over — she was on the way by the time he called me back. That was about two o'clock — two-thirty. He said, "I'll meet you at the hospital." He'd already called the ambulance himself . . . By the time I got to the hospital he was in pretty bad shape . . . They hooked him up to every damned thing they had . . . He opened his eyes one time and saw all that stuff ... He said, "They might as well save all this paraphernalia for the next fellow — it isn't going to do the job." ... "It isn't going to do the job," he said ... And he was right about that ... And that's about it, John ... He was in a coma at the last and just slipped away nice and easy.

JOHN: That was the last thing he said? About the machines?

FRITZ: He rambled some — nothing, really.

CARRIE: Something once about his morning glories, I remember.

FRITZ: You'd like something more than that, I know. A message.

JOHN: ... More a souvenir.

FRITZ: (*Reaches over and pats his knee*) They come in time — over the years. (*They sit.*) Did you want him to quote a little *Lear* at the end?

JOHN: Maybe.

FRITZ: Well, he didn't do that. (*He takes a sip of his drink.*) I'd better be going pretty soon. (*To* CARRIE.) You tired, honey?

CARRIE: The whiskey is working on me.

FRITZ: That's good. Listen, are you sure you want to stay here? Grace would love to have you over ... Does it bother you to be here?

CARRIE: No — not now. When we first got here, I couldn't believe he was gone ... even though I'd seen him die ... I half expected him to walk out of the kitchen with that apron on that Grace made for him ... But now that I'm used to the place — it's almost a comfort ... Don't worry about me ... And, anyway I need to be here. I've got to take care of all this stuff ... But you'd better go on home. You look tired.

FRITZ: You don't need a tired old man on your hands.

CARRIE: You keep saying that kind of thing. Do you want me to deny that you're old? Well, I won't. What are you? Seventy-six? You're entitled to be old at seventy-six. (*She leans over and kisses him.*) So beat it.

JOHN: When did he have morning glories?

CARRIE: In the little stone house — along the south side.

JOHN: Oh — yes.

(FRITZ *begins to laugh quietly.* JOHN *and* CARRIE *look at him.*)

FRITZ: Did I ever tell you about the time he pulled that stunt? (*Shakes his head with amusement.*) The junior class was giving its play. He only had a small part, but he always found a way ... Anyway, did I tell you about that? There's nothing so tedious as an old crock who tells the same stories over and over.

CARRIE: Tell us. John and I could use a story.

(JOHN *nods.*)

FRITZ: Well, the junior class — this was in college — the junior class was giving a play. I don't remember what it was ... I think it may have been *While the Lentils Boiled.* No — that was another time. Anyway, it doesn't matter — that part of it — Al just had a small role. He had to come down the aisle from the back of the auditorium ... (*He gets up and pretends that he is walking stealthily down the aisle.*) I think he was supposed to be a detective — something like that. He had on this silly looking hat that came down over his ears like this ... And — you remember how he could wiggle his ears — Somehow he'd secured a rubber band inside that hat so that when he wiggled his ears the hat popped up on his head. Of course, he crept down the aisle until he was sure everyone was looking. His timing was great. And, then, he wiggled his ears and that hat just went ... (*He illustrates how the hat popped up.*) No one knew how he did it ... Your dad — he was something, wasn't he? (*He sits back down.*)

CARRIE: He was.

FRITZ: I didn't want him to die, kids.

CARRIE: We didn't want him to, either. But he did, didn't he?

FRITZ: He did ... Well, he was never the most accommodating man. (*Again silence. They sip their whiskey.*) Carrie, I know you told me, but I forgot. When is Addie getting in? Did you ever get back to her after your dad died?

CARRIE: She knows. She could be here fairly soon, I'd think.

FRITZ: (*Looking at his watch*) My God! It's almost one. I'd better let you guys get some rest. And I should be getting home to Grace — I slipped her a mickey, though, so I know pretty much where I'll find her ... she won't have gotten into any trouble.

JOHN: (*Looking at his glass*) What are you, the sandman? Sending everybody off to oblivion? A little pill here — a nice glass of whiskey there ... Will there be anybody left to tend the store by the time you get done?

FRITZ: I'm your connection, boy — treat me with respect — without me we'd never have found the whiskey.

JOHN: Oh, you'll always find the whiskey — no fear on that account.

FRITZ: Yes — I guess you're right — we all have our capabilities ...
Other people see auras — one of my grandchildren does — Dottie's
Anne says she sees auras, but I have a preternatural sense of where
to find the whiskey — You're right about that, Johnny ... And,
you know, of the two abilities — I prefer mine. (*Stretches.*) I am
tired ... Do any of your kids see auras, John?

JOHN: Not yet. They're a little young. Auras start around eighteen,
I think. They probably will, though — and I suppose mine will be
the wrong color — indicating something awful about me.

FRITZ: (*Laughs*) Are they hard on you?

JOHN: They're zealous. It's wearing.

FRITZ: I remember that — At least it means they haven't given up on
you — you're worth fighting with.

JOHN: That's true.

FRITZ: Ever notice how long it takes old people to depart?

CARRIE: That theme again?

JOHN: You are kind of preoccupied with your age tonight, aren't you?

FRITZ: We're all mortal, guys, but some of us are more mortal than
others.

JOHN: (*Standing*) I think you need to deliver yourself one of your
little wonder workers and get a good night's sleep.

FRITZ: I'm going ... Good night, kids. (*They ad lib good nights.* FRITZ
exits stage right. Then — offstage.) You have to mess around with
this door if you want it to lock. I'm just going to leave it, okay?

JOHN: I'll get it, Fritz.

(JOHN *turns back toward* CARRIE *and looks at her. She raises her
glass.*)

CARRIE: You know, John, I don't think enough good things have
been said about whiskey.

(JOHN *sits down in the chair stage left.*)

JOHN: It was low of him to die before I got here. Addie — I can
see. She had to come all the way from San Francisco.

CARRIE: He wasn't thinking about you or Addie — or me — when
he died.

JOHN: ... I don't feel anything.

CARRIE: Me neither.

JOHN: You were feeling plenty when you called.

CARRIE: That was then.

JOHN: Gone, huh?

CARRIE: All gone — except a little sense of panic. All this time of having him in and out of the hospital has kept me so busy — dashing over here for two or three days at a time, then going back home — I can't remember if I have a life outside of Dad's sickness.

JOHN: He died. You didn't.

CARRIE: You're sure?

JOHN: It's a promise.

CARRIE: ... Peter's not coming until the day of the funeral. What about Diane?

JOHN: I don't see the point in her coming until then, do you?

CARRIE: No. This really is just for you and Addie and me ... God, there's a lot to do. But I'm not going to think about that tonight.

JOHN: This is going to be hard, Carrie — between Addie and me. She hasn't written since her visit — and what was that? Two months ago? I wrote her twice.

CARRIE: I know.

JOHN: She walked out of my house while I was at school—gave Diane some bull shit excuse and left.

CARRIE: You'll both just have to forget it for now. What we have to do here doesn't have anything to do with that — whatever it is.

JOHN: (*With amusement*) I have always admired the way you can put your problems on hold, Carrie.

CARRIE: You do not admire it; don't lie.

JOHN: I'm in awe of that ability.

CARRIE: It's easy. It's the easiest goddamn thing in the world. Not that it comes naturally — you learn — with practice.

JOHN: You've had practice.

CARRIE: I'm always in the middle of the room when the roof caves in ... Why were you sitting here in the dark, Johnnie?

JOHN: I'm so sorry I scared you. That was terrible.

CARRIE: I wasn't scared — it was just that I suddenly realized that I don't really know he's dead. And I saw him *die*.

JOHN: So it doesn't help that much to be there.

CARRIE: Contrary to Fritz's theory ... Why were you sitting here in the dark, John?

JOHN: Waiting for the word.

CARRIE: And?

JOHN: The usual zilch. (*Pause.*) I refuse to bury the man until I've felt at least one appropriate emotion.

CARRIE: What the hell's appropriate?

JOHN: Something.

CARRIE: Who's to say? And it's not like we *do* this all that often ... We were so young when Mother died. Do you know that next year I'll be forty-four? She was forty-four.

JOHN: Does that scare you?

CARRIE: I think about it. (*There is the sound of a car pulling up outside.* CARRIE *gets up quickly.*) That must be Addie!

JOHN: Carrie — I'm going to give Addie a chance to — take this in — (*He indicates the house — the room.*) Tell her I'm napping — if you want.

CARRIE: All right, John. (*She exits stage right.* JOHN *looks around the room, picks up a couple of magazines and exits stage left. We hear the offstage voices of* CARRIE *and* ADDIE.) Here, give that to me.

ADDIE: No. I've got it. (CARRIE *enters.* ADDIE *follows with suitcases.* ADDIE *is thirty-one — a tall, graceful woman. She puts the suitcases down.*) It's so warm here. I'd forgotten it was spring. San Francisco never heard of spring. (*She looks around the room.*) Where is he?

CARRIE: In the guestroom ... He ...

ADDIE: (*Interrupting*) Not John ... the old man ... where is he?

CARRIE: Addie ... The place gets to you at first, I know. I didn't know if I could stay — but after awhile — it's kind of comforting, in a way.

ADDIE: (*Smiling at her sister*) You'll take your comfort wherever you can find it, won't you, Car-o-line?

CARRIE: You'd damn well better believe it ... Wherever I can find it.

ADDIE: (*Looking around*) Well, I can't say I find it comforting. (*She walks over to a dictionary on a stand, opens it up and calls into it.*) Dad? (*She looks over at* CARRIE *who is watching and continues to watch her.*) "I'm hiding; I'm hiding . . . And no one knows where . . ." How did that go, Carrie? . . . "Have you looked in the ink well? And Mother said, 'Where?'" (*She sees the whiskey bottle on the coffee table and picks it up. She peers into it with one eye.*) Dad? (*She puts it down and looks back at* CARRIE *who is smiling slightly.*) Well . . . (*She flops into a chair.*) I guess if it got him it can get anybody . . . There must be something to it, after all.

CARRIE: (*Sitting down close to her*) Did you doubt that, Ad?

ADDIE: (*Reflecting*) Um . . . yeah . . . even when he was so terribly sick the last time, he seemed a very formidable entity.

CARRIE: All of a sudden I feel like I've had a great big novocaine shot delivered directly to my psyche.

ADDIE: Yeah. . . know what I'd like? To have a whole new set of emotions . . . How did she react to her father's death? . . . "She was *furious* with him!" . . . No — that's another classic response . . . "She thought he had it coming." . . . No. I guess that's another . . . See how hard it is to justice to the occasion, Carrie. (*She shrugs.*) "She didn't really care one way or the other." (*She looks at* CARRIE.) What am I doing?

CARRIE: Feeling your way, I would guess.

ADDIE: I'm glad John's asleep — I'll have to be behaving a little more sanely by the time he wakes.

CARRIE: Don't worry. All John wants is for the two of you to set aside your differences for now — if you can.

ADDIE: That will be a whole lot easier if I watch my mouth.

CARRIE: John's not expecting you to be other than you are. (ADDIE *looks at her.*) Well, is he? Is that what you think?

ADDIE: Vas you dere, Chollie?

CARRIE: No — I wasn't there.

ADDIE: Well . . . (*She looks around. Then in a loud voice . . .*) Dad!

CARRIE: He's dead, Ad. I saw him die.

ADDIE: I know he's dead. I do know it! (*She gets up.*) But what does that mean? (*She looks around the room.*) Look at this place! Where did the life go that — what's the word? . . . that actualized this place. The body — I understand — is dead. Where's the rest? (CAR-

RIE *shakes her head.* ADDIE's *tone changes.*) Well, you'd better
figure it out. You're my big sister, and I've got no folks ... I'm an
orphan now — altogether.

CARRIE: (*Simply*) So am I.

ADDIE: (*Studying her*) But you're not a lone, lorn creatur'.

CARRIE: Why not? Why don't I ever get to be that? Why just you?

ADDIE: Because you're a grown up.

CARRIE: Go to hell. (*Pause.*) You know what? I'm terribly hungry —
are you? Shall I see what Dad's got in ... (*She breaks off with a little laugh.*)

ADDIE: What are we *doing*? I want to ask you something. How are
we able to do this? Shouldn't a death be more momentous than
this? You wanted a sandwich — I'm hungry, too. (*She looks
around the room.*) The man is *gone* — and we raid his refrigerator.

CARRIE: (*Picking up a pack of cigarettes from the coffee table*)
What's more — I'm going to smoke one of John's cigarettes.

ADDIE: And you're probably glad for the excuse.

CARRIE: I am!

ADDIE: ... Are we awful?

CARRIE: ... I don't know ... You're not ... so I guess I'm not, either.
(*They sit without talking.*) How old were you when Mother died?
Eleven?

ADDIE: I was ten, wasn't I?

CARRIE: Yes, you were ten because I was twenty-two ... I don't
suppose you remember how much there is to do — after a death.

ADDIE: (*From very far away*) No, I don't remember that.
(*Coming back.*) I guess I wasn't in on that much.

CARRIE: ... Did I write? To thank you for the pictures? The kids
divided them up and hung them in their rooms. Sharon got a lot of
mileage out of them at school. My aunt — the dancer. Peter said
maybe we can fly out next season. I haven't seen you dance for so
long.

ADDIE: I'd like you to visit my classes, too. I've come to love the
teaching ... In a sense the old man got his wish — if he could only
have seen it that way.

CARRIE: I think about San Francisco. (*She looks around the room.*)
Look at all this ... Don't let me take a lot of stuff, Addie. You'll be

doing me a big favor if you keep me from finding a use for every damn thing I pick up — or keeping old letters. Let's be ruthless.

ADDIE: I'm with you. The best recourse would be to set fire to the place.

(JOHN *has been standing in the doorway. He now enters.* ADDIE *doesn't see him until he speaks.*)

JOHN: Addie.

ADDIE: (*Jumping up*) Johnnie! (*She goes to him and he embraces her. She steps back and touches him.*) I'm sorry I didn't answer your letters . . . I didn't want to write until I knew what to say . . . And I never did know. I am sorry, John. It seems inexcusable now — looking at you.

JOHN: It's all right, Ad. I had to write — so I did. I understood that you couldn't.

ADDIE: Don't be so goddamned understanding. (*Pause.*) Isn't this strange, John? The old man did it. (*Lowering her voice.*) He let them get him . . . Does this mean I have to grow up now, Johnnie? (*He touches her face. She looks at him for a minute, then goes to the sofa and sits down.* JOHN *sits down beside* ADDIE.)

JOHN: I didn't think this was going to be the time.

ADDIE: Me neither. You probably never do.

JOHN: I like knowing that he woke up here this morning in his own place.

ADDIE: Yeah — that's good.

JOHN: . . . Addie. . . .

ADDIE: Not now. This isn't the time.

JOHN: I don't mean to talk about it. Let's acknowledge it, though.

ADDIE: (*Tipping an imaginary hat*) How-de-do.

JOHN: Come on, Addie.

ADDIE: What do you want, kid?

JOHN: I can't pretend those things don't exist.

ADDIE: I wasn't pretending. I thought we had a silent agreement to let 'em ride for now.

JOHN: We do. We did.

ADDIE: So?

JOHN: (*Laughs*) I guess I didn't know we did, actually.

CARRIE: What day of the week is this?

JOHN: Saturday.

CARRIE: Can you stay until Tuesday or Wednesday?

JOHN: Sure. I suppose the funeral will be Monday.

CARRIE: Yeah, I think. If the aunts and uncles can get here by Monday. I *hope* to God we can have it then. (*She looks from* JOHN *to* ADDIE.) You two didn't always fight. (*To* JOHN.) Remember when she was a baby and you told me she was much yours as mine?

JOHN: You never believed it, though. (*To* CARRIE.) We have put our differences on hold.

CARRIE: I'm glad.

ADDIE: But the time will come....

JOHN: Oh, I know, Ad — there's no escaping you.

ADDIE: We have to finish it up.

JOHN: You left.

ADDIE: Because too much was happening that I didn't understand. I needed to get away from it.

JOHN: And now you understand?

ADDIE: Maybe . . . Some of it . . . But, what's more important, I'm ready to try.

JOHN: I'd just as soon drop it.

ADDIE: No! We're not going to drop it.

JOHN: What a relentless sort you are.

ADDIE: Only about some things. Only when it matters, Johnnie-boy. Otherwise I relent like crazy. (*Getting up and picking up her suitcase.*) I'm going to get out of these clothes. I've been in them for half a continent. (*She exits into the hall, stage left.* JOHN *gets up and goes over to the book shelves. He takes down a book or two.*)

JOHN: Do you know how long I have waited to possess some of these books? (*Gives a short laugh.*) I have such ambivalence about his death.

CARRIE: You come to bury Caesar.

JOHN: You think that's it?

CARRIE: Addie, too — for all her defiance.

JOHN: I understand Addie.

CARRIE: You mean you forgive Addie ... You know, Johnnie, it seems to me you are always accusing yourself of humanity.

JOHN: (*Studying her*) I've always wished that I found your reassurances more comforting.

CARRIE: I wish it, too.

JOHN: What about you? Are you ambivalent?

CARRIE: Always.

JOHN: But about this?

CARRIE: About everything.

JOHN: That's not the same — quite.

CARRIE: Not quite.

JOHN: You'd made your peace with him, somehow.

CARRIE: I saw, you know, his raw need when Mother died. He was never the same for me after that.

JOHN: (*Takes this in — then turns back to the shelves and takes down another book*) Here's the Shakespeare he taught from last. (*He thumbs through.*) Complete with marginalia.

CARRIE: I have a book of Mother's that she must have read for some college course because there are notes in it. One place she wrote "Delightful passage!" ... and I can hear the lilt in her voice when I see it.

JOHN: I heard it just now.

CARRIE: Am I beginning to look like her? I think I am. Sometimes when I catch a sidelong glance of myself in a mirror, I think, "Mother!" (*She laughs.*) God, it's disappointing when it's only me!

JOHN: You hear her voice. That must be nice. (*Thumbs through the book.*) A kind of rational seance. (*Continuing to look through the book.*) Listen to this, Carrie. He underlined, "O, then, beware! Those wounds heal ill that men do give themselves." And he wrote, "Read Shakespeare and Dostoevsky, and you'll have no need for Freud." ... My God ... you're right. I hear his voice! (*He laughs.*) Advice from beyond the grave, Caroline! Ignore Freud! What did he know? Allan Brennan says we have all we need in Shakespeare and Dostoevsky ... You opinionated, bombastic old fart! Did it ever occur to you that you might be *wrong* about something?

ACT II

Setting: *Same as Scene 1 except that the livingroom is stacked with boxes, books, and miscellany. The pictures and maps are still on the walls. Some pieces of furniture are gone, and the bookshelves are beginning to empty. A kitchen table has been placed center stage.*

Time: *Early evening of the next day.*

At Rise: CARRIE, JOHN *and* ADDIE *are sitting around the table. They have finished dinner; the table is partially cleared. They are drinking coffee.* LAUREN, *aged twenty, is sitting close by on the floor, looking through a box of photographs.*

JOHN: We'll invite Uncle Otis to come and look through the books — and what he doesn't. . .

LAUREN: (*Breaking in*) These are fun. I didn't know Grandpa had any pictures I hadn't seen.

CARRIE: What do you have there?

LAUREN: Some fat baby thing with a thirty-ish lady — not your mother, I think.

ADDIE: Let's see.

LAUREN: (*Comes over to the table and shows the picture to* ADDIE) Who is that?

ADDIE: I don't know them — the other side of someone's family, would be my guess. (*Handing the picture to* JOHN.) Who are these foreigners?

JOHN: (*Studies the picture and hands it on to* CARRIE) I don't know who that is — but she's got the Brennan demeanor — look at that chin line.

LAUREN: (*She has gone back to her place on the floor*) Here's Grandmother — and Grandpa. (*She looks on the back of the picture.*) August, 1930 ... She was lovely. And Grandpa had a mustache! It looks great.

ADDIE: He was a dashing fellow.

LAUREN: Oh, Mother! This is hilarious. How old were you here? (*She brings a picture over to* CARRIE.)

CARRIE: What's so funny about that?

LAUREN: Your hair! (*She laughs.*)

CARRIE: (*Studying the picture*) On the contrary — it looks perfect, and if it didn't look just like that Mother would have to shove me out the door for school. (*She wails, imitating her teenage self.*) "I can't go looking like this — everyone will *laugh.*" (ADDIE *reaches for the picture, looks at it and laughs.*) Go find some pictures of your Aunt Addie — she was *adorable* at fourteen. (LAUREN *goes back to the pictures and* ADDIE *joins her.*)

LAUREN: Here's Grandpa again. I didn't know he was such a handsome man. His eyes were so large.

JOHN: All the better to *see* you with, my dear.

ADDIE: How were his teeth? (*Makes a snapping motion at* LAUREN.) He could finish off the likes of you with one bite.

LAUREN: His eyes look like yours, Uncle John.

JOHN: Oh?

LAUREN: (*Bringing the picture over to* JOHN) See?

JOHN: (*Looking at the picture*) A most handsome fellow. (*Lightly.*) Lauren, explain to me how two people with eyes that looked so much alike could have seen things so differently.

LAUREN: You think you did?

JOHN: Don't you?

LAUREN: No.

JOHN: No?

LAUREN: For instance, that's exactly the kind of observation he would have made. But Addie's the one who's really like him.

ADDIE: (*Looking up*) I am?

CARRIE: From Lauren that's a high compliment. They were very good friends.

LAUREN: No one understood me like he did.

CARRIE: He didn't understand you at all.

LAUREN: Well, it didn't matter. I had a father to understand me. I didn't need that from Grandpa.

JOHN: Yes — you were wise in your choice of fathers, Lauren.

LAUREN: As a grandfather he was perfect — full of stories, funny. He told me things about Mother that I'm sure she never would have — and he remembered what it was like to be a kid . . . Did he understand anyone?

CARRIE: I don't know. I didn't expect that from him.

JOHN: It was enough for you that you understood him. (*With less intensity.*) He had a real bargain in you.

ADDIE: (*Coming over to the table and sitting down*) How am I like him? (JOHN *and* CARRIE *laugh.* JOHN *walks back to the table and sits down.*) No — I really want to know. I think I am, but I don't know how.

CARRIE: You have his lusty approach to life.

ADDIE: Do I? Oh, that's nice!

JOHN: What do I get — besides his eyes?

CARRIE: Lauren's right, John, you see things the way he did — some things.

JOHN: Isn't it wonderful the way we all escaped his bad traits?

LAUREN: Mother's stubborn.

CARRIE: Hey! Watch it! (*She rises.*) I suppose we should clear this away. Fritz and Grace are coming over to pick up some of those boxes they're letting me store in their basement.

JOHN: (*Rising and starting to stack up the dishes*) That was a delicious meal, Addie. (*To* CARRIE.) I suppose you and I are stuck with the dishes since Addie cooked and Lauren set the table.

CARRIE: Looks like it.

ADDIE: Fine by me. (CARRIE *and* JOHN *clear the table during the following exchange.* ADDIE *stretches out on the sofa.* LAUREN *sits on the floor close by her.*)

CARRIE: Do you still hide the crusty pans in the oven, full of greasy dishwater, John?

JOHN: Of course, why would I let go of a good thing?

LAUREN: Did you do that, Uncle John?

CARRIE: It was infuriating.

LAUREN: Did she say, "Who do you imagine is going to come along and wash those pots if you don't? Tell me that. Who?"

ADDIE: That's it — that's perfect.

JOHN: Yes, that was how it went. She was a veritable owl on the subject. Whooo?

CARRIE: Well, who did you think was going to?

JOHN: Whooo?

CARRIE: I never have understood who people imagined was going to come along and finish their work. (*She exits into the kitchen.*)

JOHN: If Dad thought she was having any trouble managing one of us, without rising from his chair in the livingroom, he'd call out, "Caroline? Problems?" (*He speaks the two words slowly, in a low, magisterial voice. Then — to* LAUREN.) And, do you know, there never were? They disappeared — destroyed by the deadly rays of his potential wrath.

ADDIE: Did Mother ever discipline — because I don't remember it if she ever did.

CARRIE: (*Coming into the room*) Mother was very likely to go out and work in her rose garden if things got out of hand.

LAUREN: What did she do in the winter?

CARRIE: In the winter?

LAUREN: When there weren't any roses.

JOHN: She would find some rosy thing to do.

CARRIE: Yes, some rosy thing to do — with her rose-colored glasses on . . . I can remember just demanding a response from her — for instance about something like John and the infernal pots.

ADDIE: (*Laughing*) You're still mad about those pots.

JOHN: Whooo?

CARRIE: And she'd say something like, "I'm sure John has every intention of washing the pots, Caddie, after they've soaked properly." Of course there was absolutely *nothing* in John's past history to indicate that.

JOHN: She spoke only of my intentions.

CARRIE: Well, I wasn't interested in your intentions — they probably were all right — you were a nice kid. (*Pointing at him.*) But you never did end up washing the damned things, did you?... She was not long on realism.

JOHN: (*Lighting a cigarette*) She had her own brand.

CARRIE: It didn't jibe.

JOHN: With what?

CARRIE: It just didn't jibe.

JOHN: With what, though? One thing jibes with another — a thing doesn't jibe or not jibe all by itself — out there in limbo.

CARRIE: Boring English teacher — it didn't jibe with other people's vision of reality. Mother marched to a different drummer — in a totally different parade.

JOHN: Mother's parade marched to the music of the spheres.

CARRIE: Some strange little tune that played inside her own head, more likely.

JOHN: We don't know yet. There are districts yet to be heard from. As she used to say, "When the dust settles...."

CARRIE: Everything is *not* going to be all right, John! Isn't that clear to you by now? Everything is not going to be all right! (*She stands. Indicating to the table.*) Come on, let's get this thing out of here. (*They exit into the kitchen with the table.*)

LAUREN: Evidently she's still mad about her mother, too. (*Stretching out on her stomach.*) Well, aren't you going to ask me how's college and all those other aunty questions?

ADDIE: I will if you want — I'm glad you came down tonight. Tomorrow won't be much of a day for visiting.

LAUREN: Mother said none of you went to the funeral home — to see him. Will the aunts and uncles think that's funny?

ADDIE: We're Al's kids. We're allowed to be funny. No, I think they understand ... Have you ever seen a body — all laid out in a funeral home? (LAUREN *shakes her head.*) Well, there is nothin' there — less than nothing ... And we didn't want to see that. You could have gone, you know. You still can, if you need to.

LAUREN: No, I don't.

ADDIE: (*After a pause*) How *is* school?

LAUREN: It's all right, but I'm sick of it . . . I'm going to take a year off.

ADDIE: What are you going to do?

LAUREN: Head west — next fall.

ADDIE: California?

LAUREN: (*Nods*) Isn't that young and foolish of me?

ADDIE: It's wonderful. Tell me your plans.

LAUREN: Well, I'll get a summer job and just not spend a dime. I can do that — I've done it before — for things.

ADDIE: The parents know?

LAUREN: Yeah. I think they almost like it.

JOHN: (*Enters from the kitchen*) Now I remember why I always left the pots. You couldn't do them to her satisfaction, anyway, so there was no use trying. She's happy as a lark — working away in there on last week's apple brown betty.

LAUREN: Last week's what?

JOHN: Maybe you know it as apple crisp. Your grandfather called it that. To Mother it was apple brown betty.

CARRIE: (*Coming in*) Dad thought that was a ridiculous name — remember, John? He said he could understand welsh rabbit — because he could imagine a Welsh rabbit — that it would be quirky and irritable like all the creatures of the British Isles who weren't born English. But he would never agree to apple brown betty because there was no such color as apple brown — or some such. Do you remember, John?

JOHN: — Only that Mother called it one thing and he called it another. (*To* ADDIE.) What do you call it?

ADDIE: I don't call it. I never make it.

JOHN: Well — you'll have to decide, Ad — it's not an issue you can let ride your whole life long. You'll have to take a stand.

ADDIE: But not yet, Johnnie. (*To* CARRIE.) Carrie, Lauren told me her California plans.

CARRIE: I didn't know things had reached the point where they could be called "plans."

LAUREN: Oh, Mother! (*To* ADDIE.) Nothing's a plan to Mother until you start making lists.

JOHN: Are you applying to a school in California, Lauren?

LAUREN: No — I'm going to play hookey for a year.

ADDIE: Isn't that wonderful, John? I'll get to show her San Francisco. (*She doesn't wait for a response and there is none.* JOHN *sits down and picks up a magazine. He leafs through it, not involving himself in what follows until he is directly addressed.*)

ADDIE: So, now, be more specific. — Is this just travel or are you going to look for a job — or what? (*To* CARRIE.) It seems such a good idea to me.

CARRIE: (*Smiling*) Well, of course. It's an Addie type plan — probably Addie inspired.

LAUREN: Mother doesn't think I'm capable of being adventuresome on my own.

ADDIE: Let's hear the details.

CARRIE: There are no details. This so-called plan barely qualified for supper table discussion up to now.

LAUREN: Mother — that isn't true. Just because I don't know every move I'm going to make doesn't mean I haven't thought about this . . . Anyway, I'm going to do it. I'm sick of school. I've been in school every year of my life for fifteen years! Can you imagine that? *Your* life has more variety than mine.

CARRIE: God forbid my life should have any variety.

ADDIE: That's not the point, Carrie.

LAUREN: Really — that's not the point, Mother.

CARRIE: (*To* JOHN) Help! They're ganging up on me.

JOHN: (*Without looking up*) You raised 'em.

CARRIE: John!

ADDIE: (*Very much caught up in* LAUREN's *plan*) I don't think you should fly.

LAUREN: No?

ADDIE: You've never seen the West. Oh! I wish I could drive with you! (*Gets up quickly and walks around as her mind works.*) Maybe I could fly back — we could rent a car. I'd love to show you the great American West.

LAUREN: We could camp out — save money that way.

ADDIE: And I have a friend in Denver. I know he'd put us up for a couple of days.

LAUREN: Oh, that would be wonderful! — Uncle John, you should let Teddy come along. He's been in school thirteen years. That's almost as bad.

ADDIE: We could have such a time. Remember, John, how sorry you felt for Teddy when they made him sit behind a desk in first grade and write his letters so straight. Well, this is your chance. . . .

(For the first time since this conversation started ADDIE *sees what is happening with* JOHN. *They exchange a long look.)*

CARRIE: *(To* LAUREN*)* I'm sure your uncle will thank you not to infect Teddy with your itchy feet.

LAUREN: Oh, I was just kidding about that, really — though it would be fun.

ADDIE: *(Quietly)* It is a good idea, John — for kids to do these things while they they are young and free.

JOHN: *(Trying to keep it light)* Probably — but I'm not sure the proper adult role is to encourage them.

ADDIE: So it's me, really, isn't it? It's not that they *do* it — but that I encourage it. I know you think what Lauren is doing is wonderful. But I'm not supposed to cheer her on!

JOHN: You should see yourself, Addie — your eyes glisten — you positively salivate.

ADDIE: *(Tightly)* So what, John?

JOHN: Why is it that you are drawn to every action that strays from the conventional?

ADDIE: What does it matter to you? Anyway, it's my *role* — you know that. I'm Addie — who strays. And you're John — who doesn't.

CARRIE: I thought you were going to wait on this.

ADDIE: I felt you following me around when I was at your house.

JOHN: I didn't follow you around.

ADDIE: In your head. *(Becoming* JOHN.*)* "Where's Addie? What's she up to? What's she saying to Diane? To Teddy?"

JOHN: Not to them. Not just them — to everybody. . . .

ADDIE: *(Just now seeing this)* To you! *(They are all silent.)*

CARRIE: I really had hoped that the two of you . . . *(Sound of the doorbell, overlapping from "hoped.")* That's Fritz and Grace.

LAUREN: I'll get it.

CARRIE: (*To* JOHN *and* ADDIE — *not seriously*) "Forget, forgive; conclude and be agreed."

JOHN: She must be the head of the family. She quotes Shakespeare.

CARRIE: No — I quote Father quoting Shakespeare.

(LAUREN *gets up and goes toward the door.* JOHN *stands.* FRITZ *and* GRACE *enter from the hall, stage right.* LAUREN *hugs them both.* GRACE *is seventy-two; she has on a light, summer dress.*)

GRACE: It's nice for your mother that you could come down early, Lauren. Here, Carrie — I brought a rhubarb pie. I always make two — it's just as easy.

ADDIE: Oh, goodie — we aren't going to wait, are we? I want mine now.

FRITZ: I'm glad to hear that. I never did hold with that business of waiting until nine o'clock for dessert.

GRACE: This isn't for you — you had yours. This is for the kids.

FRITZ: Well, they won't enjoy eating it in front of me — I wouldn't let 'em.

GRACE: You aren't hungry.

FRITZ: How do you know that?

GRACE: Because I saw you put away too much pot roast not two hours ago.

FRITZ: I guess I must have worked up an appetite helping you into the car.

GRACE: (*Laughing*) I apologize for your uncle ... Let me help you, Carrie. (GRACE *and* CARRIE *work from a sideboard, cutting the pie and handing each of the others a piece.*)

LAUREN: Uncle Fritz, are you sure you have room for me? Aren't Uncle Otis and Aunt Rose coming up tonight, too? I can sleep right here on the sofa, you know.

FRITZ: On the sofa! What kind of a night's sleep would you get on the sofa? Anyway, Grace has been dying to fuss over somebody. She got out her little rosebud soaps and put them in the bathroom. I threatened to use one when I came in from the garden. (*He laughs.*) She still is never quite sure when I am kidding her ... as if I'd use her little no-good soaps.

JOHN: Where did you get your ornery streak? It seems to me that

Grandmother was a gentle sort and Grandfather rather quiet and stern. Where did you and Dad get your — ways?

FRITZ: We had an interesting uncle. (*To* GRACE *as she sits down with her pie.*) What's that you have there?

GRACE: See, Carrie?

CARRIE: You lay off her. See the size of that piece? I insisted she join us. (CARRIE *and* GRACE *sit down and they all start to eat.*)

FRITZ: Listen, Carrie, while we're on the subject of Grace and her ways. . . .

GRACE: Do we have to pursue the subject of Grace and her ways?

FRITZ: Just this one thing, dear — Now, Caroline, you *did* feed the rest of these people supper, didn't you? Because Grace is the sort who never really believes that people have eaten sufficiently and properly unless she sees them going at it . . . but I believe she'd take your word — and she could sleep a lot better tonight if. . . .

JOHN: Well, we all know that would be a great relief to you. (FRITZ *looks at* JOHN *questioningly.*) If she got a good night's sleep. (FRITZ *starts to laugh.* JOHN *looks at him and smiles.*)

FRITZ: (*To* GRACE) John has pointed out to me that I have maybe more than the normal amount of concern about people getting their rest.

GRACE: Oh, John, I'm so glad. He does! And he loves to make out as though I'm the only one of us interested in the physical side of things.

FRITZ: No, no. Obviously if I didn't share your interest in the physical side of things we never would have had all those children.

GRACE: And, you know, John, after sending all the rest of us to our slumbers — he came home last night and sat up until three in the morning. (*She looks at* FRITZ *lovingly.*) He said . . . Do you mind?

FRITZ: Tell my secrets, Grace — I don't care.

GRACE: You're sure?

FRITZ: (*To the others*) I told Grace it was the last day I'd shared with Al — I wasn't in a hurry to end it. (*They are all touched.*) I wasn't brooding — I just got to thinking about some of the things he and I did — I started laughing out loud. (*To* GRACE.) Did you hear me? (*She shakes her head.*) Did I tell you what I was thinking about?

GRACE: Some peccadillo, I know.

FRITZ: I was thinking about a cousin of ours — Howard Farley — you kids never knew Howard. He married a girl from Texas and moved down there to ranch with her father. He died a dozen or so years ago ... But — one summer when Al and I were — oh — in our late teens, early twenties, I guess — we went down to Kansas to hire out as farm hands. We'd move along with the haying season. We spent part of that summer with our Aunt Millie and Uncle Hal...

GRACE: Howard's folks.

FRITZ: Somehow your dad began to suspect that Howard had joined the Klan ... and I don't recall ...

LAUREN: The Ku Klux Klan?

FRITZ: Now, that shocks you, but at first it didn't seem quite the awful thing it came to be later. At least, not in Kansas.

GRACE: It was hardly a wonderful organization anywhere — at best.

FRITZ: (*Impatient to get on with his story*) Oh, granted — granted. I just want these kids to understand that it wasn't the same as if one of their cousins joined the ranks ... So — Al and I decided to find out if old Howard was really one of the boys, and the next time we heard of a meeting we tailed him ... The meeting was to be in a clearing not far from the farm so we figured he'd walk — and he did — and we tailed him. When he was a good distance from the house, he donned his sheet ... Well, we — unencumbered — cut off through the woods and shinnied up a huge cottonwood along his route. Down the path he came — old Howard — and, just as he passed us, Al said — in a soft, low voice that sounded like God's own — "No, Howard." (FRITZ *laughs hard at the memory.*) Well, kids, I've got to hand it to Howard for sheer guts —

GRACE: Never looked back, did he?

FRITZ: Never changed his pace. But I swear you could see a shiver make its journey up his spine — I can see it as plain — Just like it got caught by a gentle summer breeze that sheet shook — started at the base of his spine and traveled right up to the top of his head 'til his little peak just quivered! (*Everyone laughs.*)

LAUREN: He must have known it was you and Grandpa.

FRITZ: I don't know, Lauren. Al was a magician. He said those two words so low — and yet with such authority. I kind of think Howard was never sure if he heard 'em or only *thought* he heard 'em... That man — he could make me laugh.... (*There is silence.*)

GRACE: We went to the funeral home this afternoon. I understand how you young people feel about that kind of thing. But we needed to go ... He's not there, of course — Al's not ... But something is there that we need to see. (*She smiles at them.*) We're used to the old ways. When someone died on the farm the body would be laid out in the front room until the funeral — friends and neighbors would stop by.... (*To* FRITZ.) Remember how the kitchen would fill up with casseroles and layer cakes? (*To the others.*) And the casket would be taken to the church. Why, at your grandfather's funeral there were so many people they had to stand in the church-yard ... It was a record hot day, and ladies were fainting regular-ly. You remember, Carrie — John.

LAUREN: I thought Grandpa wanted to be cremated.

CARRIE: What made you think that, pet?

LAUREN: I thought he told me that once — I'm almost sure he did.

ADDIE: He mentioned it to me once, too.

CARRIE: Somehow people just don't get around to making those kinds of plans.

FRITZ: (*Rising*) Well, Otis and Rose will be coming pretty soon, Grace. Let's help these kids with the dishes we've dirtied and be on our way.

CARRIE: We're not going to wash any more dishes tonight. We'll stack them up and do them in the morning. (CARRIE, FRITZ *and* LAUREN *clear the coffee table of dishes, exit with them into the kitchen and return.*)

GRACE: (*Noticing the box of pictures*) You children should be finding some treasures. Your father kept his possessions pretty well culled. He was selective about what he kept so what's left should be quite interesting.

CARRIE: (*Standing beside* GRACE) What are we ever going to do with the rest of this? (*To* FRITZ.) Are you sure you have taken all the books you want?

FRITZ: Let's be honest, Carrie. One of these times my kids will have to be doing this. What I need is fewer things — not more. (*To* LAUREN.) Your mother says she will bring you over later. (*He looks at* CARRIE, JOHN *and* ADDIE.) There's something I want to tell you guys. You, especially, John — because I know men are stuck with a concern about providing that is different from a woman's concern ... Anyway, it's this — I was afraid of death when I was — say — forty, forty-five ... And now I'm not ... I'm not saying it's wonderful getting old — losing people. But I'm not afraid of death ... When I was younger I was worried I'd go like a couple of guys I knew — in their prime — afraid I'd leave Grace and the kids —

wondered how they'd do. Now — well — I look forward to whatever's left ... And it's not like I've reached some certainty about things. I've never heard a conclusive case made pro or con — things continuing. But what if it is just peaceful oblivion ... That doesn't sound so bad to me ... So — that's it. I had it in my mind that I wanted to be sure to tell you that. Maybe none of you need that little tale — but there it is. (*Lightly.*) Well, I made my speech, "Mother" ... Don't you love men who call their wives "mother"? ... Why would a woman tolerate it?

CARRIE: (*Gives* FRITZ *a hug*) Listen to me. John and I are going to put those boxes in your car, and Lauren and I will take them out when I bring her over. *You* are not to touch them.

FRITZ: I'm not feeble.

CARRIE: It's got nothing to do with feeble. It's not your project. (JOHN *and* CARRIE *exit stage right with cardboard boxes.*)

FRITZ: Well, come on, Grace. I'll take you home by the scenic route.

LAUREN: What's the scenic route, Aunt Grace? I didn't know the town had one.

GRACE: Neither did I. He probably means past the Dairy Queen.

FRITZ: After all I've eaten?

GRACE: How would I know when you're going to end this binge? Two pieces of rhubarb pie — you're going to confound your digestive system. (FRITZ *laughs.*)

FRITZ: (*Ushering* GRACE *toward the exit stage right*) Well, good night all. I don't dare mention how you should sleep.

GRACE: I'm so happy that John pointed that out — After all these years that you've been trying to paint me as one of those simple-hearted women who can't think of anything but feeding people. (*She laughs.*) Lauren, we'll see you soon. Good night, Addie dear.

(LAUREN *and* ADDIE *rise and see them to the door.* GRACE *and* FRITZ *exit stage right. All ad lib good-byes.*)

ADDIE: (*Sitting back down*) That's why I never understood mean jokes about relatives.

LAUREN: (*Joining her*) Mm.

ADDIE: Are you tired? You could go with them right now — you know?

LAUREN: No, that's all right. I think Mother wants to take the rest of this stuff when she takes me over ... But I am tired all of a sudden.

ADDIE: The whole business is exhausting.

LAUREN: I don't know what it would be like to have a father die.

ADDIE: (*After a pause*) I don't, either — and I just did.

LAUREN: I can't imagine my father dying — or my mother.

ADDIE: Your mother and father are going to die at a ripe, old age — hand in hand with their children gathered around them to wish them on their way.

LAUREN: Where will you be, Addie?

ADDIE: I'll be there, too . . . We'll thank them for having lived . . . And they will give you all to me — (LAUREN *looks at* ADDIE *closely.*) You are the first and only — original happy ending family. So that's how it's got to be . . . They will tell us all how well we turned out — smile at one another — and die with joy on their faces. (LAUREN *looks at* ADDIE *with concern.*) Look! Someone has got to live happily ever after!

(CARRIE *and* JOHN *enter stage right.*)

CARRIE: Lauren, John and I are going to load up our car. You get ready to go with me. At the risk of irritating Fritz, I'd like to be there to unload both cars — or to help, anyway.

ADDIE: I'll help you carry these things out.

CARRIE: There's not that much. Why don't you help Lauren get organized? (JOHN *and* CARRIE *load up with boxes, etc.*) I know I'm being ridiculous about Fritz. And he's being a very good sport. (CARRIE *and* JOHN *exit.* LAUREN *and* ADDIE *gather up* LAUREN's *things, and* LAUREN *puts them in her backpack.*)

ADDIE: I'd forgotten how much paraphernalia it takes to be young.

LAUREN: . . . One of the nicest things Grandpa ever said to me was that I reminded him of you.

ADDIE: (*Stops short and looks at* LAUREN) You must have been fighting with him.

LAUREN: We were arguing about socialism.

ADDIE: (*Smiling*) It was a lovely misreading on your part to take that as a compliment.

LAUREN: It was a compliment; I'd just made a very good point. Anyway, I could tell by the way he said it — he'd rather have been arguing with you. And he liked me a lot.

ADDIE: That, I know, is true. (CARRIE *and* JOHN *enter.*)

CARRIE: (*To* LAUREN) Are you ready, babe?

LAUREN: Yup.

CARRIE: I don't think I'll be long. See you guys later.

(*All ad lib good-byes.* CARRIE *and* LAUREN *exit stage right.* JOHN *sits down at the desk and lights a cigarette. He starts sorting through a stack of papers, discarding some, putting others into various piles.* ADDIE *goes to the radio, turns it on and finds a station that is playing jazz. She starts to dance.* JOHN *watches her for a moment and then continues his work.* ADDIE *dances for a few minutes. Her dancing should reflect her training only in its control. It is restrained dance that she is doing. After a time she turns the radio down.*)

ADDIE: Does the radio bother you?

JOHN: No.

ADDIE: Do you ever dance?

JOHN: Not for years.

ADDIE: You should dance, John. It loosens the soul.

JOHN: Do you think I have a tight soul, Ad? (*She bursts into laughter and looks at him a long time.*)

ADDIE: No, I don't . . . That's why I don't understand why you act so — tight-assed.

JOHN: Is that how you see me?

ADDIE: That's how you've been — with me. When I was at your house, I felt that every word that fell from my lips was being shipped off to some musty little laboratory for analysis.

JOHN: What the *hell* are you talking about?

ADDIE: Everything I am seems to bug you now, John. I couldn't take your thin-lipped disapproval; that's why I left . . . I don't know one thing about you anymore.

JOHN: Only that I'm tight-assed.

ADDIE: I'm not going to feel guilty about that . . . That's how you've acted with me — I said. I didn't say you were.

JOHN: A nice distinction.

ADDIE: An important distinction.

JOHN: Maybe there's hope for me, yet.

ADDIE: (*Not responding to that*) You remind me of the old man.

JOHN: What?

ADDIE: I thought none of us was like him in that way — withholding approval.

JOHN: I have opinions, Addie. Everyone has opinions.

ADDIE: Not so many! And such negative ones. About me.

JOHN: You? You were his special project.

ADDIE: His prodigal child. Except that I never repented — didn't spend all my talents in wasteful living and come home repentant. But you two loyal sons of bitches — you never shook your fists in his face! (JOHN *stands and they confront one another.*)

JOHN: I don't think Carrie needed to . . . And I — didn't.

ADDIE: Why not? Why not, John? I needed you to do that!

JOHN: I stood up for you — for your right to do things your own way.

ADDIE: Yes, you did. But I needed you to stand up for yourself. You got around him — that's not the same.

JOHN: I don't love a fight the way you do.

ADDIE: You had to fight him. There was *no other way.*

JOHN: You chose to rebel. There are other methods for coming to terms with things.

ADDIE: You have not come to terms with anything.

JOHN: When you're forty you'll still be doing things as a reaction against the old man — and he'll have been dead for nine years.

ADDIE: I won't listen to you — because you have not come to terms with *shit!* (*Covers her ears.*) No more. No more of your reasonable sounding voice saying all those lies. What's happening in your life? You did used to stand up for me against the old man, but you didn't stand up for yourself. You tamed your beast, and now everyone else has to tame theirs — or cage it — or kill it . . . Did you kill your beast, John? . . . He wouldn't have wanted you to do that. (*Pause.*) You tamed your beast, and we all have to pay. It doesn't matter so much with me, but what about your kids — and what about Diane? (*In a loud voice.*) What's up with you? *Where are you?*

JOHN: (*Coldly*) I am here.

ADDIE: Nah. You're just not!

JOHN: I've had about enough of this.

ADDIE: (*Throwing her hands out*) Of this? This is nothing.

JOHN: Well, then, surely we can end it.

ADDIE: Something is going on in your life and you are making me pay
— It's bad enough that Padre isn't here to finish what he started. I
really can't stand your judgments raining down on me. Get off my
back. I haven't done anything wrong.

JOHN: He pulled out and left a lot of unfinished business — not just
with you.

ADDIE: I know that.

JOHN: Anything's possible now, Addie. There's an intense smell of
freedom with him gone. And I don't know if I can *take* it . . . I've
been holding my life together with fingernail parings. The last thing
I needed when you came was the stink of freedom that wafts
around you wherever you go! It's all becoming unstuck — and now
that he's dead . . .

ADDIE: (*Interrupting*) Nothing changes because he's dead. There is no
more freedom on this side of his death! There's really very little
goddamn freedom anywhere, John! And certainly no more in my
life than in anyone else's . . . I knew there was something in me — I
don't want to be one of the things you're afraid of.

JOHN: The list is long. You'll barely notice yourself.

(JOHN *leaves.* ADDIE *stands for a bit. Then she moves some of the
boxes and furniture back and dances. This time she dances without
music, not particularly emotionally, movement for its own sake.*)

ACT III

Setting: *The same.*

Time: *An hour later.*

At Rise: ADDIE *is lying on the sofa reading.* CARRIE *enters stage right.*

CARRIE: Well, that's that. I've got my assignment for the next decade, sorting through those boxes. (*She sits down.*) Oh, do I feel irritable. Doesn't that seem like a strange reaction to you? You wanted a new response to death — there's my offering. I'm irritated.

ADDIE: With the deceased?

CARRIE: Who was that again?

ADDIE: (*Laughing*) What?

CARRIE: I've forgotten what it is we are all doing here. I swear to God, this afternoon when Grace was wanting to talk about plans for the supper — after — I couldn't remember for a minute what we were planning this event for!

ADDIE: So I guess you're not irritated with him.

CARRIE: No. No, it's not his fault. He would have thought this was all ridiculous ... He probably did want to be cremated.

ADDIE: I'd have loved to have taken his ashes to that place on the river where he used to fish ... Wouldn't that have been something, Carrie?

CARRIE: Yes, I'd like that.

ADDIE: Had Uncle Otis and Aunt Rose arrived?

CARRIE: They were sitting on the glider. The house was unlocked, of course, but Rose wouldn't let Otis go in. (*She reflects.*) I knew something was wrong with me when I looked at Otis's big, sad face and didn't know whether to cry or push him off the porch. (ADDIE *laughs hard.*) I even got annoyed with Fritz, that dear man.

ADDIE: What did he do?

CARRIE: Nothing — absolutely nothing — but, Ad, do they ever seem to you like a husband and wife act?

ADDIE: (*Still amused*) No.

CARRIE: See? I'm just a mean-spirited, middle-aged witch.

ADDIE: It's been a long, hard time for you.

CARRIE: Don't let me off the hook so easily.

ADDIE: All right. You're a mean-spirited, middle-aged witch.

CARRIE: You think that, too?

ADDIE: I think you're one tired mothah.

CARRIE: Why did you stop dancing when I came in?

ADDIE: I stopped awhile ago. How did you know I was dancing?

CARRIE: Your face is still flushed . . . Would you dance for me? Soothe my nerves?

ADDIE: Nah.

CARRIE: Please? (ADDIE *moves the furniture back.* CARRIE *stretches out on the sofa.*)

ADDIE: This is called *An Ode to Grief* or *Ain't Life Sad.* (*She does a broad parody of a maudlin interpretive dance.* CARRIE *watches with weary amusement, but this is not what she wants. When* ADDIE *stops,* CARRIE *claps, but not with noticeable enthusiasm.*)

ADDIE: That's all I get for my creative effort? (*She sits down on the floor.*)

CARRIE: I wanted to see you really dance.

ADDIE: Not tonight, Caddie. I'm sorry — but I just can't.

CARRIE: Okay, babe . . . So — Johnnie went to bed?

ADDIE: John went out.

CARRIE: For a walk?

ADDIE: I guess so.

CARRIE: Didn't he say?

ADDIE: We had words.

CARRIE: (*Disbelieving*) Words? You had a fight? (ADDIE *makes a gesture — a shrug of assent.* CARRIE *sits up — is silent awhile — then —*) The gingham dog and the calico cat — except that there is supposed to be scarcely a sign of either of you.

ADDIE: What does that mean?

CARRIE: It means why were you here, dancing — and John is gone.

ADDIE: Say what you mean, Carrie.

CARRIE: What did you say to John to make him go? ... And why couldn't the two of you leave this time in peace! Why do we have to have all these extra *feelings* floating around? Why can't we just *grieve* like other people? (*Very angrily.*) I don't want to deal with this.

ADDIE: No one asked you to. Leave it alone. It's between John and me.

CARRIE: But he's gone!

ADDIE: He'll be back.

CARRIE: This should not have been — It isn't the time.

ADDIE: It happened.

CARRIE: You could have prevented it.

ADDIE: How do you know that? You can't always orchestrate things, Carrie.

CARRIE: This is a time to lay all that aside — I thought you'd agreed.

ADDIE: It's not so simple. People aren't like that.

CARRIE: (*Getting up*) Well, I can't stand it.

ADDIE: You'll have to stand it.

CARRIE: I can't stand it! Where's John? Will you stop hurting each other? Father is dead! (*Pause.*) Every time he'd get sick, I'd think, "When he dies — then I'll have time to *feel*." I need to feel his death, and I can't get ahold of anything. It almost comes, and then there's some ridiculous decision to make — I can't believe the things I've been asked to think about these past two days! Someone asked me what color shirt he should wear! Someone asked me that! ... And now you and John — fighting. And he's dead! (*She pulls the words out.*) *Mourn him.* Let *me* mourn him — I *need* that. (*She starts to* cry hard. ADDIE *rises and tries to comfort her, but she will not be held.*)

ADDIE: What can I do for you? ... Anything? Is there anything I can do for you? Do you want me to call Peter? (*This stops* CARRIE.)

CARRIE: (*Angrily*) Peter? Why should you call Peter? What's he got to do with this? Hand the mess over to Peter!

ADDIE: I thought you might want him.

CARRIE: (*Sits down. Then, quietly*) I want Mother.

ADDIE: Carrie....

CARRIE: I want Mother ... She should be here. She is absolutely the only person I want right now.

ADDIE: (*Looking at her sister with compassion*) What would she do for you?

CARRIE: (*Thinking*) She'd put me to bed with a cold, wet cloth over my forehead, and she'd send John to the store for ginger ale. (*She starts to cry quietly. They are quiet for a time.*)

ADDIE: Would whiskey do?

CARRIE: It would be lovely.

(ADDIE *exits into the kitchen.* CARRIE *pulls her feet up under herself.*)

ADDIE: (*Offstage*) Where did you put that bottle of whiskey?

CARRIE: In the refrigerator.

(ADDIE *returns with the bottle and two glasses.*)

ADDIE: Would Mother have joined you in your ginger ale? (*She sits down.*)

CARRIE: I don't remember ... When will John be back — do you think?

ADDIE: I don't know, Carrie ... You don't have to concern yourself with everything. No one asks that of you — but you.

CARRIE: Well, I've heard that before, of course. Peter calls me a meddlesome twat.

ADDIE: (*Laughs*) He does?

CARRIE: Mm.

ADDIE: You know something?

CARRIE: What, Ad?

ADDIE: If mother were here, she'd be a little, old lady — like Grace.

CARRIE: Oh, — she would, wouldn't she?

ADDIE: She'd be a little, old lady — and bereft.

CARRIE: And I'd be thinking I should take her home with me — to fill the void.

ADDIE: Will you miss Dad so much?

CARRIE: Over the years — yes. But the void . . . There's nothing like someone else's serious illness to give your life a sense of purpose. And I love that, Addie — that illusion of purpose — and order.

ADDIE: I haven't met very many people whose lives were more purposeful than yours.

CARRIE: (*She gives a short laugh*) And that doesn't make you the least bit suspicious? (*She gets up and walks over to the window.*) Did you find anything good in those old letters?

ADDIE: One very funny letter from Mother to Dad — early in their relationship, I'd guess. It was so ridiculously cagey! She made it clear that she missed him — but not too much. That he was first in her affections — or, at any rate, a close second.

CARRIE: Read one from the summer they were engaged. When did we decide that would be? 1929?

(ADDIE *looks through the pile of letters from a small box beside her on the sofa.* CARRIE *sits down on the floor close by.*)

ADDIE: (*Holds up a letter*) Look at that hand — that person knew his duty to God, country, and family. (*Looks at the letter.*) Grandfather Harris. (*Picks out another.*) Here's one from Mother — and it's that summer. August 17. (*She reads.*)

Dearest Allan,

This will not be long. I promised Mother that I would help her can today, and the peaches just *will* ripen. Besides that, there are more string beans in the garden than any human family should be expected to consume. Mother isn't terribly pleasant when she is canning, either. But your lovely letter just arrived, and I have permission to answer it if I do so quickly.

I was terribly lonely after you left last Sunday night, but as I was lying in bed, the rain started up again, and I thought how very obliging the weather had been, with the rain stopping long enough to allow us to escape the house, and then starting again just as we approached the shed up on the hill. I'll never feel the same about that old shed. Love, Your Stell.

(ADDIE *puts the letter down. Both women are quiet for a minute.*)

They made love in that shed.

(CARRIE *nods.*)

How wonderful. It was no "wifely duty" to her then.

CARRIE: Oh, no. It was always a strong physical bond. I knew that.

ADDIE:: She gave us that, anyway, but she didn't pass on that romantic turn of mind, did she?

CARRIE: What's the matter with us? Why didn't we fall in love like that?

ADDIE: Too much our father's children. What about John? Did he?

CARRIE: Don't you remember his passions?

ADDIE: With Diane.

CARRIE: When he was younger, too ... And he still has pain of that kind — coming from somewhere ... But with you and me it seems to be all mixed up with Dad's skeptical approach.

ADDIE: You shouldn't be skeptical about love.

CARRIE: Yeah, kid. Tell it to the judge. Anyway, we're talking about romance. Train whistles in the night.

ADDIE: (*Reflecting*) Romance. And yet I do believe in it — and so do you, sucker.

(CARRIE *laughs.*)

CARRIE: Find me one of his from that summer.

(ADDIE *looks through the letters.*)

ADDIE: (*Taking a letter from the box and reading the post mark*) August 3, 1929.

(*She takes the letter from the envelope and reads.*)

My dear Stell,

The only bright spot in my week was your letter. I love hearing about your days. I see home anew through your eyes.

I had heard about your heat wave, but at least in Iowa the heat smells like clover and freshly cut grass. We aren't so lucky in Chicago. And I swear that the city conspires to store up the heat all day so that it can give it back to you all night. I often walk along the lake shore until well after midnight, knowing that it's useless to try to sleep before that.

But, for all that, I love Chicago. And I never thought I could care for a city. I want to bring you here someday take you into one of the smart shops, and buy you one of those little hats all the Chicago women wear. No one will know you're a small town girl unless you start talking pickles and preserves.

I will be seeing you a week from this weekend.

(*She looks up.*)

He's talking about that same time!

(*Going back to the letter.*)

Tell your mother I am bringing her a surprise. And you, Miss Stell, powder your knees and meet the 8:10 Rocket because what I am bringing you from Chicago is one lonely man. All my love, Al.

(ADDIE *puts the letter down.* CARRIE *gets up, swings the blanket around her shoulders, and walks to the window.*)

CARRIE: I wonder where John went.

ADDIE:(*Sitting up*) He's okay. Can't you go to bed? Shouldn't you?

CARRIE: Pretty soon.

ADDIE: (*Standing*) Come, stretch out here, and I'll read to you. I'll find some of your letters from college.

CARRIE:(*Turning from the window*) That is not an irresistable offer. (*She goes to the sofa and stretches out, covering herself with the blanket.* ADDIE *sits in a chair.*) What's the matter between you and John?

ADDIE: John's running scared.

CARRIE: I know that, but what does that have to do with you?

ADDIE: I'm not sure. He seems to see me as some kind of unfettered spirit ... Sometimes I think John has chosen a safety he doesn't believe in. Or he thinks he's done that, which is just as bad. (CARRIE *doesn't respond.*) Do you know what I mean?

CARRIE: Like me?

ADDIE: You chose *with* your fate.

CARRIE: I chose with my fate. What a lovely idea, Ad—and how full of crap you are. Look here at me. My life is a very long way from perfect—how many times do I have to tell you that? ... And next year I'll be forty-four—did you know Mother was forty-four when she died?

ADDIE: You're not going to die.

CARRIE: Good. Ever since she died I've been telling myself that they'd have a cure for cancer by the time I got to be forty-four ... What are they *doing* with all that money? I send them money all the time!

ADDIE: (*Laughing*) You do?

CARRIE: Sure. Are you kidding?

ADDIE: Why don't you go on to sleep — none of that is going to happen.

CARRIE: (*Curling up*) In my cowardly moments, Ad, I do wish that I were what you think I am—what a marvelous, able, fulfilled. . . .

ADDIE: Well, that's a tired old tale. I know you're really only Caroline Brennan Newell, a mean-spirited, middle-aged—what was all that? (*She looks at* CARRIE.) Asleep, by God. (CARRIE *murmurs an unconvincing denial.* ADDIE *gets up quietly and goes to the window. She stands there a minute, looking out, and then goes back to her chair. She pours herself a little whiskey.*) Father's whiskey. (*She takes a sip. Then she picks up the box of letters and starts looking through them. Soon there is the sound of the front door opening.* ADDIE *looks up as* JOHN *enters from stage right.*) You're back. You were a long time about it.

JOHN: About what?

ADDIE: Whatever you were doing out there ... What were you doing, John?

JOHN: Wandering around town—pretending I was fifteen.

ADDIE: Oh, yeah, I've done that. It's fun.

(*There is an awkward silence.*)

ADDIE: Sit down. Have some of Father's whiskey. (*She rises.*) I'll get you a glass—and water, isn't it?

JOHN: Yes — just water. (ADDIE *exits into the kitchen.* JOHN *sits down in the other chair.* ADDIE *returns and hands him his glass. She sits back down in her chair. They look at one another for a minute.*) I don't recall that you were ever spanked. And yet I remember that you needed it from time to time — something clean like that and unequivocal.

ADDIE: I don't think I ever was. You think it would have made a difference?

JOHN: It might have convinced you that there were some things you didn't know — that there was another side to the truth and that just because you didn't understand it didn't mean you weren't going to have to do business with it.

ADDIE: (*Shrugs*) Might make sense. If you're saying there are things about your life that I don't know — and that they'd make a difference to what's been between us — then it seems to me you should let me in on them.

JOHN: Everybody spills his guts these days. I'm going to start reversing the trend. I insist on my right to keep a few hidden places in my soul.

ADDIE: But if you won't tell me what's up, you can hardly blame me for not knowing.

JOHN: You're old enough now to take it on faith that everyone has elements in his life — facts of his existence — that you can't know.

ADDIE: You don't think I do that?

JOHN: I think you have a little of the spoiled child in you, Addie.

ADDIE: Now you're ready to fight? Too bad, John. You waited too long. I'm tired.

JOHN: No. I don't want to fight. I just wanted to make that observation.

ADDIE: One question. Don't you think you should have told me — when I was at your house — not the details, but that your life was in a bad way? It wasn't nice — the way you treated me.

JOHN: I know. I apologize for that. You seem to think I understood what was happening. I was entirely crazy — you must have noticed.

ADDIE: Yeah. You were nuts. (*They both laugh.*) And I don't think you are all that wonderfully well now, to tell you the truth. I wish I could help.

JOHN: . . . I never seem to know what I am entitled to, Addie. I don't know why that is.

ADDIE: Well, it has to be the old man — let's blame everything on him! (*Pause.*) Hey, John, I'm sorry I said you were like him. What I meant, really . . .

JOHN: I knew exactly what you meant.

ADDIE: But I *didn't* mean it.

JOHN: I don't think there's much you say that you don't mean — or much you think that you don't, eventually, say.

ADDIE: That's an awful trait, right?

JOHN: It's not always comfortable.

ADDIE: It's an awful trait, I know. (*She leans forward.*) The thing is, Johnnie, you're nothing like Padre in the way I was saying. He always held such strong opinions, you know? From the way you should make an omelet to how you should conduct the crucial affairs of your very soul. (JOHN *smiles.*) Didn't he? It was everything I could do to stand up to him. And I never, never felt I could let down my guard. So when someone seems to have an opinion about my life, that's scary enough — and if they don't approve — well, you saw.

JOHN: I approve of your life, Addie. It's a quality life.

ADDIE: Listen. I'll take back that you're tight-assed if you'll take back that I salivate.

JOHN: Let's let it stand. There's some truth in both charges.

ADDIE: And you say *I'm* relentless. (*Pause.*) Try to understand this, John, because I need you to. If I rejoice at something like Lauren's plan, it's because I see her as a comrade, taking up arms against a sea of fathers. (JOHN *nods.*) And you? You don't think you needed to do that?

JOHN: I'm not combative.

ADDIE: You've come to terms in your own way.

JOHN: To put it as prettily as you did — I don't suppose I've come to terms with shit ... And I haven't killed my beast, Addie.

ADDIE: I know. I'm glad.

JOHN: I don't even think I've tamed it.

ADDIE: It prowls?

JOHN: It prowls, Addie. It bays at the moon. (CARRIE, *who has begun to stir, moans and then says something indistinguishable.*) Go back to sleep, Carrie. (CARRIE *opens one eye and sits up partially.*)

CARRIE: And what kind of beast is Addie?

ADDIE: What are you talking about?

CARRIE: (*Flopping back down*) Your game. I thought you were playing a game.

ADDIE: Well, we weren't. Go back to sleep. No one belongs in this conversation who can only keep one eye open at a time.

CARRIE: I don't want in your silly conversation. (*She sits up.*) I thought you were deciding what kind of animal everybody was like.

JOHN: (*To* ADDIE) Determined, isn't she?

ADDIE: Well, if you must know, we were. And John had just said that you were like one of those lovely sows they used to have at the country fair that always seemed to have one more piglet than she had teats. (JOHN *laughs.*) But I said — no — that really you were...

JOHN: I said no such thing, of course.

CARRIE: Oh, John, I recognize Addie's touch. (*She looks at their glasses.*) If we're having a party you should have woken me.

JOHN: Don't you need ice? (*He gets up.*) I'll get it. You, Ad?

ADDIE: (*Looking in her glass*) Okay, yeah, a couple of cubes. (JOHN *exits into the kitchen.*)

CARRIE: (*Watching him leave*) He seems fine.

ADDIE: (*Laughing*) Of course he's fine. If anything, he's better off for being yelled at.

CARRIE: Sure, that's just the ticket. (*She stretches.*) How long did I sleep?

ADDIE: Not long at all. I suppose we should all go to bed soon. (JOHN *returns with the ice.*)

CARRIE: We did used to play a game like that, you know. (JOHN *and* ADDIE *laugh.*) I remember one time when Dad said that Dr. Ellis, the head of the department at Fairfax, was like an altered lion. I loved that.

JOHN: (*Reflecting*) He was. It's nasty — but wonderfully apt.

ADDIE: What kind of animal am I? (JOHN *starts to respond, but* CARRIE *interrupts.*)

CARRIE: You're one of those yappy little terriers with bows on its ears. (*She loves this.*) Isn't she, John? One of those noisy, persistent little terriers.

ADDIE: (*Amused at* CARRIE'*s delight*) I am? I thought I was a doe.

CARRIE: (*Gleeful by now*) You see? That's what makes it so entertaining. You think you are a doe. If you knew you were a terrier it wouldn't be nearly so — fun.

ADDIE: Say something mean about John.

CARRIE: That's not mean, Ad. The truth shall set you free.

ADDIE: Oh, well, I don't care. I always kind of liked those spunky little dogs — thought they could take on the world just because their toenails were painted. (*She starts leafing through the letters.*)

CARRIE: (*Taking up her knitting*) Where did you walk, John?

JOHN: I wandered around — At night the town smells the same ... I always go back to the big house when I'm here. And tonight I walked out to the little stone house we lived in when Addie was born. (*To* ADDIE.) Do you remember that house? I think you were about three when we moved.

ADDIE: I guess I don't.

CARRIE: You walked out there? Along the river?

JOHN: Um.

CARRIE: That was a nice house. Wonderful, secret places ... We lived in that house when we had Sugar Puss. You don't remember that cat, Addie. John named her Sugar Puss — we had her for years. (*She is taken back to those years.*) She came from a litter the Lumblatt's cat had just before they moved ... Really — if I'm like any animal — in my heart of hearts — I'm like that cat. Every spring she'd have a huge litter, and by the end of three weeks she'd had it with motherhood. You might find the kittens anywhere. She tried to give them to Dad many times. It became a standing joke. Remember, John? ... He used to say, "Send that cat out and have her maternal instinct repaired!" She left her litter in his bedroom slippers once ... Sugar Puss....

JOHN: And that's your true self, is it, Caddie?

CARRIE: Will you take 'em, John? Let me run away from home and realize myself?

JOHN: Give them to Addie. It will add another dimension to her dancing.

ADDIE: People will say, "What is that new element in the dance of Adelaide Brennan?"

JOHN: "There is a restraint we hadn't noticed before. That almost airborne quality has been replaced by a subtle feeling that borders on the mundane...."

(ADDIE *gets up and goes over to the bookshelves. She looks through them and pulls down a book or two, reading cursorily.* JOHN *picks up some of the old letters, and* CARRIE *continues knitting. They are silent for a time.*)

CARRIE: That was a good thing you did, John — visiting your lost youth ... I haven't been out past that little house for years. How does it look?

JOHN: It looks well loved.

CARRIE: I'm glad. That was a cozy little house.

ADDIE: (*Looking up from her book*) I always felt that every warm and wonderful thing that happened in our family happened in that house — before I was born. I never met the Lumblatts, but you've all been talking about them my whole life long, and I am sure — to this day — that they must be the most marvelous people in the world — and that no friendship I ever had compared to yours with Sue Ann Lumblatt.

CARRIE: Poor Addie, John, she missed out on everything.

JOHN: It's just the name, Ad. Lumblatt. Pretend you had a friend named Audrey Lumblatt. I give her to you — Audrey Lumblatt. The two of you used to set up your tea parties under the lilac bush at the corner of the house.

ADDIE: (*Coming back to the sofa*) Mother used to talk about that house in a special way, too. "The house we lived in when Addie was born." (*She looks at* CARRIE *and* JOHN.) Now that Father's dead I suppose we'll film him in soft focus — like the little stone house.

JOHN: Let's don't do that.

CARRIE: Have we done that with Mother?

ADDIE: The myths start before they take their last breath.

CARRIE: John's right. Let's don't do that. Let's make a pact.

JOHN: No myths.

ADDIE: Let's do Father the honor of remembering him as he was. (*To* CARRIE.) Already you're quoting him.

CARRIE: I always quoted him. He was a funny man.

ADDIE: But it's different now that he's dead. It's beginning to sound like a collection — the humorous side of Chairman Mao. (CARRIE *laughs*.) I'm going to watch myself. I just will not sentimentalize the man. He was caustic — sometimes he was cruel. More than once I saw him level some person just because he'd thought of the perfect cut. He loved words more than people . . . I swear to God that I will not let him slip out of focus. I want to remember him funny and flawed — egocentric — opinionated — loving in his way, but blind as a bat about so many goddamned things!

(*For a moment they are all silent. Then* ADDIE *puts her hand to her mouth, and a kind of gasping cry escapes. This is her first real awareness of the finality of her father's death.* CARRIE *looks at her quickly, but* ADDIE *wards off any comforting gestures with her other hand, shakes her head and exits down-stage right.*)

CARRIE: . . . I miss Dad. I want him to walk out of the kitchen right now. (*She looks toward the kitchen door.*) If he did, what would he say, Johnnie?

JOHN: (*Becoming his father*) "I've been thinking about what kind of animal you are, Caroline... We had a lovely little female dog once — mixed breed — but she carried herself as if she came from a long line of whatever she was. Looked like it, too — interesting markings. People used to stop your mother and me on the street and ask about her. We'd give her a new heritage each time." (JOHN *laughs — an imitation of his father.*) "My favorite response was — I have to admit — one of my own. I said she was a Baskerville terrier. But — you remind me of that dog. She had a lot of style. Everyone assumed she'd inherited it, but her pedigree was her own."

CARRIE: (*She is touched*) There is more of John Brennan than Allan in that.

JOHN: Allan Brennan! Coming right up! (*He gets up and goes to the kitchen door, turns, and walks back toward* CARRIE.) "No! No, John! Why, in the name of thunder, when there are five perfectly reasonable interpretations of a passage, do you *always* manage to find a sixth that is indefensible! Why must the tree be a phallic symbol! What's wrong with it — just this once — being a tree? It *is* a tree — damn it! I know it's a tree. I blame Freud. I blame him entirely. It's not your fault. I blame Freud."

CARRIE: Can you ever forgive him? Will you miss him at all?

JOHN: I can start missing him now — and I can bury him. Because I figured out what I felt when you called. It was release, Carrie — a heady sense of release ... I could never quit caring what he thought ... It was humiliating. The man had no business having a son — he didn't leave enough room in the family for a second male.

CARRIE: I suppose you feel bad, John, that you were relieved.

JOHN: After the release I panicked. I haven't had time for guilt. (*With amusement.*) I'm sure it's on its way. (*They are quiet.* JOHN *picks up a stack of letters.*) Were you and Addie sorting these?

CARRIE: Reading them. I can't throw them away, John.

JOHN: You can't keep them all. Let's burn them — tonight.

CARRIE: You think so?

JOHN: Yes. Come on, Caddie. We've taken what we really want — let's burn the rest.

CARRIE: The pictures too?

JOHN: Sure — why not? We'll have a ceremony.

CARRIE: (*Nodding*) All right.

JOHN: What a strange time ... Caddie, I haven't told you what's up with me because I don't see the point. You've had so much to think about, and it wouldn't help me yet to talk about it ... Try not to worry about me. (*He smiles at her.*) "When the dust settles. . . ."

CARRIE: If only she'd been right about that, John.

JOHN: ... I harbor a childish hope.

CARRIE: Sure. Me, too.

JOHN: And I don't want you to worry about this thing between Addie and me — I learn from Addie.

CARRIE: She should learn from you, too. She has things to learn.

JOHN: She learns.

CARRIE: What were you talking about, anyway? About beasts.

JOHN: Addie had said I'd caged my beast — some such thing as that.

CARRIE: That *you* had? I don't see that.

JOHN: (*Getting up*) Maybe you'll give me a note to that effect. (*He moves around the room restlessly.* CARRIE *goes back to her knitting.*)

CARRIE: No, I don't see that in you, at all. And if she thinks you've caged yours — what must she think of me? I'll bet she thinks I was born without one! (JOHN *laughs.*) Crippled from birth!

JOHN: Can you imagine the horror of the attending physician? (*They are both laughing when* ADDIE *appears in the doorway. She smiles slightly.*)

ADDIE: I'm done. (CARRIE *gets up and goes to* ADDIE, *who has advanced into the room.* CARRIE *puts her arm over* ADDIE's *shoulder and pulls her over, kissing her on the cheek.*)

CARRIE: John thinks we ought to burn the rest of the letters and the pictures — have a ceremony ... You can dance and John will read poetry. (CARRIE *and* ADDIE *walk toward center stage with* CARRIE's *arm still flung over* ADDIE's *shoulder.*)

ADDIE: You can be the keeper of the flame.

JOHN: There's just enough whiskey left to serve as a libation.

ADDIE: (*Sitting down*) Don't you have to pour it out on the ground if it's a libation?

(CARRIE *picks up the bottle, pours a little whiskey into the palm of her hand and puts the bottle back. Dipping her right hand into her left palm, she sprinkles some whiskey around the room.)*

CARRIE: That — for the gods — and the rest for us.

ADDIE: Where are we going to burn these things?

CARRIE: Let me see what I can find. (*She exits into the kitchen.*)

ADDIE: Oh, I dread tomorrow. I hate funerals! They're so solemn. (JOHN *laughs.*) But they're not tragic — you know, John? I don't want to go there and sniffle into my hankie. I want to keen and wail. We grow big, fat cancers in our guts because we don't wail enough. (CARRIE *enters with a large crockery bowl which she puts down in front of the coffee table. She sits down on the floor.*) Let's all sit together at the funeral — cling to one another — and rock — and weep.

CARRIE: Let's not go.

ADDIE: They'd come after us. A posse of Brennans.

JOHN: We can get away from them — they're old.

ADDIE: Let's — steal — the — body.

CARRIE: And have him cremated, after all.

ADDIE: I wanted to take his ashes up to the top of Rainbow Lookout and scatter them to the winds.

JOHN: Or to the river. (*He puts a handful of letters into the bowl and touches a match to them. During the rest of the scene, each of them occasionally adds to the fire.*)

ADDIE: Or divide them up and send them, anonymously, to his adversaries— one last joke.

JOHN: Would we have enough for that? (*They all laugh very hard.*)

CARRIE: I wonder if we had the same parents. You two seem to see him so differently from me...

ADDIE: Oh, yeah? Then why were you laughing so hard?

CARRIE: Well, I know he was autocratic and ...

JOHN: We didn't have the same parents, of course. (*He lifts his glass.*) Here's to the parents we had — whoever they were.

CARRIE: To Estelle Brennan — of the smile and the roses ... And to Allan ... We observe his death with sadness — his life with joy ... And to our separate, most personal ceremonies, we'll assign no — name.

ADDIE: (*Lifting her glass slowly*) To the parents. (*They all drink.*)

End

Signs Of Life

Joan Schenkar

To the ladies

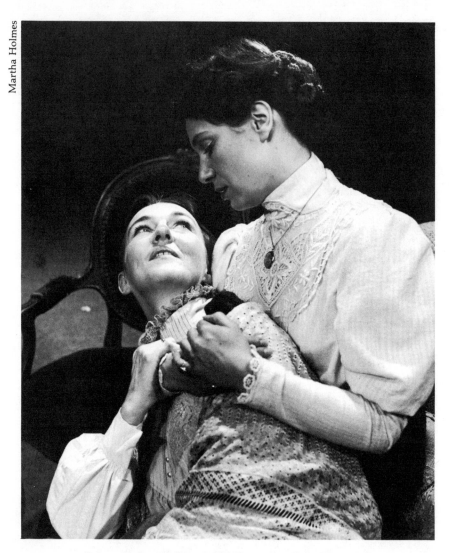

left to right: Kathleen Chalfant, Caroline Thomas

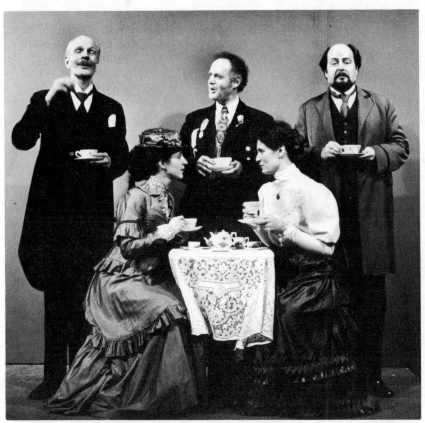

Martha Holmes

left to right: Gwyllum Evans, Susan Stevens, Barton Heyman, Caroline Thomas, K. Lype O'Dell

Author's Note

Signs of Life was composed as much as possible as a piece of music. It has movements, developed themes, arias, duets, etc. I had hoped to mark it for performance much the way music is marked—for prose language does not offer us the nice distinctions of pitch, stress, and juncture that music does—but the designs of publishers do not often match the intentions of authors and the piece goes unmarked. A particular loss for this author is the use of italicized words instead of underlinings to indicate stressed words or syllables. Italics, in their *insubstantiality*, make a word disappear; underlinings, in their unbroken emphasis, resemble crescendo marks in music—which brings us exactly back to the point.

Art made from extreme situations can often find its "facts" (i.e., the hinges upon which certain of its circumstances swing) in history. Thus, the Uterine Guillotine expertly wielded by Dr. Sloper in *Signs of Life* was invented and named by the founder of American gynecology, Dr. J. Marion Sims—a man who "performed" countless clitoridectomies and referred to himself in writing as "the architect of the vagina." Thus, too, Alice James's "companion" really was Katherine Loring, Jane Merritt, the Elephant Woman, had a male counterpart in the narrative of the Elephant Man by Sir Frederick Treves, and Henry James's burning of his sister's journal happened just as it does in *Signs of Life*.

Characters

P.T. BARNUM
DR. SIMON SLOPER
THE MOTHER/THE NURSE
HENRY JAMES
KATHERINE PEABODY LORING
THE WARDEN
JANE MERRITT
ALICE JAMES
THE FREAKS: WORKHOUSE INMATES/THE BLIND

Signs of Life was given a rehearsed reading by The Women's Project on March 12, 1979, directed by Esther Herbst, with the following cast:

P.T. BARNUM . . . . Barton Heyman
DR. SIMON SLOPER . . . . Gwyllum Evans
THE MOTHER/THE NURSE . . . . Katina Commings
HENRY JAMES . . . . Thomas Ruisinger
KATHERINE PEABODY LORING . . . . Kathleen Chalfant
THE WARDEN . . . . Barbara Le Brun
JANE MERRITT . . . . Joan MacIntosh
ALICE JAMES . . . . Cynthia Harris

It was performed as a studio production May 29 through June 7, 1979, directed by Esther Herbst, with sets by Henry Millman, lighting by Pat Stern, costumes by Whitney Blausen and Walker Hicklin, and the following cast:

P.T. BARNUM . . . . Barton Heyman
DR. SIMON SLOPER . . . . Gwyllum Evans
THE MOTHER/THE NURSE . . . . Susan Stevens
HENRY JAMES . . . . K. Lype O'Dell
KATHERINE PEABODY LORING . . . . Caroline Thomas
FREAKS . . . . Ethan Kane Dufault, Nancy Mainguy,
                                                                     Lisa Rifkin
THE WARDEN . . . . Barbara Le Brun
JANE MERRITT . . . . Kathleen Gittel
ALICE JAMES . . . . Kathleen Chalfant

Note to the actors: It might be helpful to imagine the characters in this play as each an aspect of a *shared* consciousness, rather than each an exponent of a *separate* consciousness. They do have in common certain prejudices and inclinations which make even the most opposed characters seem to share—however stealthily—a kind of identity. The effect this identity (or these identities) should have on the audience is a constant and nervous recollection of familiarity; a shudder of recognition in the most incongruous places. The actors must do everything possible to increase the audience's discomfort in this respect.

The Lobby

An actor in the costume of P.T. BARNUM *struts and frets and twirls a cane beside the ticket booth. As the audience buys its tickets,* BARNUM's *voice is amplified throughout the lobby. His spiel continues—improvised, syncopated, outrageously hokey—until every person has entered the house. The actor who speaks* BARNUM's *part can address individual members of the audience by, for instance, what they wear— "Mr. Red Shirt, Miss Brown Bag"—but he must never be abrasive or accosting. Good-humored lubricity is the tone to take. Here are some of the things* MR. BARNUM *might say:*

BARNUM: Ladies and gentlemen, gentlemen and ladies, welcome to P.T. Barnum's American Museum! Please have your money ready.

We have a fascinating bit of exotica here for you tonight. The lady you've all heard so much about is with us at last! That's right, folks, it's Elephant Woman! Queen of the Curiosities! Empress of the Awful! *The* most extraordinary female freak of the decade, just returned from a triumphant tour of Western Europe!

Ladies and gentlemen! Elephant Woman *walks*, she *talks*, she even *laughs* like a human being, but due to a dreadful accident of birth she appears to be part pachyderm. That's what I said, Madam, the lady looks just like an elephant. She's got an arm the size of an oak tree! A nose like an elephant's trunk! And other features too horrible to mention!

Come on in sir, don't hesitate. Line forms to the right. You *know* P.T. Barnum wants to please the people.

Folks, I've combed the world to bring back attractions the American people want to see! Remember Mme. Clofullia, the Bearded Lady from Belgium? I know you *do*, Ma'am. The in-credible Chang and Eng—the Siamese siblings who couldn't bear to be separated? *You* were here on their opening night, Sir. I remember your face. How about the famous Mermaid from Feegee? The renowned Gen. Tom Thumb? All these and many more have made their debuts right here in P.T. Barnum's American Museum.

But I tell you, ladies and gentlemen, there's never been anything here like the young lady you're about to see tonight. Those of you with conditions of the heart—I'd advise you to have your glycerin tablets ready. Ladies, if you're subject to fainting fits, reach for your smelling salts now. We have a physician in attendance, but he can't be everywhere at once.

That's right, friends, move right along. Have your money ready. P.T. Barnum guarantees you'll never have an experience like this one again. Believe me folks, it's the best bargain in the solar system! Etc., etc., etc.

The Apron

As the seats begin to fill and until the house lights go down, the following scene is played on the stage apron over the sounds of an arriving audience. The scene must be repeated continuously (with, perhaps, certain attitudinal changes) until the last person to arrive has seen it at least once through:

At a tea table, stage left, HENRY JAMES, DR. SLOPER, KATHRYN LORING, *and* JANE ELIZABETH MERRITT *(the* MOTHER*) are serving each other in an abstracted and ritualistic way.* BARNUM *comes from the lobby to join them. The table must be very small, so that the characters are at some* *pains to avoid touching each other. The scene should induce in those members of the audience who actually listened to* BARNUM's *spiel and therefore expected something salacious, a sharp feeling of disappointment. If it puts them in an unreceptive mood—so much the better. The actors will only have to work harder at seduction. As each character speaks, she/he turns from the tea ceremony and addresses the audience.*

BARNUM: (*Elegiac*) In the middle of the hottest summer I can remember, the summer of 1864, the summer I began my American Museum, a female child was born to Jane Elizabeth Merritt of the city of New York. That child made almost as much money for me as General Tom Thumb did.

DOCTOR: (*Clinical and breezy*) The child was born a monster and that's the simple truth of it. Clinically, she suffered from an extreme form of a disorder diagnosed by me twenty-four years after her birth. The name of the disorder is multiple neurofibromatosis. The name of the child was Jane Merritt. It was not until Mr. Barnum discovered her, that she became known as ... um ... (*Distastefully*) the Elephant Woman.

MOTHER: (*A sense of wonder and protest*) Joan, I named her Joan, after ... someone. At birth, her skin was only a little roughened, only a little thick. When she smiled at me she was like any happy child. Her mouth moved a little ... strangely, that was all. (*Slowly.*) She *was* slow to walk. Very slow. (*Quickly.*) But there was no reason to imagine what she would become ...

HENRY: *I* saw what she became. I saw it only once. Of course, I never told Dr. Sloper what I saw. Why take the story out of a good man's mouth? At any rate, one autumn afternoon in 1889, while temporarily eluding the febrile demands of my sister Alice, I walked into Mr. Barnum's American Museum. And there she was, the Elephant Woman. Surrounded, it seemed to me then, like any youthful heiress, by a small, but significant circle of admirers who blocked her face from my view. It was not until I'd made my way to the front of the crowd, that I saw the tears on her ... terrible cheeks.

(*Pause. A general muttering of tea service language.*)

"*Won't* you have more?
"*Will* you have a little?
"One lump or two?
"No thank you."
"Yes I believe I will."
"Petit fours are *so* bad for the figure."
"An unusual day."
"A *most* unusual day."

(*Pause.*)

BARNUM: The year that I was clerking in a drygoods store in Bridgeport, Conn.—1851 it would have been—the three sons of Henry and Mary James were treated to an awful surprise. A girl child came into the James family. A baby sister. In her Newport, Rhode Island home, Mary James produced a healthy daughter, Alice by name. (*Sits back, amused.*) I understand the James boys never forgave her.

HENRY: (*Disgusted*) A *daughter*? A *sister* for William, Wilkie, Robertson and me? What an in*d*ignity. Girls didn't have much of a chance in our family, I'm afraid. Alice became a life-long invalid.

KATHYRN: (*Tenderly*) I took her to my bosom as though she were my own child. We were the same age, but I saw the damage they had done to Alice as clearly as I saw the color of her eyes which were, incidentally, slate blue. She had *beautiful* eyes. I loved her eyes.

DOCTOR: Alice James was the most accomplished neurasthenic I have ever treated. Her fits were a *marvel* of patient orchestration. She had a genius for the well-timed disease. A real genius. What a performer she would have made.

(*The characters look at each other, relinquish their grip on the tea service, and* KATHRYN, MOTHER *and* BARNUM *rise and move off stage;* BARNUM *allowing the ladies to rise first and trailing huckster's phrases, good-naturedly, experimentally, almost to himself:*)

BARNUM: That's right, ladies and gentlemen. You heard what I said. The Elephant Woman. A gen-u-wine, home grown, American freak.

(HENRY JAMES *and his protagonist from the novel* Washington Square *are left alone at tea. Their actions are precisely those of two late-Victorian gentlemen at a tea table; that is, murderously banal. The actors' voices must be intimate and possessive when discussing facts and feelings, and bored and correct when asking for butter or more tea.*)

HENRY: A pleasure to see you again, Dr. Sloper.

DOCTOR: It must be five years since we've taken tea together, Mr. James.

HENRY: Surely not that long, sir.

DOCTOR: Five years, Mr. James and I still remember where our conversation left off.

HENRY: Let me see. I believe I had just said that the similarities between my sister Alice and your . . . um . . . *patient* Jane Merritt were striking.

DOCTOR: And then the Spanish-American War was declared.

HENRY: (*A little confused*) Oh yes, of course. The war. (*He begins to re-*

settle the tea things and he and DR. SLOPER *both rearrange themselves in the attitudes of their conversation of five years ago.*)

HENRY: (*Energetically*) It *is* a striking coincidence, doctor.

DOCTOR: Both women being my patients, you mean.

HENRY: I mean both of them being what they *were*. So ... limited.

DOCTOR: My dear Mr. James. How can you compare *your* brilliant sister with *my* freak of nature? More tea?

HENRY: No, no more thank you. My brilliant sister, dear doctor, spent twenty years in bed and produced nothing more than a cancer of the breast. If *that* isn't freakish ... (*Shrugs, drinks tea.*) The *butter,* Dr. Sloper.

DOCTOR: Certainly, Mr. James. (*Forgets it.*) And my poor *freak*, Jane Merritt ... in *her* twenty years, I suppose you could say she produced nothing more than *me*. It was those experiments on (*corrects himself*) uh ... *with* the Elephant Woman that made me famous, you know. (*Butters a scone energetically.*) She was to me what most humans spend their *lives* seeking out. My perfect *sub*ject, my sublime *ob*ject, my ... inspiration! (*Decrescendo.*) Uh ... sugar, Mr. James?

HENRY: Thank you doctor, I never take sugar.

DOCTOR: In the whole of my association with Jane Merritt, I could never *bare* to take my eyes from her. The *attr*actions of such repulsiveness ...

HENRY: (*Visibly irritated*) The ... *but*ter, Dr. Sloper.

DOCTOR: Certainly, Mr. James.

(*Slight pause. Sounds of butter transfered to scones and other tea table business.*)

HENRY: Well, doctor, I couldn't say that Alice had a *repulsive* physiognomy, but she *did* come into the world with her Mother's architectural forehead and her Father's flamboyant chin. (*Pause, shakes his head.*) A discouraging combination. (*Pause.*) I could scarcely ... tolerate the sight of her. (*Sighs.*)

(*Pause. They muse.*)

DOCTOR: (*Suddenly a toast*) The ladies, Mr. James?

HENRY: (*Roused, raises his cup*) Indeed, Dr. Sloper.

(*Pause. Again tea sounds. The moment the* DOCTOR *begins to speak,* HENRY *begins to sleep, nodding precariously into the scones.*)

DOCTOR: More hot water? Faces *do* have a terrible effect on us Mr. James. Careful, these scones are *piping* hot. I've often wondered what it was in Jane Merritt's expression that moved me to explore the secrets of her bones.

HENRY: (*Awakens abruptly*) Doctor, doctor, life's cup is *brim*ming with imponderables. (*Holds his cup up.*) I *will* have a touch more water, if you don't mind. My own dear Alice presented *me* with a similar question. (*Drinks his tea.*)

DOCTOR: Go on, Mr. James.

HENRY: Well ... I've always wondered what it was in Alice's eyes that drove me to pursue the secrets of her journal. She wanted that journal published, you know. Released into the world from the miasmal swamp of her opinions. (*Examines a toasted scone.*) Naturally, I ... burnt it to a crisp.

DOCTOR: Hmmmm.

HENRY: Yes.

(*Pause. They muse.*)

DOCTOR: (*The toast.*) Ahh, the ladies, Mr. James.

HENRY: (*Raises his cup*) Indeed, Dr. Sloper.

(*An appreciative pause. They both lean back. Then they both lean forward.*)

HENRY: Strong tea, doctor.

DOCTOR: I send to England for it.

HENRY: It has a distinctive ... *taste*, doctor.

DOCTOR: *Does* it, Mr. James.

HENRY: A peculiar ... *color* as well.

DOCTOR: Everyone says that.

HENRY: A certain ... cloying consistency.

DOCTOR: Ummmm.

HENRY: One might say an almost ... sacramental quality.

DOCTOR: (*As though paying a compliment*) The quality is in your imagination.

(*Pause.*)

HENRY: I believe I'll take a biscuit.

DOCTOR: Please do, Mr. James.

HENRY: What a dry taste.

DOCTOR: Really.

HENRY: Dusty, a dusty sort of dough.

DOCTOR: They're made in my kitchen, Mr. James.

HENRY: It tastes . . . ossified, it tastes . . . god help us . . . it tastes like *bone*.

DOCTOR: Impossible, Mr. James.

HENRY: (*A rising panic*) Dr. Sloper. There is blood in my cup. And there is bone in my biscuit.

DOCTOR: *Just deserts*, Mr. James.

HENRY: (*Calming*) Ahhh yes. Quite right, doctor.

(*Pause. He muses majestically.*)

DOCTOR: (*The toast*) The ladies, Mr. James.

HENRY: (*Remembering*) Ah yes, the *ladies*, Dr. Sloper.

(*They raise their cups. The house lights go down. They lower their cups. The stage lights come up. They remain at tea throughout the play, moving in and out of the action as indicated.*)

The Stage:

Any set you like so long as it is mostly vacant, clearly confining, and entirely out of the light. A few objects are possible, but they must be innocent ones: broken and/or remnants of other, wholler objects. What is present throughout the play is a bed, a sort of chiffonier (its mirror is covered when it's JANE MERRITT's *chiffonier, uncovered when it's* ALICE JAMES's*) and a bedside chair. These props are seen from one angle when they are in* JANE MERRIT's *room and from another angle when they are in* ALICE JAMES's *room. It's always the same room, the arrangement is always the same; it is merely our axis of vision that must appear to change.*

All the scenes centering on JANE *are played in her room; all the scenes centered on* ALICE *are played in her room.*

Jane Merritt's Room in the Workhouse

Stage lights come up on JANE's *room in the Workhouse.* JANE's MOTHER *and the* WARDEN—*a large and imposing southern woman—are upstage right, in close conversation. An earlier* JANE (*earlier than we see through the rest of the play*) *is center stage, hidden from view by a cluster of Workhouse inmates. An ancient hag, a pair of idiots, a deformed young man, a stammerer, a spasmodic adolescent all crowd around her staring*

and pointing, lifting her garments, removing her cloak. She remains
hidden until the WARDEN *ends the following scene, each of whose lines*
can be randomly assigned:

"It's a monster."

"A real monster."

"Did you . . . did . . . did . . . did . . . didyou . . . didyou . . . did you
  see the *skin*?"

"That's not *skin*."

"It's *tree* trunk."

"It's *e*lephant hide."

"Touch it go ahead."

"I dare you."

"How does it *stand* with legs like that."

"Never mind standing, how does it *eat*."

"The mouth looks sewed shut."

"Nobody's gonna make me sit next to that thing."

"It's a *her*, it's a *her*, look at the chest!"

"It's an elephant woman."

(One of the idiots takes what appears to be a hat and mask from JANE,
puts them on and capers around the stage.)

"Can she *walk*."

"Poor thing."

"Can she *hear*?"

"Poor *thing*."

"Can she *speak*."

"The *poor* thing."

(More punching and poking of the unseen JANE: *the inmates are having*
a wonderful time.)

"I hear they're going t' set 'er up in a room here."

"Haw haw. I'd set 'er up in a jar of formaldehyde, that's what I'*d* do."

"Ohhh Christ, hush your mouths, here comes Warden."

"Ssssh,ssssh, she'll beat us."

"Quick, quick *dress* the thing."

"Put her cloak on. *Hurry*."

"Sssh for gawd's sake."

"The *hat*. Get the *hat*."

"It's *Warden*."

*(*WARDEN *and* MOTHER *move toward the cluster of freaks,* MOTHER *in*
mid-conversation.)

MOTHER: And I named her after that woman who led the army in
  France. I thought, when I saw . . . what she was, I thought she would
  need a strong name.

WARDEN: Back! Stand back you motherless children or I'll beat you black and blue! (*As the* DOCTOR *speaks, she charges the crowd, swatting indiscriminately.*)

DOCTOR: (*At tea, to* HENRY) Jane, of course was her name. Elephant Woman came later. I often imagined that plain name was the source of her attraction for the novels of that other Jane, Miss Austen. Can you believe it, Mr. James? That missbegotten, deformed creature fancied herself the heroine of an Austen novel, sitting in some sunlit corner of a rectory garden, embroidering antimacassars for her father, the vicar! As if those horrible hands could hold a needle!

(WARDEN *subsides, breathing heavily. The inmates are strewn about the stage, momentarily subdued. The figure of* JANE MERRITT *draped in dark cloth is exposed; an icon center stage.*)

MOTHER: (*To* WARDEN, *to everyone*) At birth her skin was only a little roughened, only a little thick, it was ... there was no reason to imagine what she would be*come*. She smiled at me like any baby, she smiled frequently. She loved bright bits of color and she would ... always have me by her.

(*The inmates regroup, a skirmish is imminent.*)

WARDEN: (*To* MOTHER *as she terrorizes the freaks into a corner*) You just keep talkin', honey, while I take care a my children here.

DOCTOR: Bright bits of color. Oh yes indeed. Mother's *rouge* pots. The mother was a common whore, the child born a monster and that's the simple truth of it.

WARDEN: (*Mopping her brow*) Now you all calm down, all a you! (*To* MOTHER.) They just silly little children and they got to be treated as such.

MOTHER: Oh I knew something wasn't right about her mouth. I'm a seamstress and I know what it is to make a good fit. Her mouth didn't fit right. There was an extra piece on it, a flap of skin, that just grew and grew until she couldn't nurse or cry or even smile. So I sewed the cape and mask and we made a game of it. Hiding from the light, we called it. And now my ... customers won't come for their fittings as long as that "monster" is there. And that monster is my only child and we are starving together ... Life is a terrible thing, Warden. Sometimes it's a terrible thing.

WARDEN: (*To* JANE, *ignoring* MOTHER) And *this* here's mah new child. Well, darlin', let's have a look at you.

MOTHER: (*Moves in front of* JANE) Warden, it's *too soon*. She *shrinks* from the eyes of ... other people. In all her life, she's hardly ...

been in the light.

WARDEN: (*Hands on hips*) Lady, this here's the Workhouse. You leavin' your daughter here, you got to leave *all* of her. Now move yourself on outa here. And let me do mah duty. We're holdin' a class today. You just git along and leave her to me.

(JANE *stands stolidly until her mother embraces her, then the one good arm, the left one, comes up and touches the* MOTHER's *face.*)

WARDEN: Here now let's have a look at you.

(WARDEN *takes off* JANE's *cloak. Then her hat and mask.*)

WARDEN: Oooooo mah *gawd.* Is that a human *bein'*?

(*Everyone on stage freezes; an awe-full moment.*)

MOTHER: (*As though in explanation*) She was born at a carnival. I was at a carnival . . . standing near the Elephant. He turned towards me, I began to bleed . . . and she was . . . born *right there* in the . . . sawdust.

WARDEN: (*Transfixed, gentler*) Go 'long now Miz Merritt. It's gonna take quite a while to get her in-tegrated in with the rest of 'em. It'll be easier if you go along.

MOTHER: (*A list*) They *stone* her, they *shout* at her, they knock her down, and now a *carnival* wants to *buy* her from me. (*Shudders.*) I am her mother and I cannot stand the sight of her. *Some*one has to protect her . . .

DOCTOR: Jane Merritt was abandoned to a workhouse when she was very young. I presume her mother's lovers couldn't tolerate the sight of their mistress's little monster.

MOTHER: (*Takes a miniature of herself from her reticule and puts it in* JANE's *good hand*) Try to keep this longer than I've kept you. (*Exits quickly.*)

(JANE *releases one horrible wail. It is literally released —like a bird from a cage —and is as suddenly gone.* WARDEN *and* JANE *face each other,* WARDEN *still transfixed, as we are, by what* JANE *looks like.*)

WARDEN: (*Loudly, to break the horror*) Alright, the rest of you get on ovah here, we gon' have a class. We gon' have a class in lookin' and seein' and (*Another look at* JANE) bein' a freak. Cause you all freaks and you might bettah learn to be what you are. Now pick up them books. (*Inmates stoop to a pile of tattered periodicals.*) You now (*To* JANE), *what* did she say yo' name was. *Jane.* You, Jane Merritt, you stand here. Least you can do is learn to *hold* a book.

(*The inmates assemble in front of* WARDEN, *weaving, bobbing, slobber-*

ing, some with their books upside down. Throughout WARDEN's
*monologue they listen as intently as their various handicaps allow them
to, and respond to her commands as well as they can. The staging here
is surreal: a parody of all parodies.*)

WARDEN: Now the first thing you want to learn in this class is HOW TO
LOOK. You bettah know you all look *real* disgusting. Ready now?
The lesson is HOW TO LOOK. Look to the side. Keep your head
straight. Not up in the air. When you look to the side see what's
there. Just see what's there. To the *side*, to the *side*, to the *side*. (JANE
looks down.) In a freak class there's no reason to look *down*.
Everybody in the *world* already down on *you*. Just look to the side
and *see*. See. *See* that bastard sneakin' *up* on you. *See* his knife. Be
AWARE. See that nice lady gon' give you some money. *See* her look.
She just *waiting* t' see you smile. *Limp* on up to her now and hold out
your hand. Good. Look to the side, to the side, to the side, to the
side. *See*. In a freak class you got to be awake. You in training for
your life. If you're *real lucky*, one a them carnivals yo' Mama was
talking about might pick up on you.

(JANE *might seem to register the word "Mama".*)

Now the last thing you got to learn in this class is how to laugh ac-
cordin' to an audience. Most a you gonna end up bein' looked at by a
lot a people, and you got to learn to laugh real big so people think
you're happy. Nobody's gonna pay to see you if you can't be happy
for 'em. C'mon children. C'mon now. Let's show her how to laugh.

(FREAKS *and* WARDEN *laugh.*)

AH HA HA HA HA HA HA HA HA HA HA HA HA HA HA.

(*The laughter degenerates into scuffles among the inmates and* WARDEN
moves in to swat them.)

"It's *her*, Warden. It turns my stomach standing in front of her."
(*Points to* JANE.)
"She smells terrible."
"She looks awful."
"She's a real *freak*."

WARDEN: Hush yo' mouths now. We gon' have Dr. Sloper in to look at
her. She's some kind of a scientific curiosity.

"Dr. Sloper!"
"He's no doctor."
"He's a *ghoul*."
"A *grave*-robber."
"A *butcher*."
"He's always bringing those knives around."

"Lost his own little girl on the operating table."
"Stomach-trouble, I heard."
"Appendicitis."
"Whatever *that* is."
"He's the . . . he's the . . . he's . . . he's . . . he's the *freak*!"

DOCTOR: (*His most urbane, organ-like tone*) I love all swelling things, Mr. James. Buds in spring, women's bellies before they come to term, the waxing moon, and, yes, one of my . . . specialties, the vermiform appendix before it bursts.

(WARDEN *herds the inmates offstage with cuffs and threats:* "Classtime! Get a move on monsters! Let's go! Classtime!" *etc., etc., and* JANE *is left alone. She limps toward the bed, examines it, pulls herself up on it, seems content.*)

JANE: (*With great difficulty, the mouth is virtually sealed*) This, my home. I have it. (*Takes out* MOTHER's *miniature.*) This, my mother. I . . . lose her. No mother . . . no home. Now I . . . have . . . nothing. (*And the wail flies again like a bird from her throat.*)

DOCTOR: (*Largely*) Well, Mr. James, Jane had *everything*. One short examination of her disordered body and the weight of all my interests amassed a gigantic precipitation and rained down a shower of gold into her lap. (HENRY *yawns hugely.*) She was the *real thing*, an anatomist's *dream*, a *true case* of congenital deformity! My first examination of her was a scientific revelation . . .

(*And the* DOCTOR *moves from his tea table into* JANE's *room, carrying a satchel filled with scalpels.*)

DOCTOR: (*His most patronizing and mellifluous tone to* JANE) Now my dear, I'm going to speak very gently. I know you don't understand me, but the sound of my voice will calm you as it calms all my patients. (*Seeing her see his scalpels.*) No, no, don't worry, I bring these with me as a matter of course. There will be no cutting, certainly not yet. I simply wish to examine you for a greater cause. Um . . . Mother Science, my dear, Mother Science.

(*As he examines* JANE, *he speaks to* HENRY *as though he were an entire anatomy class taking notes. The lights come up very bright.*)

The subject of this disorder is a woman aged twenty-four. The disorder concerns both the cutaneous and the osseous systems of her body. With the curious exception of the . . . um . . . genitalia and the left arm and hand, the subject has tubercles covering the whole of her integument. The subcutaneous tissue has greatly increased in amount and density; the surface of the integument itself shows a papillomatous condition, particularly exuberant over the dorsal region and the gluteal districts. The entire bone structure is enormously hypertrophied. Huge dewlaps hang from her outsize skull; bands of connective tissue seal off her mouth and left ear. Are there any questions so far?

HENRY: Can she speak, doctor?

DOCTOR: Her power of speech, if she had it, would be totally impaired.

HENRY: How does she move?

DOCTOR: Articulation of all joints (*He moves her right knee, she jerks away.*)—oops, sorry my dear—is extremely difficult. There appears to be an old injury to the right hip which has resulted in a painful (*He touches her hip, she jerks away.*) —tch, sorry again, *very* painful and extremely restrictive displasia.

HENRY: (*Reaching for a biscuit*) And eating. What about eating?

DOCTOR: A liquid diet is . . . barely possible. (*Carelessly.*) More than likely we'll run a tube down her nasal passage and feed her that way. It's easier on the staff.

HENRY: What about . . . evacuation?

DOCTOR: (*A little professional laugh*) What *about* it?

HENRY: (*Embarrassed*) How does she do it?

DOCTOR: As best she can, sir, as best she can.

HENRY: (*Changing the subject*) What is your prognosis, doctor?

DOCTOR: Death at an early age, I'm afraid. Though, certainly, it's far too soon to rule out the possibility of a surgical cure. I have great faith in my little knives gentlemen, *great faith.*

HENRY: You intend to operate, then?

DOCTOR: I intend to examine the subject (*Ominous*) *much more thoroughly.* And *then* make my decision. No further questions? (*Pause.*) In sum, then, the subject before us can barely walk, eat, speak, or eliminate, and it is to be profoundly hoped that the god who invested her with this condition, also withheld from her the power to perceive it. Thank you very much, gentlemen. (*To* JANE.) And now, my dear, a few daguerrotypes for Mother Science. I want you to hold very still, yes, very good, that's right. I know you can't understand me, but there will be a flash of light . . .

(JANE *registers horror at the word "light," the light when it comes is blinding, there is a blackout, and the* DOCTOR *is back at the tea table.*)

DOCTOR: She was a world, I tell you Mr. James she was an entire universe . . .

Jane Merritt's Room in the American Museum

BARNUM: (*Offstage, picking up where he left off in the lobby*) "That's right, folks, she's the best bargain in the solar system."

(*The lights come up on* JANE, *now dressed for display as Elephant Woman, sitting on her bed, looking at the miniature of her mother. As* BARNUM *enters, she hides the picture.*)

BARNUM: Bargain! The joke's on Phineas T., my dear! You're a bargain for everyone but me. Elephant Woman costs more to keep than a whole *herd* of elephants. (*Goes to a liquor bottle on the chiffonier, pours a drink.*) That gilt cage of yours alone took six weeks profits right out of my pocket. (*Starts to smell the liquor.*) My god! What a stench! You're beginning to smell the way you look. (*Drinks.*)

HENRY: (*Extremely irritated*) The *butter*, doctor.

DOCTOR: Oh certainly, certainly.

(BARNUM *drinks again. Sounds of satisfaction.*)

JANE: (*With difficulty, but clearer than before*) I'm . . . hungry.

BARNUM: Now Jane, you know you can't eat before a show. You'll spoil the performance. (*Regards the bottle.*) Expensive brand. But worth it. Well worth it. (*He drinks.*)

JANE: I'm . . . cold.

BARNUM: The admiration of the crowd will warm you, my dear. (*Regards the bottle.*) Nothing like a little refresher in the middle of a day. (*Pause.*) Or at the beginning of a day. (*Pause.*) Or at the end of a day. (*Pause.*) For that matter drinking all night long is a wonderful experience.

JANE: The light . . . bothers my eyes.

BARNUM: The light is for the people. The people *like* to see what they're paying for. (*Holds bottle up to the light.*) Shines just like gold . . . (*Raises bottle to his mouth.*)

JANE: My mouth is bleeding again.

BARNUM: (*Stops cold*) What! Blast that doctor! We can't have *blood* for the performance! The people won't put up with *blood*! He guaran*teed* there'd be no blood!

JANE: The knives he used . . . were not clean.

BARNUM: *Damn* the fool! I'll have his diploma. *Doctors.* Licensed scoundrels! *That's* what they are. Legal murderers! (*Calming.*) How's your speech. Any better?

JANE: As you hear it.

BARNUM: (*As though noticing it for the first time*) It *is* better, *much* better. Before he cut that flap back all you could do was slobber. There's an improvement, alright.

JANE: It's . . . easier to speak. When I want to.

BARNUM: (*Anxious*) And you can laugh? Can you laugh yet?

JANE: (*Patiently*) He made me try. I can laugh a little.

BARNUM: (*Relieved*) Good, good, people love to see a freak laugh. (*Pause.*) God knows why. Well, we'll just have to put up with the bleeding for a while. Maybe the crowd won't notice it.

JANE: There . . . *is* no crowd.

BARNUM: (*Self-important*) There will be, my dear. This is P.T. Barnum's Museum. There are *always* crowds here.

JANE: There were five people in the audience this afternoon . . .

BARNUM: Afternoon's are slow . . .

JANE: . . . but their eyes were awful. One man especially . . .

BARNUM: (*Definitively*) There will be an enormous crowd here tonight. I can promise you that. The name of P.T. Barnum does not produce dead houses, my dear.

(*Slight pause.*)

JANE: I think . . . *I'm* dead.

(*Pause.*)

BARNUM: (*Breaks it, malevolently*) You had better not be, my dear. You have a show to do in ten minutes.

JANE: I mean . . . I think I'm dying. When I look into the eyes of the people I think I'm dying. *You* never look at me anymore, but they . . .

BARNUM: (*His speech becomes more inebriated, coarse, and colloquial; he drinks throughout*) They better be looking at you, by God, that's what they're *here* for! Ach! The fools! They live with their eyes sewed shut and they come to P.T. Barnum to clip the stitches for 'em. And when I show 'em something it has to be so *shock*ing that it'll last 'em til the *next* time they come to me to show 'em something—because they won't see a *thing* til I SHOW IT TO 'EM. NOT ONE THING. ME! I HAVE TO DO IT! P.T. BARNUM! I HAVE TO SHOW ONE HALF OF THE WORLD TO THE OTHER (*Drinks*) half. *God* what a responsibility. (*Drinks, subsides slowly, notices that* JANE *has put her mask on. Speaks quietly.*) And what are *you* doing?

JANE: I'm . . . dreaming.

BARNUM: (*Drunken dignity*) Y' don't say.

JANE: I'm dreaming I'm with people whose eyes are in their hands.

BARNUM: (*Drunken largesse*) Go right ahead, m' dear.

JANE: The hands are touching me in every part of my body. There are hands on the bones of my feet. Now I feel them melting the muscles of my upper arms. They are rubbing the nerves of my throat. There is a hand inside my stomach. There are hands reaching for my kidneys. Fingers are straightening my ribcage. There is a hand holding my heart. Hands are between my thighs. Wait. Something has happened. The hands are . . . (*Stops.*)

(*Pause.*)

BARNUM: (*Coarsely*) *Hands*? On *your* body? Hah! That's no dream, that's a *night*mare. Haw haw haw. (*Stops.*) Freaks. (*Dejected.*) I never had one yet that didn't dream. (*Pauses, bottle in hand.*) Life's a terrible thing. Sometimes it's a terrible thing. (*Drinks.*)

JANE: (*Takes mask off*) What happened to your other freaks? The ones you tell the stories about?

(*Slight pause.*)

BARNUM: (*Bluster.*) Why they all went on to illustrious retirements my dear, just as *you* will. (*Pause. He drinks. A grim litany.*) Mme. Clofullia, the Bearded Lady, lost her beard. Some kind of gland disease. She cut her throat in Schenectady, the year I took you out of the Workhouse. The Siamese Twins hated each other so much, they hunted up some phony doctor in Tennessee to cut 'em apart. *They* died on the operating table. Tables, I should say. They insisted upon separate operating tables . . . Let's see. Tom Thumb. Poor Tom Thumb. He fell in love with a large lady from Louisville who took his money and ran a toy sword right through his little heart. What a loss *that* was. That boy was the biggest money-maker I ever had. The Mermaid from FeeGee was nothing but a papier-mache doll . . . As to the rest of 'em . . . (*Pause.*) . . . I really don't remember.

(*Pause.*)

JANE: (*Slowly*) Life must be a terrible thing.

(*Noise.*)

BARNUM: Shh! Listen! Do I hear people?! (*Excited.*) There are *people* out there. What do y' know. I told you, P.T. Barnum always produces. We're going to have a *real show* tonight, by God. I've got to get out there and work that crowd. (*Turns back, ominous.*) Now listen, my dear, I want a big laugh out of you when we bring the lights up. Do you understand? A *very* big laugh. That's what the people want and that's what they're going to get! We're not here to disappoint the people! (*Exits. Offstage we hear him: "Ladies and gentlemen. We have a fascinating bit of exotica here for you tonight."*)

(*As soon as Barnum's voice dies away, the Blind people of* JANE'*s dream enter. There should be seven of them, as in the story the Persian poet Rumi tells about the seven blind people confronting an elephant. They all move slowly towards* JANE, *groping the air in front of them. One of them begins a modal hum—in, say, the mixolydian mode—and the others take it up, with variations always in the mode of the theme, until* JANE *is surrounded by the Blind and surrounded by the sounds of the Blind. Each of the Blind concentrates on touching a different area of what passes for* JANE'*s body. The movement of the hands of the Blind must be precisely choreographed so that the icon becomes one of Elephant Woman being created as a sculpture by the hands of the Blind. The music, the modalities, should seem to come out of what the hands are touching. A real effort must be made by the actors to receive and transmit the vibrational frequencies of Elephant Woman's body. At the moment the icon is complete, that is, at the moment the Blind have created a sculpture of sound to enclose the sculptured form of Elephant Woman—they must seem to vanish from her room. Lights dim to darkness.*)

DOCTOR: After that first examination at the Workhouse, Jane Merritt passed completely from my life. (HENRY JAMES *is soundly sleeping.*) Mr. James, forgive me, but your elbow is in the creamer. (DOCTOR *shakes* HENRY *who wakes, startled and mumbling: "I wasn't asleep, I wasn't asleep."*) Oh, I'd hear of creatures like her, here and there, exhibited in small towns on the Chattaqua Circuit—Mme. Monster this and Elephant Woman that—but I could never be sure it my *my* freak they were talking about. Only if I heard that Mme. Monster could not bear the light, or that the famous Elephant Woman was remarked by the crowds who viewed her to have had tears running down her terrible cheeks—only *then* was I certain that this was the creature I'd examined in the Workhouse on that fateful day. For that poor, stunned specimen displayed the most painful aversion to any form of light . . . She broke down completely during the last series of daguerrotypes. I have treasured a few prints that show her tears. See here and here Mr. James—imagine tears from such a creature!

HENRY: (*A brave show of wakefulness and response*) Tch tch shocking. Perfectly shocking. (*Snoozes immediately.*)

DOCTOR: Yes, yes it *was* shocking. Something about the blinding flash of the gunpowder . . . terrified the *life* out of her . . .

Jane Merritt's Room Inside Her Mother

Lights come up slowly on JANE, *alone in her room. She is remembering what it was like to be inside her mother and, remembering, speaks about it:*

JANE: It is dark in here. I am crowded by walls of flesh not my own. My eyes—shut. My ears—useless. Folded tight against my head. My thick skin is wrinkled. My tusks are little buds. My trunk is rolled up. Every part of me is curved or curled against every other part. I am in a prison to grow. But I grow strangely. I can feel it.

Suddenly I hear my father's voice, speaking from another place. He is loudly calling my Elephant name. The soft clotted blood on which I rest is sucked away. Flesh not my own begins to press and release me. I am in a terrible pain of pressing back. I push past this pain to other pain. Flesh not my own closes around me. I give up. I am renewed. I push again. Flesh closes around me again. I give up again. I am little. I do not move. Then I push again. In a river of liquids not my own, I push out into blinding light. Now the walls are not the walls I know. I hear my father calling my Elephant name nearby. The light is like a loud noise. Something . . . has happened. (*With wonder.*) My . . . trunk is gone. The buds of my tusks . . . retreated. My large ears . . . no more. In their place, lumps of bone, strings of flesh. I am . . . not what I was. Something has happened. I am not what I am supposed to be. My mother sees me between her thighs. She *knows* something has happened. When she sees me, her scream . . . is as loud as the light.

(*Blackout and back to the* DOCTOR *and the drowsy* HENRY. *Before the lights come up fully on the tea table,* HENRY'*s voice issues defensively from the darkness: "I'm not asleep. Doctor. I heard every word you were saying."*)

DOCTOR: Well, I found her again of course. I couldn't let a prize like that escape me. I installed her right here in my hospital. Under my protection. In sight of me, always in sight of me. Naturally, she was a trifle . . . reluctant to expose herself to science at first. Just the . . . tiniest bit inclined to refuse certain . . . necessary treatments. But I was very convincing and, of course, she had no place else to go . . .

Jane Merritt's Room in the Hospital

A pile of books is on the floor. DOCTOR SLOPER *sits in the bedside chair, examining and writing. His knives are with him, gleaming sedately in their box.* JANE *is asleep sitting up, her back propped by pillows, her heavy head resting on her knees. When she wakes, she speaks more clearly than she has before.*

JANE: It's always the same dream.

DOCTOR: The Blind again, eh? Turn just a little to the right, please.

JANE: The dream of people whose eyes are in their hands.

DOCTOR: (*Pleased*) Really, Jane, your articulation is superb. How is the lip this morning?

JANE: It won't stop bleeding. I think you shouldn't have cut it again.

DOCTOR: Don't be ridiculous, my dear. You know you're much happier speaking.

JANE: I spoke before. You couldn't understand me.

DOCTOR: And now I can. That's important, my dear. Head up now. By God, we'll have you smiling yet. Now if we could only get you to sleep lying down like other people . . .

JANE: I could try. I would love to try.

DOCTOR: But of course we know that's not possible. Your head is far too heavy. If you were even to lie back for a moment, your windpipe would snap like a straw. (*Visualizes it.*) Just like a straw.

JANE: I have thought of it that way many times.

DOCTOR: Don't bother to, my dear. We have enough pillows here to keep you propped up forever. (*Pause, writes.*) You've finished all your books, I see.

JANE: Miss Austen is my favorite. She fits things together so . . . nicely.

DOCTOR: (*Busy with writing*) A peculiar taste for you.

JANE: Oh I *like* a good fit.

DOCTOR: Odd that you should . . . I have another patient with tastes like yours. The sister of a famous novelist. (*Musing.*) She's been dying for years . . .

JANE: (*Suddenly*) Life must be a terrible thing.

DOCTOR: (*Abstracted*) So it is, my dear, so it is. (*Pause while he checks a list.*) Now we're going to palpate that hip.

JANE: (*Speaking over the pain of the examination*) I'd like to read more of the Bronte sisters. Sometimes I think I can hear my father in their books, calling my Elephant name across the moors.

DOCTOR: (*Not listening*) What? Oh anything you like Jane. Shift your weight a little, please.

JANE: And sometimes I see him in Miss Austen's parlor scenes, swinging his trunk back and forth, just as he did the day I was born.

DOCTOR: Good, Jane. Hold that position.

JANE: Then often he comes to me when I read Miss Emily Dickinson. She only describes an inch of him in each of her poems. But that inch is enough.

DOCTOR: (*Irritated*) Hold *still*, Jane. How can I examine you if you *move* every minute?

JANE: (*Experimentally*) This morning he spoke to me directly for the first time. (*Imitates him.*) "Come to me, daughter," he said. "My thick skin will protect you, my heavy legs will shelter you, my trunk reaches out to embrace you, my memory will conserve you—come to me and be healed."

DOCTOR: (*Ignoring her and looking at his watch*) Well, we'll have to suspend the usual examination this afternoon. I have an engagement for tea and (*Looks at his watch*) I see that I'm already late. To-morrow at the same time, my dear.

(JANE *slowly sinks into her sleeping position.* DOCTOR *exits in a hurry to the tea table. Sits down with a thump.* HENRY *seems to waken.*)

HENRY: Dr. Sloper?

DOCTOR: Mr. James?

(HENRY *starts to sleep again, but pulls himself awake.*)

HENRY: Did I understand you to say that you annexed that poor creature for your own purposes?

DOCTOR: Never in this world, Mr. James.

HENRY: I'm relieved, Dr. Sloper.

DOCTOR: I'm delighted, Mr. James.

(*Pause.* HENRY *begins again to sleep, than rouses briefly.*)

HENRY: Doctor?

DOCTOR: Sir.

HENRY: Whose purposes *were* they?

DOCTOR: Mother Science's, Mr. James, Mother Science's.

(HENRY *nods, then rouses again. They muse.*)

DOCTOR: (*The toast*) Shall we drink to the ladies, Mr. James?

HENRY: (*Roused*) Ah yes. Of course. The ladies.

(*Cups are raised, complete blackout on both sets.*)

* * * * *

Alice James's Room in Henry's House

The lights come up on ALICE JAMES's *room. The mirror on the chiffonier is now uncovered.* ALICE, *who does indeed have her mother's architectural forehead, is reclining on her bed-chaise, propped with five pillows and blanketed with three shawls. She is rifling the pages of her journal irritatedly.*

ALICE: Damn! Where is it? It's bad enough keeping a journal without losing track of what you've written in it. (*Reads a passage mockingly.*) "Anyone who spends her life as an appendage to five cushions and three shawls is justified in committing the sloppiest kind of suicide at a moment's notice." Hmmm. Not very cheerful, are we? Ahhh, I remember *this* one " . . . it used to seem to me that the only difference between me and the insane was that I had not only all the horrors and suffering of insanity but the duties of doctor, nurse and straight-jacket imposed on me too." Oh Alice, Alice, what an inhos*pi*table temperament. Ahhh, *here* we are. (*Reads slowly as though experiencing it.*)

"On the morning of my thirteenth birthday, and I remember still how sudden the impulse was, I walked into my brother Harry's bathroom, and I carefully removed his razor from its box, and I carefully stropped it back and forth as I'd seen him do so many times, and I carefully shaved off every hair on my body except the hairs growing on the top of my head. I was so careful that although it was the first time I had used a razor *in that way*, I did not experience a single cut. Every morning for months after that I would walk into Harry's bathroom and repeat the same performance before his mirror. Fear and embarrassment made me careless, and each morning fresh cuts followed the razor over my skin. I was able to stanch the cuts on my face with small pieces of lambswool which I wet under the faucet as I had seen Harry do. Until it dried, the wool blended nicely with my skin. The cuts on my arms were deeper, somehow, and harder to stop from bleeding. There is something in the conformation of an arm that does not . . . lend itself to the razor. The most I could do with these cuts was to conceal them under the awful, long-sleeved middy blouses that Aunt Kate so persistently sewed for me. At odd moments during the school day, I would look down to see the white sleeves of my middy dotted and stained with blood from the cuts on my arms. I began to develop complicated rituals that kept my arms below the level of the school desk . . . so that I would not have to see what my brother's razor had done to me."

(HENRY *moves from the tea table into* ALICE's *room and stands at her bedside. She quickly closes the journal.*)

ALICE: (*Surprised, it's a first meeting*) Harry. You're so . . . sneaky.

HENRY: My dear. How are you.

ALICE: (*Cheerfully*) Dying, as usual.

HENRY: Alice, I wish you would concentrate more on cheerfulness.

ALICE: Ah Harry. What does it matter. I'm here at last, with you and Kathryn to care for me. (*Ominous.*) Until the end.

HENRY: (*Uncomfortable*) You don't . . . plan to go back to the old house in Cambridge, then?

ALICE: My dear, you should have *seen* them dragging my carcass between Boston and New York! I'll never have the courage to attempt *that* trip again. Really, if it hadn't been *my* body bumping around in that railway car, I would have enjoyed the spectacle immensely. As it was, (*Ominous*) I had an attack.

HENRY: Oh good god. Not again.

ALICE: (*Cheerfully*) Again *and* again. I had two of them, actually. The one in Grand Central Station was the most interesting. (*Coyly.*) Several old friends of the family happened to be catching trains at just that moment, and so were able to watch me thrashing about on the floor of the grand concourse.

HENRY: Alice, Alice! And the sentence. I suppose you couldn't have an attack without saying that sentence.

ALICE: Kathryn tells me I was in full voice. She never heard me articulate it so clearly, she said. Although Mary Cabot insisted that *she* missed the last two words.

HENRY: (*Horrified*) Mary *Cabot* was there!

ALICE: (*Happy as a clam*) And Bay Lodge. Who complimented me on my performance.

HENRY: If the James family has a social position left, Alice, it's no thanks to you. I suppose you were examined by a physician?

ALICE: They called in that Dr. Sloper again. You know. The one who operated on his own daughter and killed her. (*Admiring.*) He has such an . . . *extensive* collection of scalpels.

HENRY: Well, Alice. What is it this time? Neurasthenia? Hyperaesthenia? Nervous prostration? You always inspire doctors to such impressive diagnoses.

ALICE: (*Dimpling as for a compliment*) Nothing of the kind, Harry. Dr. Sloper said I was quite strong enough to go on having attacks for years if I wanted to. He made me very happy. He *did* want to examine a little further a lump he found on my right breast.

HENRY: On your right b.....delicacy was never your strong point, Alice. How did Dr. Sloper manage to find a *lump* on your *chest* in the middle of the Grand Central Station!

ALICE: Well, *naturally* I was carried to the ladies' room. They stretched me out on the cosmetics counter. And the doctor noticed the blood stain on my ... um ... *bodice*. Kathryn said I was quite a sight laid out amongst the powder puffs and the eau de colognes.

HENRY: And where *is* the redoubtable Miss Loring? She's usually not more than two inches from your right elbow.

ALICE: Kathryn's gone to Barnum's Museum. You know her taste for curiosities.

HENRY: And is she come to stay here forever also?

ALICE: You know, Harry, that Kathryn is *devoted* to me.

HENRY: I see. It *is* forever then.

ALICE: Take comfort, brother. I may not last the year.

HENRY: Alice. If I have one certainty in this diseased and distracted world, it is the strength of your constitution. You've survived the constant treatment of at least ten reputable physicians. It's quite a testimonial.

ALICE: I won't need much in the way of attention, brother. Your devotion, all of Miss Austen's books—I haven't read her in at least a year—and some of the Brontes', will do me very nicely.

HENRY: (*Pouting*) Alice, it's plain to see you prefer the books of those scribbling females to mine. You haven't asked after the new novel at all.

ALICE: Nonsense, Harry. I like your novels enormously. Especially the ones you steal from me.

HENRY: (*Stiffly*) I have no idea what you're referring to.

ALICE: Brother. Year after year you have entered my sickrooms armed with paper and pencil or with your prodigious memory and you have taken careful note of my valetudinarian ramblings. And then six months, eight months, a year later, I find embedded in your narratives the subjects we've turned over.

HENRY: Oh that. Perfectly justifiable, sister. It's all in the family.

ALICE: Certainly, Harry. Certainly. And if I ever turn my hand to writing, I'll feel as free to use you as a resource.

HENRY: (*Pompously*) I think I'm quite safe on that score.

ALICE: Ah! I hear Kathryn in the foyer. Leave me brother. I'd like to greet her alone.

(*Blackout on stage, lights up on the tea table.* HENRY *now sits in the host's seat.*)

HENRY: Alice was the most severe trial of my entire life, Dr. Sloper. And yet, she fascinated me, utterly fascinated me. I believe the tea is ready now.

DOCTOR: Thank you, I never take tea at this hour. It has a desperate effect on my sense of time.

HENRY: (*Not at all interested*) Really? Have some marmalade then, the biscuits are pure poison without it. Well, as I say, my sister Alice nearly drove me mad. (DOCTOR *consults his timepiece.*) First she resisted getting sick. Then she resisted getting well. *Then* she resisted dying. *God* how she resisted dying. The family used to say it was your diagnosis that killed her, not the tumour. Your diagnosis . . . and the scalpels. (*Slyly.*)

DOCTOR: (*Shakes his watch*) I . . . (*Shake, shake.*) . . . never had the occasion to use *any* of my instruments in treating your sister, Mr. James. It was a *great* disappointment to me. (*Shake, shake.*)

HENRY: I meant her *obsession,* with scalpels, of course, doctor. Any physician in the Adams Nervous Asylum can tell you about the hundreds of butter knives and nail scissors Alice had secreted in her dresser drawers—and the *pages* of comparisons between the pains in her body and the kinds of cuts different blades can inflict. (*Grim.*) I saw them *all* before they were incinerated.

DOCTOR: What is this nonsense about *my* scalpels, then? And do you have the *time,* Mr. James?

HENRY: It's *tea* time, Dr. Sloper. Have another biscuit. Well it seems that when Alice first saw *your* scalpels in that railway station, it set the seal on her obsession. She had never seen anything quite like them before. And to make matters worse—will you have some tea *now,* doctor?

DOCTOR: (*Shaking his timepiece*) Thank you, it's not time yet.

HENRY: To make matters worse she began to insert the word "scalpel" into that disgusting sentence she used to say when she was having her attacks.

DOCTOR: Oh yes, you mean . . .

HENRY: (*Quickly*) Never mind, doctor, I heard quite enough of that phrase while Alice was alive. The family calculated once, that from the time she was nineteen, Alice averaged five major attacks per month, day in and day out, good weather or bad, until her demise. That is to say, by conservative estimate, my gently reared and modest sister Alice spewed out that horrible sentence of hers at least seventy times a year. Seventy times!

DOCTOR: (*Still shaking the watch*) Tea-time.

HENRY: I beg your pardon?

DOCTOR: Tea-time. Alice was always "taken" during tea-time. She always had an attack between the hours of four and six in the afternoon.

HENRY: Yes ... yes ... I think you're right. I'm *sure* you're right. She loved to catch those dowagers with their hands on their tea cozies.

DOCTOR: (*Stretches complacently*) I *will* take some marmalade. These biscuits are disgusting.

HENRY: (*Hand on marmalade*) I can't hold it back any longer!

DOCTOR: (*Hopefully*) The marmalade?

HENRY: No, no doctor, the *truth*. The truth is that Alice *was* a great trial to me, but not the greatest one.

DOCTOR: (*Dully*) The marmalade, Mr. James.

HENRY: (*Hand on the marmalade again*) The greatest trial of my life was Kathryn Peabody Loring.

DOCTOR: (*Brightens*) Ah, I remember, the Amazon.

HENRY: Amazon? The colossus. The skyscraper. The *mon*ument. The moment Alice met that woman, she took to her bed prostrate with love. She was so fond of Miss Loring's *nursing* that I—her own brother—was treated entirely as a superfluous appendage.

DOCTOR: You were superfluous, Mr. James. You certainly were superfluous.

(*They muse.*)

DOCTOR: (*Sighs, reaches for the marmalade, raises it*) The ladies, Mr. James.

HENRY: Ah yes. The ladies. (*Deeply depressed.*)

Alice's Room in Henry's House

Dimout on the tea table. Lights up on ALICE *and* KATHRYN *who is competently arranging flowers in a vase.* KATHRYN *moves constantly throughout the play; a woman of intense, palpable vitality.*

KATHRYN: There you are, my dear. Some signs of life.

ALICE: Harry does keep a dismal house.

KATHRYN: Sepulchral. Positively sepulchral.

ALICE: He keeps a dismal house because he was a dismal child. The only way I could stir him up was to have a nervous attack in some public place.

KATHRYN: I hope you made the most of your opportunities.

ALICE: Oh, I did reasonably well.

KATHRYN: (*Smiling in remembrance*) You should have *seen* Mary Cabot's face this morning after you delivered your sentence.

ALICE: It does seem to be what they call a real "show-stopper." The last thing I remember is Miss Cabot's tiny red eyes fixed on me in horror. (*Smiling in remembrance.*)

KATHRYN: Is it always like that Alice?

ALICE: Always. (*As though it's happening.*) Someone's eyes in a crowd catch mine, I feel the . . . censure or the disgust, or I invent it, I abandon a certain portion of my consciousness and as I fall, I speak . . .

KATHRYN: Always the same sentence?

ALICE: Ever since I can remember.

KATHRYN: (*Admiring.*) What an exhibitionist you are, my love.

ALICE: It used to drive the family insane. (*With some satisfaction.*) Father spent years dragging me from eminent nerve doctor to eminent nerve doctor. And they all told him the same thing.

KATHRYN: That you would either die or recover.

ALICE: Exactly. Well, I've been at this for the last twenty years or so, and I am neither dead nor recovered.

KATHRYN: (*To the bed, carrying a counterpane, smiling*) It's a miracle we met, Alice.

ALICE: (*A hand on* KATHRYN) A *miracle*?!   I spent *months* arranging it.

(*Embrace. Release.*)

(*Pause. The mood recedes.*)

ALICE: It's peculiar about that doctor, don't you think.

KATHRYN: The one who treated you this morning.

ALICE: Yes that one. Dr. Sloper.

KATHRYN: He reminds me of Harry.

ALICE: It's peculiar about those knives of his.

KATHRYN: Well you know, dear, physicians are not the most balanced class of people.

ALICE: But to carry them *everywhere* like that . . . in a little leather box . . .

KATHRYN: Rather unsanitary, if you ask me. You ought to show him your collection of nail scissors and hat pins, my love. *That* would quiet him down.

ALICE: (*The staged equivalent of a blush*) Umm . . . Where are they?

KATHRYN: I put them in the drawer there (*Points to chiffonier*) so that we'd be spared Harry's reaction. The last time you came to visit he found the pen knives.

ALICE: (*Laughing*) I'll never forget his face when he saw my *sketch*book.

KATHRYN: And I'll never forget his *actions*. Three month's commitment to the Adams Nervous Asylum.

ALICE: (*Nonchalant*) It was comfortable. And they gave me all the drawing paper I wanted . . . (*Inconsequently.*) Massachusetts has more mad houses than any state in the union. (*Pause.*) I ought to know.

KATHRYN: (*Definitively*) Harry's a monster.

(*Pause.*)

ALICE: Kathryn.

KATHRYN: What is it, love.

ALICE: (*Tentatively*) Do you really suppose Harry thinks I don't know what a terrible life he leads?

KATHRYN: A brain surgeon might be able to uncover your brother's thoughts, Alice. I'm not qualified.

ALICE: Guilty exchanges on docks. That vast sensibility of his brought to bear on the bodies of adolescent sailors. (*Laughs a little.*) How surprised they must be if he talks to them.

KATHRYN: And how bored.

ALICE: Poor fellow. At least I've retired into the kind of friendship the world is still forced to support. (*To* KATHRYN.) The Woman's Home Companion. (*Reaches for her, and we have the sexual connection for the first time powerfully.*) With your *breast* still spotted red from my love-making.

KATHRYN: (*Intimate*) I want you well Alice.

ALICE: I've never been well, Kathryn.

KATHRYN: Then I just . . . *want* you.

ALICE: Ah! That's different.

KATHRYN: But when you *are* well, we'll go to the country.

ALICE: (*Taking it up*) And the sun will warm our bodies.

KATHRYN: (*Slyly*) And the wind will cool our ardour.

ALICE: (*Glumly*) And then Harry will appear.

KATHRYN: He always does, doesn't he?

(*Pause.*)

ALICE: (*Experimentally*) We might . . . poison him.

KATHRYN: With the tea *he* serves, he must be immune to everything by now.

ALICE: Well, I *could* have another attack.

KATHRYN: That would kill him on the spot. (*Grimly.*)

ALICE: (*Musing*) What a carnival . . .

KATHRYN: Life, you mean.

ALICE: (*Purposefully*) I had my first attack at a carnival. Did you know that?

KATHRYN: At a carnival! Oh, Alice, what a performer you are.

ALICE: It *was* a carnival. They had taken me to a carnival for my thirteenth birthday. (*As though experiencing it.*) I was standing near the largest Elephant, watching him. Suddenly he turned and seemed to come straight at me, trumpeting wildly and swinging his trunk like an ax. The woman next to me fell to the floor of the tent and began to bleed between her legs. The last thing I remember is her horrified eyes on my face . . . (*Pause.*) When I woke up, I found that I had suffered the fit, said the sentence, and nothing was in its proper place.

(*Pause.*)

(*Ascendant.*) And ever since that summer, I have dreamt constantly of monsters; inhuman shapes, all hung with lumps of bone and strings of flesh . . . And ever since that summer, I have yearned to watch the blood of my father and all my brothers run a red river through the halls of our childhood home.

(*Pause. No one moves for a while.*)

KATHRYN: (*Slowly.*) You write these things in your journal, Alice?

ALICE: Everything is in my journal.

KATHRYN: Everything about Harry?

ALICE: Everything I can think of.

(*Pause.* KATHRYN *considers.*)

KATHRYN: We had better put it in a safer place.

(*Lights dim on the stage.* ALICE *and* KATHRYN *on the bed, barely visible. The twining of their figures produces on the wall behind the bed an image like an elephant moving. The elephant must absolutely seem to be the shadow of their shadows—no matter how awkward the image is. As* HARRY *and the* DOCTOR *begin to speak the shadow world deepens to black, all lights on the stage are extinguished . . . Lights up on the tea table.*)

HENRY: Yes I burnt Alice's journal, but I couldn't burn Alice's friend.

DOCTOR: You should have given her to me, Mr. James. I would have found a use for her.

HENRY: I never thought of it. What a pity she wasn't mine to give.

DOCTOR: So many times I had to visit the cemeteries to carry on my researches . . .

HENRY: Well, I can't say that Miss Loring was in any condition to be researched, doctor.

DOCTOR: *I* thought she was in perfect condition. I *will* have some tea now, if you don't mind.

HENRY: Ahh, at last. I think you'll find this to your taste . . . I meant that Miss Loring was *alive*. You don't generally . . . um . . . experiment on the living, do you doctor?

DOCTOR: Not . . . generally. (*Changing the subject.*) And yourself, sir?

HENRY: *Only* on the living. Though there are certain publishing scoundrels—critics I mean—who would deny it. Well, well, the house of fiction has many windows. Hasn't it. Doctor, what's the matter?

DOCTOR: (*Sputtering into his tea*) What have you done to the tea?

HENRY: Done to the tea?

DOCTOR: Ptui! It tastes like old medical journals!

HENRY: Old . . . literary reviews.

DOCTOR: What did you say? Ptui.

HENRY: Not medical journals, Dr. Sloper. Literary magazines. I have them ground and roasted.

DOCTOR: (*Disgusted*) Good god.

HENRY: Then I brew them up. (*Some satisfaction.*) And *then* I drink them. An old family custom. Alice was devoted to it.

DOCTOR: (*Back to shaking his watch*) De-votion. That's what they give us, Mr. James. Devotion.

HENRY: Who does, Doctor?

DOCTOR: The *ladies*, Mr. James.

HENRY: (*Rousing himself*) Ah yes, of course, the *ladies*, Dr. Sloper.

(*Blackout.*)

Alice James's Room in Henry's House

KATHRYN *reclines, unrecognizable, on* ALICE's *bed. She's covered with* ALICE's *shawls, propped by* ALICE's *pillows, and she looks just like* ALICE *until she moves.* HENRY *bursts in from the tea table.*

HENRY: Alice, damn you Alice, there isn't a butter knife left in the whole house! How can I offer people biscuits without butter knives? What did you do with them *this* time! Oh! Miss Loring. (*Embarrassed docility, nervous laugh.*) Wherever is Alice?

KATHRYN: She had another fit this afternoon. (*Bitterly.*) Dr. Sloper took her to the hospital.

HENRY: (*Exasperated*) God, what an inconvenience. (*Collects himself.*) I mean, how is she? Is she . . . recovering?

KATHRYN: She always recovers, Mr. James. No thanks to the doctor. She never would have gone to the hospital if she'd been conscious. She can't *bare* waking up in a white room.

HENRY: (*Nods*) Yes, I understand. It's . . . too much like death.

KATHRYN: (*Bitterly*) I couldn't stop him from taking her. He insisted upon his medical rights. (*Bursts out.*) Medical rights, when all my darling needs is to be held and spoken softly to! (*Pause.*) But he was adamant. (*Pause.*) I think . . . I did manage to . . . scratch him a bit, though.

HENRY: Miss Loring, you're joking.

KATHRYN: And just possibly, the tip of my right boot came into rather painful contact with the middle portion of his left shin.

HENRY: (*Horrified*) A brawl? Here in my house? With my honored friend? Over the prostrate form of my sister? (*Looks like he's going to faint.*)

KATHRYN: Here, Mr. James, why don't you lie down. I'm sure that Alice, if she were *here* and not in some *horrible hospital*, would invite you to use the chaise.

(HENRY *staggers to the chaise, muttering*, "This is too much, really this is too much," *etc.* KATHRYN, *with an evil intent, begins to settle him on the pillows and cover him with the shawls so that, finally, he looks very much like* ALICE.)

KATHRYN: (*An evil intention*) That's *fine*, Mr. James. You just rest here awhile. *Alice* won't mind. *She's* probably still unconscious, anyway. I'll go into the kitchen and fix you a cup of camomile tea. I'll make sure it's camomile and not that dry tea you've been serving lately. Alice and I haven't enjoyed *that* tea a bit.

(KATHRYN *exits*. HENRY *wriggles around trying to get comfortable, there is a clanking sound behind him and he reaches under the pillow and draws out an entire set of butter knives tied up with a ribbon. He holds them up in disbelief. Blackout.*)

(*Lights dim on stage; tableau of* NURSE *massaging* ALICE *in* DR. SLOPER's *hospital, during the following scene between* HENRY *and the* DOCTOR. *Lights up on the tea table.*)

HENRY: I've been thinking very hard about hands, Dr. Sloper.

DOCTOR: Have you, Mr. James.

HENRY: I've been thinking . . . without hands, what would we have?

DOCTOR: (*Dourly*) A nation of double amputees, no doubt. Please pass the butter.

HENRY: (*Unstoppable*) If we have no hands, then we have no art. If we have no art, then, certainly, we have no life. Think of it. (*Pause.*) . . . The natural cause of *death*. Well sir?

DOCTOR: (*Finally lured into it*) Death *has* no natural causes, Mr. James.

HENRY: I hoped you'd say that, doctor. More tea?

DOCTOR: (*Unstoppable*) Death, Mr. James, is almost always the result of an unnecessary exploration. *This* gentleman, seeking the pleasures of youth, pushed his heart too hard. *That* one, pursuing wealth, worked his only son into the grave. *That* lady's compensatory drinking exhausted her liver; *this* one's consumption of tonics destroyed her bladder. (*Pause.*) Etcetera.

HENRY: (*Slyly*) *This* doctor, seeking fame, cut too deeply into the deformities of a friend . . .

DOCTOR: (*Immediately*) *That* writer, pursuing immortality, drew too painfully upon the life of a sister . . .

(*Pause. They regard each other.*)

HENRY: Ahh! What would we do without the ladies?

DOCTOR: I haven't the slightest idea.

(*Pause. A new rhythm.*)

HENRY: I think I'll order more tea.

DOCTOR: A fine idea.

HENRY: Something a little less dry.

DOCTOR: What about a Japanese tea.

HENRY: I have one right here, doctor. Just let me reach it for you.

DOCTOR: (*Uncertainly*) Tea makes everything . . . clearer.

HENRY: Here we are, doctor. Japanese tea.

DOCTOR: Ummm. It smells very fine.

HENRY: (*Beaming*) Doesn't it. Nothing like a good Japanese tea—made from the subjects of the Emperor Hirohito.

(*Pause. They drink a kind of agreement.*)

DOCTOR: (*Looking at his hands*) This is the hand that invented the Sloper speculum . . .

HENRY: Really, doctor.

DOCTOR: And this one fashioned the Sloper scalpel . . .

HENRY: A famous instrument.

DOCTOR: In this hand, my daughter's appendix burst like a bag of water . . .

HENRY: I wish you wouldn't.

DOCTOR: And with these hands I have opened all the organs of the female pelvis . . .

HENRY: (*Warning*) Doctor.

DOCTOR: Picked the rare flowers of a lady's garden: the polyps, the fibroids, the cysts . . .

HENRY: Let me warm your cup.

DOCTOR: (*Magisterial*) Scooped up ovaries without question, extracted uteri without number. Ahh, Mr. James. The signs of life are closer to the bone than you imagine. And when you find them, there's no stopping until you're covered with blood . . .

(*Slight pause.*)

HENRY: One sugar or two?

DOCTOR: (*Impassioned*) Two please. When you find them you must cut and cut . . . (*Tastes the tea, calms instantly.*) Ummm, A very good tea, indeed. Your health, sir.

HENRY: Thank you doctor. This is the finger that poked Alice's right eye all through our childhood.

DOCTOR: You don't say.

HENRY: And this is the hand that stopped her mouth the second time she said her sentence.

DOCTOR: My my.

HENRY: This one signed her commitment papers to the Adams Nervous Asylum . . .

DOCTOR: A noble sacrifice.

HENRY: And this one plunged the pen deep into her bosom and produced life with her heart's blood.

DOCTOR: Well *done*, sir.

(*Pause.*)

HENRY: It *is* an excellent tea, doctor. Is it time for the toast yet?

DOCTOR: Goodness yes, it *is* time. (*Raises his cup.*)

HENRY: (*Enthusiastically*) To the *ladies*, Dr. Sloper.

(*Blackout on the tea table and the stage.*)

Alice's Room in the Hospital, again.

DR. SLOPER *stands by* ALICE's *bedside, showing his scalpels to* ALICE, *who is propped up with pillows.*

DOCTOR: And this one here is so light, it can slip through the gluteus maximus virtually without resistance.

ALICE: God knows why you'd want to do *that*. (*Placatingly.*) But it *is* an amazing instrument. I have nothing in *my* collection to match it.

DOCTOR: (*Horribly disappointed*) Oh? I didn't know you had a . . . collection.

ALICE: (*Self-deprecatingly*) A ... small one. Pen-knives, poignards, stilletos, hatpins, razor-blades—*household* items. Nothing *serious*. Nothing like *yours*, doctor.

DOCTOR: (*Visibly relieved*) Well. In that case, let me just show you the latest of the Sloper scalpels. The one I hope to be remembered for. (*Pulls out a horrible, three-pronged instrument of torture.*)

ALICE: *I'll* certainly remember you for it.

DOCTOR: It's the Uterine Guillotine. I designed it to separate the organs of the female pelvis from their moorings. No rending, no tearing, no post-operative oozings. Just a quick cut and it's all over.

ALICE: For the woman.

DOCTOR: (*Dismissing it*) In a manner of speaking. (*Pause. A sly look.*) Uh ... Miss James. Have you ... ever considered ... having the operation?

ALICE: The tumour is in my *breast*, doctor. Not *below* it.

DOCTOR: It's an operation every woman should have at your time in life.

ALICE: I think ... not, Dr. Sloper.

DOCTOR: (*Inspired*) We could begin with the vesico-vaginal fistula operation. Quite unnecessary, in your case, but a beautiful operation, nonetheless. It collapses the vagina and makes those ... monthly infirmities you women suffer entirely unnecessary.

ALICE: I haven't menstruated in years.

DOCTOR: Then we could move on to a simple ovariotomy. It's taken me hundreds of attempts to perfect that one. I wish we could keep you conscious for it. You would so appreciate the precision.

ALICE: I have a certain ... attachment to my organs, doctor.

DOCTOR: Then, of course, if you're willing — and so many of my female patients are — we could (*Dramatic tone*) strike at the root of the evil. We could cut *everything out*. We could have a FULL HYSTERECTOMY. (*Appreciative pause by the* DOCTOR.) What do you say, Miss James.

ALICE: I say ... CERTAINLY NOT. What about my breast tumour. Isn't that what I'm *here* for?

DOCTOR: Oh *that*. It's completely inoperable. If I cut you for *that*, you'd bleed to death in twenty minutes.

ALICE: (*A little smile*) *Now* you're beginning to tempt me.

DOCTOR: (*Horrified*) Miss James! I'm a physician, not a *murderer*.

ALICE: (*Mock-surprise*) Ohhh. Well . . . (*Considers*) since I'm so clearly about to leave this life, I think I'd like to go out more or less intact. *Female organs, tumour and all.* (*Looks at her breast.*) Ahhh the stain. Do you see the stain? Funny how . . . it begins to bleed whenever you come near me. (*Looks up at him.*)

(*Pause. An exchange of hard looks.*)

ALICE: Who are you hiding upstairs. Doctor.

DOCTOR: What do you mean?

ALICE: And how long has she been there?

DOCTOR: How do you know it's a "she."

ALICE: I saw the nurse carrying the works of Jane Austen into her room. The only male in America who reads Jane Austen is my brother Henry. And *he* does it for competitive reasons.

DOCTOR: The woman upstairs is being treated for an incurable disorder.

ALICE: How is she being treated?

DOCTOR: *Surgically*, Miss James.

ALICE: I'd like to speak to her.

DOCTOR: That's impossible. She can't speak without bleeding.

ALICE: I'd like to see her then.

DOCTOR: That's out of the question. You can't move without fainting.

(*Pause.*)

ALICE: What is the woman's name, doctor.

DOCTOR: She's called . . . Jane Merritt.

(*Pause.*)

ALICE: (*A long sigh*) I think I'd like to read now, doctor.

DOCTOR: I'll speak to Nurse about it. We're here to make you . . . comfortable, Miss James. I hope you remember that.

(*An incredulous look from* ALICE, *then the* DOCTOR *exits.* ALICE, *alone, shifts uncomfortably, looks around. Each group of sentences, after the first one, should be spoken with a different voice as though coming from different parts of her body.*)

ALICE: Such . . . a . . . white room.

(*Pause.*)

From just behind the eyes, my head feels like a dense jungle into which no ray of light has ever penetrated.
(*Pause.*)

This unholy granite substance in my breast enlarges daily, consuming cell by cell, all the living tissue that surrounds it. I can feel its appetite increasing.
(*Pause.*)

Sometimes when Kathryn is out of the room, or always when the doctor approaches, I feel every pointed instrument I own turning its blade against me. And then this uninvited lodger in my breast begins to leak and seep.

(*Pause.*)

I feel ... (*Stops, then in her normal, acerbic tone.*) I feel that one has a greater sense of intellectual degradation after an interview with a doctor than from *any other human experience.*

(*Blackout. A match strikes at the darkened tea table, two cigars are lit, then the lights come up.*)

HENRY: (*Puffing importantly*) I have always thought that Alice's tragic health was, in a manner of speaking, the only solution to the problem of her life.

DOCTOR: (*Puffing reflectively*) The only solution we could *accept* ... Mr. James.

(*Blackout.*)

* * * * *

The Apron

It is later than it was, both at the tea table and on the main stage, but tea-table time is much later than main-stage time. P.T. BARNUM *stands alone in a circle of light, stage left. He leans against the proscenium, bottle in hand.* HENRY *and the* DOCTOR, *dimly visible stage right, are still at tea, but their exchange has lessened—now it's a breath or two faster than what a slow motion camera might record. As* BARNUM *begins to speak, he makes short, staggering forays in and out of the circle of light. He might describe circles with his movements or he might describe ellipses. Whatever shape his choreography takes, there must be a clear literal and metaphoric play between* MR. BARNUM, *the dark and the light. The words he speaks are a half-drunken reminiscence, his style much more careless now, in the manner of one who sinks into "himself" when unobserved.*

BARNUM: Well she's dead, poor freak. What's her name's dead. My old Elephant Woman. I heard it on the street this morning. Or was it . . . yesterday morning? Strangled to death in her sleep, they say. (*Drinks.*) Poor freak. I didn't make a dime off her. (*Shakes head. Drinks.*) Wonder what happened to that gilt cage of hers. (*Examines his frayed cuffs.*) It cost me six weeks' take. (*Examines his bottle, then straight to the audience.*) Life's a terrible thing. You know that? *You* know that. Sometimes it's a terrible thing.

(*Blackout on* BARNUM.)

Jane Merritt's Room in the Hospital

Same set, the mirror still covered, the tea table very dim. JANE *is standing slightly off center, center stage. Her diction will be clearer than ever and her form much less in focus as a thing of horror. She is dressed as a Victorian lady, and stands quite straight. Jane is in a circle of light, a cone of light if possible. In her good hand she holds the small picture of her mother which she looks into as though it were a mirror.*

JANE: I am looking at my face in the mirror—a thing the doctor has forbidden—and I do not believe what I see. The sight of my own skin makes me scream. (*A scream begins and stops.*) I look at my body, and it's . . . a costume, a bad fit, the hide of some animal that will live a long time. I cannot live a long time. I cannot hold this heavy head up any longer. (*Pause.*) Every night in my dreams I lie down with the blind. (*Pause.*) Everyday my lip bleeds in a new place. (*Pause.*) No matter how often I look at myself, I still do not know what I really see.

(*As* JANE *speaks the next line, she shrinks into what she was at the play's beginning.*)

The image blurs, the ugliness fades, and the face of a woman my

mind can live with covers my own face. (*Looks, long pause.*)
I read somewhere... that Charlotte Bronte was a very small and
plain lady. And I think Nurse told me that George Eliot was the
ugliest woman in England.

(*Blackout on* JANE MERRITT. *Lights up on the tea table.* BARNUM, *hair
white and carrying, once again, his cane, has joined* HENRY *and the*
DOCTOR. BARNUM'*s diction in company is precise and "observed."*)

BARNUM: Well, gentlemen, that's how it's always been with me.
Profit and loss, profit and loss.

HENRY: Some tea, Mr. Barnum?

DOCTOR: Do have a biscuit. They're made in Mr. James' kitchen.

BARNUM: (*Horrified*) I never drink ... tea, thank you. Tans the
stomach. (*Counting on his fingers.*) Yes...Tom Thumb.
Mme. Clofullia, Chang and Eng. I lost 'em all and I mourned 'em
all. (*Looks at his bottle.*) In my fashion. (*Slight pause.*) But the
worst of it—gentlemen (*Calls to* HENRY *and the* DOCTOR *who are
separately musing*), the worst of my losses was Jumbo, the
Elephant. *You* remember Jumbo.

DOCTOR: I don't believe I recall him...

HENRY: I don't think I ever saw him....

BARNUM: (*The showman, now*) Why gentlemen, Jumbo was the most
expensive pachyderm in the en-tire world. He created an
e-normous sensation wherever I exhibited him. Frightened the
ladies into fits. (*Chuckles comfortably.*) Anyways I lost Jumbo just
before your dear sister died, Mr. James. Remember how hot that
month was?

HENRY: I do not.

DOCTOR: I thought it was unusually cool.

BARNUM: Well, it *was* a hot month and Jumbo stepped up on a railroad
track to get a little air just as the four-forty from Chicago was pulling in. It was a terrible meeting. Poor Jumbo had to be shot in the
head. A three thousand dollar elephant. (*Shakes head and drinks.*)
I cried like a baby. Three thousand dollars. (*Pause.*) I think they cut
him up for cat food. (*Pauses, drinks, looks at bottle, drinks.*)

(*Pause.* HENRY *and the* DOCTOR *ignore* BARNUM.)

HENRY: You know, doctor, I've been thinking.

DOCTOR: Marvellous exercise, Mr. James. I prescribe it whenever
possible.

HENRY: I've been thinking of making a play out of certain...um...
past events.

DOCTOR: Ah, Mr. James. To make a play. That *would* be the distin-
guished thing.

BARNUM: Seems to me I once owned a theatre somewhere....St.
Louis, was it? Birmingham? (*Drinks largely.*)

HENRY: (*Irritated*) I've been thinking of making a play about *Alice*,
Doctor.

BARNUM: Ah! your dear sister. Wonderful idea, Mr. James. (*Slight
pause.*) I saw quite a bit of her...um companion in those last
months.

HENRY: (*Surprised*) *Did* you, Mr. Barnum.

DOCTOR: How...un*usual*.

BARNUM: Oh yes indeed. Why she used to... (*Pause.*) Whatever happened to Miss Loring? (*Pause.* BARNUM *embarrassed at the silence.*)
I mean after Miss James's...uh demise. Where did she go?

DOCTOR: I haven't the slightest idea.

HENRY: I can't remember.

BARNUM: (*Trying to cover the chill*) I thought I heard she was trying
to get a manuscript published. (*Muses.*) Could it have been
something of Miss James's?

DOCTOR: (*Quickly*) Highly unlikely.

HENRY: (*Finally*) Utterly impossible. (*Pause, softer.*) My dear sister
could scarcely put a sentence together. She never wrote a word in
her life.

DOCTOR: She was a *collector*, Mr. Barnum, not a *writer*.

HENRY: (*Firmly*) She had a *large* collection of *small* household items.
(*Pause. The subject is sealed.*)

BARNUM: I...

DOCTOR: *Do* have some biscuits, Mr. Barnum.

HENRY: A glass of milk, perhaps.

BARNUM: No, no...(*Trails off.*)

(*Pause.*)

DOCTOR: In this...play you will write, Mr. James, what will you do
with Miss Loring? How would you treat a character like Miss

Loring?

HENRY: An early death, I think. Somewhere in the first act.

(*Smiles of satisfaction by both gentlemen.* BARNUM *is ignored, asleep or befuddled.*)

HENRY: More tea, doctor?

DOCTOR: More *sugar*, Mr. James.

(*Freeze and blackout. Lights up on* ALICE *and* KATHRYN.)

Alice's Room in Henry's House

ALICE *is on her bed-lounge reading from a newspaper;* KATHRYN *is near the chiffonnier.*

ALICE: "And the old couple, poverty stricken, homeless, without hope, was found bound together, with stones in their pockets, at the bottom of the Hudson River early this morning." (*Admiring pause.*) What a *beautiful* story.

KATHRYN: Alice, you're a ghoul.

ALICE: (*Carefully cutting out the article*) It runs in the family. Put it in the journal, will you darling?

KATHRYN: (*Grimly*) Right next to the story of the woman who took poison on the eve of her marriage to the mail clerk.

ALICE: She certainly made the better choice. (*Slight pause. Realizing something.*) You know I've kept that journal ever since I had my first attack.

KATHRYN: (*Obliging, indulgent, but fatigued*) You have the most unusual hobbies, Alice.

(*Pause.*)

ALICE: (*Looks at* KATHRYN, *a cold, indifferent tone*) Aren't you ever tired of my hobbies?

KATHRYN: (*Looks, stops*) Certainly, I am.

ALICE: And aren't you sometimes bored by my symptoms? Disgusted by my brother? Drained of your vital energy by my demands?

KATHRYN: (*Dead serious*) Continually, my dearest.

(*Pause.*)

ALICE: (*Satisfied, more alive*) I thought so. You've been a nurse too long, Kathryn.

(*Pause.*)

KATHRYN: All my life, I have moved from the illness of one woman to the illness of another. My mother's long disease, my sister's unending complaints, your own unusual symptoms...(*Back to whatever normal is.*) Life is a terrible thing Alice. (*A patient pause.*) Why don't you go on reading, it will calm you.

ALICE: (*Numbly takes the paper and begins to read*) Here's something ...*This* one. What a sad story. The largest Elephant in Mr. Barnum's Museum—Jumbo the Giant—was run over by a railroad train. It says here that he died in agony, over a period of eighteen hours. "The animal was finally dispatched amid cries of terrible suffering by a well-placed bullet in the brain. Prior to the shooting of the elephant, Mr. P.T. Barnum, owner and exhibitor of the animal, was observed to be selling sarsparilla and collecting coins from the large and raucous crowd that had gathered to watch the death-throes of its favorite circus star."

(*Blackout on Alice's room. Just in back of the tea table, stage right, we see a corner of* JANE MERITT'*s room in* DR. SLOPER'*s hospital.* NURSE *and* DR. SLOPER *are lighted in consultation.*)

DOCTOR: She's ... *dead!* Jane's *gone!* I don't believe it! We were going to operate again tonight!

NURSE: There'll be no more cuttings on *that* body, doctor. It's gone beyond all of us.

DOCTOR: It's impossible that this could have happened now! She made a *complete recovery* from the last operation. I examined her myself! She's in *perfect health!*

NURSE: That's right, doctor. Perfect health. And she's lying there dead as a doormouse.

DOCTOR: *Lying.* What do you mean *lying there!* Jane Merritt does not lie down!

NURSE: You haven't seen her? You didn't go in?

DOCTOR: Of *course* not. I ... the sight of a newly dead body is ... disturbing to me.

NURSE: Well she's lying there, the poor thing, flat on her back. I heard this awful sound coming from her room. Like someone blowing on a trumpet for the first time. I rushed right in and all her pillows were on the floor—can you imagine—and there she was lying flat on her back, her windpipe snapped like a straw. Just like a straw in the wind.

DOCTOR: (*Furious*) One more operation! One more cutting and she would have been able to look in a mirror like other people!

NURSE: She looked in mirrors all the time, she told me so.

DOCTOR: One more operation and she could have laughed like other people.

NURSE: Go and look at her laid out on that bed, doctor. There's a smile on her face that's nearly splitting it.

(*Instant blackout. Lights up on the tea table.* HENRY *and the* DOCTOR *are present.* MR. BARNUM *is absent, but represented by his cane which is hung over the back of his chair. It's later than it was.*)

HENRY: (*In mid-sentence*) . . . and the writing of this play has taken over my entire life.

DOCTOR: (*Buttering and pouring*) Is that a fact, sir?

HENRY: It's more than a fact, doctor. It's virtually an obsession. There *was* a time when my evenings were spent in healthful promenades along the docks of New York . . .

DOCTOR: (*Looks up sharply at* HENRY, *who continues obliviously.*)

HENRY: . . . stopping, now and then, to have a chat with a sturdy young seaman, or an occasional glass of hock with a naval officer.

DOCTOR: Really, Mr. James. I never would have thought you had interest in the *navy*. I always assumed that Herman *Mel*ville had exhausted *that* subject.

HENRY: (*The subject is uncomfortable*) In any case, doctor, my evenings now are consumed entirely by dreadful dreams. Even the act of writing has become a kind of constriction on my impulses.

DOCTOR: Nerves, Mr. James, nerves. The use of the chamomile flower brewed in a tea is very effective in these instances. Just let me put up a cup for you. . .

HENRY: All I imagine now are the eyes of this hideous audience fastened upon me as though my writing were a kind of performance. Front row, center, amongst the hundreds of pairs of undistinguished irises, are the unwavering orbs of my sister Alice, trained upon me the way a gun is trained upon a target in the moment before it is fired. I tell you doctor, I see my own death in those eyes! My own death!

DOCTOR: Chamomile, Mr. James. Chamomile. Let us drink to your tranquility. (*Raises cup.*)

HENRY: (*Correcting*) To the *ladies*, Dr. Sloper. We must always drink to the *ladies*.

(*Blackout on the tea table. Lights up on . . .*

Alice James's Room in Henry's House

ALICE *lies back, noticeably weaker.* KATHERINE *in silhouette, her back to* ALICE. ALICE *is writing in her journal.*)

KATHRYN: They were at tea again together yesterday. Thick as thieves.

ALICE: I overheard them, I'm sorry to say. Henry was advancing that repulsive theory of his that Emily Dickinson had a distant passion for William Wordsworth.

KATHRYN: Wordsworth! Good god, Alice. Have you ever seen a *picture* of Wordsworth?

ALICE: I have, yes, unfortunately. He had a *very* short neck.

KATHRYN: Wordsworth! Your brother had better look to the tattered remnants of his *own* love life.

ALICE: I'm afraid he is, my darling. Haven't you noticed how . . . um . . . *lengthy* his evening absences have become?

KATHRYN: I was too relieved with his going to count the hours. (*Slight pause.*) Though now that I think of it, Mr. Barnum mentioned to me that Henry is often seen . . . perambulating the docks of lower New York.

ALICE: My, my. It must be a fairly public perambulation for Mr. Barnum to know about it.

KATHRYN: Not necessarily. Mr Barnum has quite a talent for acquiring bizarre bits of knowledge.

ALICE: And so do you, my dear. I've noticed how your visits to Mr. Barnum's establishment have lengthened as the predictions for my life span have shortened.

KATHRYN: Even a nurse needs comfort, Alice. Those oddities in Barnum's Museum help to remind me that your early death is not the only freakish and terrible thing in this world.

ALICE: Kathryn, my love. When will you remember that it's *life* that is the terrible thing! Life is such a tragedy, that it *requires* a happy end. And mine, thank god, is coming soon.

KATHRYN: (*Picking up* ALICE's *journal*) When I think of what you might have written . . .

ALICE: (*Disgusted*) Oh good god Kathryn! I might have written what Harry writes. Novels like dry deserts! Endless *Saharas* of insinuation and inference with scarcely an oasis or a sign of life in them. At least I have the satisfaction of knowing that I never put anything parched and dead into the world.

KATHRYN: But Alice, to die away from *me*! What will I do without you?

ALICE: Oh, you'll mourn me very prettily for a while. And then I imagine you'll find another selfish and interesting woman with a sentence to say.

KATHRYN: Never.

ALICE: Of course you will, Kathryn. It's your fate. (*Pause.*) You know, my love, the only thing I regret about dying is that the experience will occur in New York City.

KATHRYN: (*Recovering herself*) You're not serious.

ALICE: No, really. I'd *love* to die in New England. Those flinty faces, the granite inflections, the stone-cold eyes. Why Kathryn, being in New England is the next best thing to being dead. I'd hardly notice the transition.

(*Blackout. Lights up on a corner of . . .*

Jane Merritt's Room in the Hospital

We see only DOCTOR SLOPER's *back, in its white surgical coat slightly on-stage as he performs an autopsy on the off-stage body of* JANE MERRITT. NURSE *is behind him handing him instruments from a surgical tray.*)

DOCTOR: *What* did you say? Dammit, hand me another surgical clip. Oh Jane, Jane. Alive, you were a wonder. Dead, you're miraculous! Where are those clips, dammit!

NURSE: (*Craning her neck to see*) Why do you cut her so deeply? I thought you already knew everything there was to know about her.

DOCTOR: Ah so did I, Nurse. And maybe I do, maybe I do. But this dissection will tell me for sure, for certain. Oh my god, look at that! Just look at that!

(*Blackout. Lights up on the tea table. Henry is yawning uncontrollably.*)

DOCTOR: It used to be, Mr. James, that you could understand how a thing worked by looking at it. A locomotive, a steam shovel, Theodore Roosevelt—none of *them* hid anything from the mind. But Jane Merritt!

HENRY: (*Bitterly*) Jane Merritt and my sister Alice have their place in love's darkest night, doctor—way down in the bottom of the sandman's bag. They're what gets sprinkled in your eyes along with the sweeter dreams.

DOCTOR: (*Reaching for the creamer*) You're having bad dreams again?

HENRY: I am. I write monstrous things in the day and dream dreadful ones at night.

DOCTOR: A good way to lose your audience, sir. I threw your last novel across the room three times before I'd finished the first chapter.

HENRY: (*Glumly*) I must say you're in the company of every critic in America with that opinion. (*Brightly, with malice.*) Now your monograph on Jane Merritt's disorder . . . That business about the poor creatures . . . um . . . private parts was revoltingly unnecessary.

DOCTOR: (*A cautionary finger*) Ah, but she *was* amorous. Yes, Mr. James, Jane was amorous. She would have liked to have been a lover. The signs were unmistakeable. I saw great significance in the fact that the skin of her vulva was virtually the only area of her body untouched by the disorder.

HENRY: (*Choking slightly on his tea*) A disgusting piece of work, doctor.

DOCTOR: I had to do it, Mr. James. Mother Science required it. It was certainly no choice of mine. God knows, if there's anything I hate, it's exploring the organs of the female pelvis.

HENRY: (*Genuinely shocked*) My god, sir. Your're a *woman's doctor*.

DOCTOR: (*Raises his cup*) Let's have a toast to the ladies, Mr. James. *This* one is for the ladies.

HENRY: (*Raises cup glumly, sighs profoundly.*)

(*Blackout. Lights dimly up on* KATHRYN *and* ALICE. ALICE, *much weaker now, and supported by many pillows.* KATHRYN *sits by her, holding her hand and head. There is a spot on* ALICE's *mouth, so that it is outlined, accentuated; its movements providing the only "action" in this short scene. Beginning with* ALICE's *monologue and continuing through the* DOCTOR's *and* HENRY's *monologues, whatever is said should be spoken very fast as though to disintegrate the forms surrounding it.* ALICE's *monologue must be a tableau with only* ALICE's *mouth moving — almost a Pieta.*)

ALICE: I saw the most beautiful thing last night, Kathryn. I saw a slender, perfect arm, white as lambswool, rising up from a rotted lump of flesh. (*Her body is taken by pain, she contracts sharply; the next few words are in a stentorian voice.*) Kathryn, Kathryn, give me that morphine! I cannot bare the pain! It leaks and seeps into every corner of my life! (*Again, a spasm.*) I yearn for my death but I haven't the strength to go to it alone. Kathryn! I beg you, give me that drug! You did it for your mother! (*Accusing and very loud.*) You did it for your mother!

(*Blackout. Lights up on that corner of* ALICE's *room in* HENRY's *house which represents the operating room. The* DOCTOR *in his white coat is still performing the autopsy on the body of* JANE MERRITT. *The* NURSE *is not present.*)

DOCTOR: (*Back still to us*) Oh Jesus Christ! What a thing to witness! Oh horror, horror, horror! Who is the god that could leak life into such a form! Look at her ovaries! Look at her stomach! (*Calls in horror.*) Nurse, Nurse, for godssake Nurse come here and look at her breast!

(*Instant blackout. Lights up on* HENRY *who is pacing the stage in* . . .

Alice's Room in Henry's House

HENRY: She followed me for spite, pure spite. I know very well she wanted to die in New England. (*Pause.*) But how my writing soared when she was with me. All the eyes at all the windows in my house of fiction were open wide. (*Pause, a shudder.*) Ugh! That forehead! The eyes underneath! (*Pause.*) Every night I dream lumps of bone and strands of flesh. Every day I struggle to disentangle the meaning of what I write from what I am writing. (*Pause.*) I can't go on without Alice. I know that now. (*Pause.*) I wonder . . . how I ever thought I could?

(*Blackout. Lights up again dimly on* KATHRYN *and* ALICE. ALICE's *body is almost gone, now, but the voice is still alive and speaking.* KATHRYN *is taking dictation.*)

KATHRYN: Alice, darling . . . will you speak louder. I can scarcely hear you.

ALICE: (*Broken speech, the words constantly intersected by pain*) This . . . block of stone in my breast . . . has moved to fill my throat, Kath . . . I cannot push the words past it . . . very well.

KATHRYN: Try . . . Alice . . . oh can't you try. I'll write everything down, *everything . . . everything.*

ALICE: It is . . . too late to expect anything . . . important of me, now, my darling . . . Just let me say my sentence once for you. I cannot . . . hold my head up any longer.

KATHRYN: Say it, Alice, speak it to me. It will be the last thing I write in your journal.

ALICE: (*Raises herself up with her arms around* KATHRYN's *neck and speaks her sentence in* KATHRYN's *ear.* KATHRYN's *face in great pain,* ALICE *falls back smiling, and speaks with great difficulty*) Remember me to Mr. Barnum.

(*Lights quickly down on* ALICE *and* KATHRYN, *then up for a moment very bright and blinding on the corner of the hospital where* JANE MER-RITT's *autopsy is being performed; the* DOCTOR's *white jacket is now entirely covered with blood.* NURSE *is present, but mute and stationary. She holds the Uterine Guillotine in one hand.*)

DOCTOR: (*In an ecstasy*) The blood, the *blood*, the *blood covers* me!! Oh it's red, it's *human's* blood! I've found the thing I needed to know. Nurse, Nurse, who would have thought it. *Joan* Merritt, *Jane* Merritt, the *Elephant Woman* . . . has blood . . . as red . . . as *yours!!*

(*Instant blackout. Quick return to the tea table where* HENRY *and the* DOCTOR *sit.* MR. BARNUM's *cane hangs casually over the middle chair. They are whiter, older, more crotchety. Parts of the tea service are missing, now, from the table. The characters' interaction with the missing parts should be a silent one.* HENRY *might reach for the creamer and register its lack; the* DOCTOR *could begin to pour tea into an absent cup; some one of them might turn to ask* MR. BARNUM *again if he could tolerate a biscuit. The charade must gradually run down and* HENRY *and the* DOCTOR *should be left facing each other for a moment. A silence in which each one in turn leans forward to begin something, gives it up, and drops back in his chair.* HENRY *pulls himself together first.*)

HENRY: Alice wasn't buried until a full week after she died. It took the railroad five days to carry her body from New York to Cambridge. The train was struck by a horse cart in New York State, derailed in Western Massachussetts, and stopped for half a day in Brookline when it ran out of coal. The railway conductor told me that he had never in his life had such a journey. (*Pause, slowly.*) During all that time Kathryn Loring sat up with Alice's body in the baggage car. She sat dry-eyed and stony-faced, she spoke to no one, she seemed, from time to time, to be writing sentences in a small black book. (*Pause.*) When the train finally reached Boston and Alice was . . . um . . .unloaded and carried to the platform, a careless porter set her down clumsily and the lid of her coffin sprang open. Kathryn Loring had walked on ahead, so no one with sufficient authority was present to push down the coffin lid. And so Alice remained there on the platform of the second largest railway station in the Northeastern United States for quite a while. . .

DOCTOR: Her last public performance, you might say.

HENRY: It seems that a large crowd gathered —how often, after all, is such an exhibition presented in a public place? I was told that before Miss Loring returned, a man in a tattered coat began to offer refreshments for sale and even to sell tickets for what he promised were further revelations about the dead woman. My sister, Alice. (*Pause.*) The ticket seller was later driven from the railway station by Kathryn Loring who seemed to recognize him.

DOCTOR: (*A look at* BARNUM's *empty chair*) Mr. Barnum left his cane here.

HENRY: (*Carefully*) I noticed that he had.

(*Pause.*)

DOCTOR: (*A fresh energy*) Of course all I heard about your dear sister's death were the medical rumors. That, in her coffin, her fingernails were observed to have grown an inch.

HENRY: (*Nods*) They did grow. It was a most amazing thing. Alice's last collection of pointed instruments. You might say . . . that she was buried . . . armed to the teeth.

(*Slight chuckles from both men. Pause.*)

DOCTOR: (*Tasting*) The tea is quite cold.

HENRY: (*Tasting*) The biscuits are . . . *very* dry. (*Glumly.*) The butter is gone.

DOCTOR: (*Irritated*) Where's my . . . tea cup?

HENRY: (*Testily*) I could have *sworn* I had a saucer . . .

(*Pause.*)

DOCTOR: You know . . . (*Stops.*) . . . I haven't really performed a successful operation since Jane Merritt's autopsy.

HENRY: My books have sunk like stones in still water since Alice died.

DOCTOR: (*Ostentatiously checking his watch*) Face it, my dear sir. Life is far too crowded an experience to have in it a room for your happiness. (*Slight pause.*) Or mine, for that matter.

HENRY: (*Sighs heavily*) I'd better ring for more tea things. Let me see, we need a saucer, another cup, the jam, the cream and (*looks around the table*) hmmm . . . everything else.

DOCTOR: Don't bother ringing, Mr. James. I've lost my appetite.

(*Suddenly* P.T. BARNUM *sticks his head into* ALICE's *room.*)

BARNUM: Ladies and Gentlemen, Gentlemen and Ladies, welcome to
P.T. Barnum's street museum. Please have your money ready.
That's right, folks. A whole new concept in the presentation of
curiosities. See the cucumber man, see the human frankfurter from
Fiji, see the incredible contortionist from the Carolinas. And make
sure you see the most fascinating bit of exotica we have. Yes, that's
correct, she's just behind the curtain. The child you've all heard so
much about is with us at last! That's right, folks, it's Rhinoceros
Woman. *The* most extraordinary female freak of the decade. Her
elder sister cut quite a figure here and abroad a few years ago, but
she was nothing compared to this little girl. *This* little girl is a *real*
freak. That's right, folks, line forms to the right. Rhinoceros
Woman walks, she talks, she even laughs like a human being, but
due to a dreadful accident of birth she appears to be part rhino.
That's what I said, Madam, the girl looks just like a little
Rhinoceros.

(*A long, long laugh from* BARNUM *and his head disappears. Pause.
During* BARNUM's *spiel* HENRY *has found his way back to his seat at the
tea table and he and the* DOCTOR *have twisted around to look at* BAR-
NUM. *In the pause between the end of* BARNUM's *spiel and the re-
grouping of the tea ceremony, much is indicated, nothing said. Then*
HENRY *and the* DOCTOR *resume, as though nothing has intervened
since their last complaints at the missing parts of the tea set.*)

DOCTOR: I was sure you said your saucer was missing.

HENRY: It *is* missing, doctor, and I'm not happy about it.

DOCTOR: Oh, well, *happiness* . . .

HENRY: Why that's odd.

DOCTOR: *What's* odd. Could you hand me whatever's left of those
biscuits. My appetite seems to be returning.

HENRY: That's *very* odd. The butter-knives are gone. Every . . .
damned . . . one of them.

DOCTOR: (*With some asperity*) My, my. Is there anyone *else* in your
household who collects pointed instruments? *Please* pass the
biscuits, Mr. James.

(HENRY *has taken the plate of biscuits in hand and continues to hold
them.*)

HENRY: This is most upsetting, doctor. (*Gets up with plate of biscuits
which the* DOCTOR *is now grabbing for, and begins to pace.*) I can
tolerate *bone* in my biscuits. I can put up with *blood* in my cup.
But, doctor, I warn you, I will not do without my butter-knife. No

sir, I will *not* do without my butter-knife.

DOCTOR: Dammit, Mr. James, give me those biscuits immediately! I don't care *what* you've ground up in them — book reviews, Japanese citizens, give them here, sir! They're *mine!* Give them *here!*

(DOCTOR *and* HENRY *both on their feet now. They begin to struggle trance-like over the plate, come out of their separate reveries and relapse into horribly embarrassed, self-exculpatory chuckles.*)

HENRY: Heee heee heee.

DOCTOR: Aha ha ha.

HENRY: After *you*, sir.

DOCTOR: No *no*, after *you.*

HENRY: I insist.

DOCTOR: (*Angry.*) Be *seated*, Mr. James.

HENRY: (*Vicious*) You *first*, doctor.

DOCTOR: *I will not.*

(*Pause. They look at each other and begin the embarrassed laughing again.*)

HENRY: (*Conciliatory*) I think we might sit down together, doctor.

DOCTOR: What a good idea, Mr. James.

(*Plunk. They sit down exactly together.*)

HENRY: Well, sir, I see we have only one cup between us.

DOCTOR: That's all we need for the *toast*, Mr. James. We certainly don't need more than one cup for the *toast.*

HENRY: Quite right, doctor. (*Slight pause.*) *Which* toast is that?

DOCTOR: (*Slightly puzzled*) Why ... our *usual* toast, Mr. James. (*Raises his cup high.*) To Jane Merritt and Alice James and all ladies everywhere. (*Ringing tones.*)

HENRY: (*Raises his hand, tentatively, and puts it on the cup also. slowly*) To the ladies, doctor. Who would have thought their blood ... could be ... so ... *red.*

(*Freeze. Instant blackout.*)

End

Appendix A

THE WOMEN'S PROJECT PLAYWRIGHTS AND DIRECTORS

PLAYWRIGHTS

Joyce Aaron
Lynne Alvarez
Sallie Bingham
Patricia Bosworth
France Burke
Sophy Burnham
Kathleen Collins
Martie Evans-Charles
Penelope Gilliatt
Rose L. Goldemberg
Gloria Goldsmith
Roma Greth
Momoko Iko
Diane Kagan
Susan Lukas
Carol K. Mack
Gail Kriegel Mallin
Honor Moore
Lavonne Mueller
Sally Ordway
Sybille Pearson
Phyllis Purscell
Joan Schenkar
Adele Edling Shank
Patty Gideon Sloan
Luna Tarlo
Nadja Tesich
Joan Vail Thorne
Sharon Tipsword
Dorothy Velasco
Elizabeth Wray

DIRECTORS

Joyce Aaron
Joanne Akalaitis
Billie Allen
Julianne Boyd
Patricia Carmichael
Tisa Chang
Geraldine Court
Terese Hayden
Esther Herbst
Gitta Honegger
Anita Khanzadian
Sue Lawless
Susan Lehman
Cassandra Medley
Caymichael Patten
Livia Perez
Gaby Rodgers
Victoria Rue
Betsy Shevey
Dorothy Silver
Joan Micklin Silver
Joan Vail Thorne
B.J. Whiting

Appendix B

CHRONOLOGY OF READINGS
AND PRODUCTIONS

1978-79 SEASON

REHEARSED READINGS

Aug. 8   *Choices* by Patricia Bosworth, directed by Caymichael
             Patten
Oct. 16   *A Little Going Away Party* by Sybille Pearson, directed
             by Caymichael Patten
Oct. 23   *Tom, Dick and Harry* by Sharon Tipsword, directed by
             Susan Lehman
Oct. 30   *Warriors from a Long Childhood* by Lavonne Mueller,
             directed by Betsy Shevey
Nov. 6   *The New World Monkey* by France Burke, directed by
             Sue Lawless
Nov. 13   *Years* by Honor Moore, directed by Victoria Rue
Nov. 20   *Penelope* by Sophy Burnham, directed by Terese Hayden
Dec. 4   *African Interlude* by Martie Evans-Charles, directed by
             Billie Allen
Dec. 11   *Billy and the Rainbow* by Susan Lukas, directed by Susan
             Lehman
Jan. 15   *Separate Ceremonies* by Phyllis Purscell, directed by
             Geraldine Court
Jan. 22   *The Corridor* by Diane Kagan, directed by Patricia Car-
             michael

Jan. 29	*S.W.A.K.* by Sally Ordway, directed by Caymichael Patten
Feb. 5	*Broken Borders* by Elizabeth Wray, directed by Gitta Honegger
Feb. 12	*The Guitarron* by Lynne Alvarez, directed by Livia Perez
Feb. 19	*My Mother, My Daughters and Me* by Gloria Goldsmith, directed by Joan Vail Thorne
Feb. 26	*Holy Places* by Gail Kriegel Mallin, directed by Victoria Rue
Mar. 5	*A Safe Place* by Carol K. Mack, directed by Cassandra Medley
Mar. 12	*Signs of Life* by Joan Schenkar, directed by Esther Herbst
Mar. 19	*Letters Home* by Rose Leiman Goldemberg

STAGED READINGS

Dec. 18	*Alfred Jarry Loves Oscar Wilde* by Dorothy Velasco, directed by Gaby Rodgers
Apr. 23	*Separate Ceremonies* by Phyllis Purscell, directed by B.J. Whiting
Apr. 30	*A Little Going Away Party* by Sybille Pearson, directed by Caymichael Patten
May 14	*The New World Monkey* by France Burke, directed by Sue Lawless

STUDIO PRODUCTIONS

Nov. 30 through Dec. 17—*Choices* conceived by Patricia Bosworth, directed by Caymichael Patten and adapted by Ms. Bosworth, Ms. Patten and Lily Lodge

May 17 through May 27—*Warriors from a Long Childhood* by Lavonne Mueller, directed by Betsy Shevey

May 29 through June 7—*Signs of Life* by Joan Schenkar, directed by Esther Herbst

May 31 through June 10—*Letters Home* by Rose Leiman Goldemberg, directed by Dorothy Silver. Based on Sylvia Plath's "Letters Home," edited by Aurelia Schober Plath.

1979-1980 SEASON

REHEARSED READINGS

Oct. 22	*Quotations from Other Lives* by Penelope Gilliatt, directed by Gaby Rodgers
Oct. 29	*Dancing in the Dark* by Sallie Bingham, directed by Joan Vail Thorne
Nov. 5	*Night on Bare Mountain* by Patty Gideon Sloan, directed

by Caymichael Patten

Nov. 11   *Killings on the Last Line* by Lavonne Mueller, directed by
             Dorothy Silver

Nov. 19   *The Greatest Day of the Century* by Roma Greth,
             directed by Anita Khanzadian

Jan. 14   *After the Revolution* by Nadja Tesich, directed by Joyce
             Aaron

Jan. 21   *Flowers and Household Gods* by Momoko Iko, directed
             by Tisa Chang

Jan. 28   *Acrobatics* by Joyce Aaron, directed by Joanne Akalaitis

Feb. 4   *In the Midnight Hour* by Kathleen Collins, directed by
             Billie Allen

Feb. 25   *Winterplay* by Adele Edling Shank, directed by Joan
             Micklin Silver

Apr. 8   *Terms* by Joan Vail Thorne, directed by Gaby Rodgers

Apr. 9   *Snowstorms* by Sophy Burnham, directed by Susan
             Lehman

Apr. 10   *Haze* by France Burke, directed by Pat Carmichael

STUDIO PRODUCTIONS

Dec. 6 through Dec. 16—*Holy Places* by Gail Kriegel Mallin,
            directed by Victoria Rue

Feb. 28 through Mar. 9—*Milk of Paradise* by Sallie Bingham,
            directed by Joan Vail Thorne

May 9 through May 18—*Personals: An Improvisational Revue,* music
            by Michael Ward, directed by Julianne Boyd, with Cyn-
            thia Bostick, Stephen Mellor, Molly Regan

AMERICAN PLACE MAIN-STAGE PRODUCTIONS—
DEVELOPED IN THE WOMEN'S PROJECT

Oct. 12 through Nov. 9—*Letters Home* by Rose Leiman Goldem-
            berg, directed by Dorothy Silver

May 29 through June 15—*Killings on the Last Line* by Lavonne
            Mueller, directed by Dorothy Silver

Authors' Biographies

Joyce Aaron, an original member of Joseph Chaikin's Open Theatre, collaborated in the creation of *Terminal*, *The Serpent*, and Brecht's *Clown Play*, among others, and performed them throughout the U.S. and Europe. She is a member of Mr. Chaikin's Winter Project, which last year created *Re-Arrangements*. She wrote, directed, and performed in *Acrobatics* at the Interart Theatre, for which she won an Obie for best actress in 1975-1976. Other acting credits include the original productions of Jean-Claude van Itallie's *The Fable* and *America Hurrah!*, both in New York and in London and Sam Shepard's *La Turista* at The American Place. She also worked as a visiting artist in Paris in Peter Brook's International Research Laboratory. She has acted, directed, and written for The Women's Project.

Kathleen Collins is Professor of Film History and Aesthetics at City College; worked for several years as a film editor, assistant director, associate producer in the film business; has just produced and directed her first movie, *The Cruz Brothers and Miss Malloy*; has written several screenplays; has written several critical articles on film; worked as a translator for the French film journal *Cahiers du Cinema*; translated books from the French; published several short stories and is presently at work on a novel.

Penelope Gilliatt is a London born novelist and script writer. For the last eight years she has written for *The New Yorker* magazine. She has published novels and collections of short stories both here and in London, and is a fellow of The Royal Society of Literature. Her screenplay for *Sunday, Bloody Sunday* received awards from The National Society of Film Critics, The NY Film Critics Circle, and The English Film

Critics Circle, and received an Oscar nomination for best original screenplay. She has just finished a play for the BBC, *In the Unlikely Event of an Emergency*, an original three-act opera libretto commissioned by the English National Opera Company, and a new book of profiles called *Three Quarter Face*. Her new play, *One Asks Oneself*, is to be done in England, and a fourth collection of short stories is coming out in the autumn of 1980. She is also working on a new novel.

Rose Leiman Goldemberg has written for television, radio, and film, as well as the stage, and started out her life writing poetry. Her play *The Rabinowitz Gambit* was premiered at the Cleveland Playhouse and later produced in New York; *Gandhiji* was chosen for the O'Neill Conference and later produced at the Back Alley Theatre in Washington, D.C.; *Rites of Passage* was produced at the New Dramatists and later at the Astor Place Theater in New York City. Other plays produced in New York include *The Merry War*, *Love One Another*, and *Marching As To War*. For television, she created and wrote the widely acclaimed special about immigrant life, *Land of Hope*, and more currently *Mother and Daughter* and the CBS five-hour mini-series, *A Celebration of Women*. Her feature film credits include *Doubles*, for Time-Life.

Lavonne Mueller has written ten plays in the last three years. Last spring she had *Warriors from a Long Childhood* produced as a studio production as part of The Women's Project. *Crimes and Dreams* has been optioned for Off-Broadway and *Mutiny In the Silence After the Last Sniper* has been optioned for The Yale Repertory Theater. Her children's play, published by Baker's Plays, has been performed in community theatres throughout the U.S. She has published articles and poetry in such magazines as the *New York Quarterly*, *English Journal*, *West Coast Review*, *Caribbean Review*, *Psychology Today*, and others. She has also written two text books. Ms. Mueller grew up on army posts, lived all over the world, and has finally settled, with her husband and daughter, in DeKalb, Illinois, where she has taught English. She is the recent recipient of a Rockefeller Foundation Playwright-in-Residence Grant.

Phyllis Purscell was born in Iowa and attended college there, later completing her B.A. at the State University of New York at New Paltz. She lives in Red Bank, New Jersey, with her husband and children. She has written two screenplays, *Will They Be All Right, I Wonder?* (an adaptation of her play of the same title) and *The Original Chicken of Scottstown*. She is currently working on a third screenplay and the book and lyrics of a musical.

Joan Schenkar has had plays produced in New York, Paris, Los Angeles, Colorado, Florida, etc. Her work has been shown at The Public Theatre, WPA Theatre, St. Clement's, La Mama, Studio 17,

Florida Studio Theatre, Theatre of the Open Eye, The Changing Scene Theatre, The American Place Theatre, etc. She was playwright-in-residence for Joseph Chaikin's experimental Winter Project for two years, has been a visiting fellow at artists' colonies in the east and midwest, and is a member of New Dramatists. *Signs of Life* won a N.Y. State CAPS grant award and has been produced by The Women's Project of the American Place Theatre and by The Changing Scene in Denver.

Luna Tarlo, a Canadian, has written several novels including *The Bear Garden* and *The Tourist*. She has recently completed *Coming to Earth*, a novel concerning a woman's response to the death of her father. *Acrobatics* is Ms. Tarlo's first theatre piece. She is presently at work on her second, once again an exploration of the relations between women. For the last few years Ms. Tarlo has been living and writing on a small island in the Caribbean.

Julia Miles is a graduate of Northwestern University and began her career as an actress. In the early 1960s she co-founded Theatre Current in Brooklyn Heights, whose production of Arnold Weinstein's *Red Eye of Love*, directed by John Wulp, was moved to Off-Broadway. She then co-produced a season of new plays Off-Broadway and in 1964 joined The American Place Theatre on its first production, Robert Lowell's *The Old Glory*. Ms. Miles is currently Project Director of The Women's Project and Associate Director of The American Place Theatre. She is also president of "Four Women Productions" and a partner in "Tolan-Miles Productions," which is Executive Producer of Steve Tesich's forthcoming film, *Four Friends*, directed by Arthur Penn. Ms. Miles is married and has three daughters.

PERFORMING ARTS JOURNAL PLAYSCRIPTS

General Editors: Bonnie Marranca and Gautam Dasgupta